Coronary Heart Surgery

A Rehabilitation Measure

Edited by
H. Roskamm and M. Schmuziger

With 203 Figures

Springer-Verlag
Berlin Heidelberg New York 1979

Professor Dr. med. Helmut Roskamm
Benedikt Kreutz, Rehabilitationszentrum
7812 Bad Krozingen, Federal Republic of Germany

Dr. med. Martin Schmuziger
Benedikt Kreutz, Rehabilitationszentrum
7812 Bad Krozingen, Federal Republic of Germany

ISBN-13: 978-3-642-67297-2 e-ISBN-13: 978-3-642-67295-8
DOI: 10.1007/978-3-642-67295-8

Library of Congress Cataloging in Publication Data. Main entry under title: Coronary heart surgery. Papers presented at the international symposium held under the auspices of the European Society of Cardiology, Mar. 17–18, 1978, on the occasion of the inauguration of the Dept. of Heart Surgery at the Rehabilitation Center in Bad Krozingen, Ger. Bibliography: p. Includes index. 1. Coronary heart disease--Surgery--Congresses. I. Roskamm, Helmut. II. Schmuziger, Martin, 1936- III. European Society of Cardiology. IV. Benedikt-Kreutz-Rehabilitationszentrum für Herz- und Kreislaufkranke. [DNLM: 1. Aortocoronary bypass--Congresses. 2. Heart surgery--Congresses. 3. Coronary disease--Rehabilitation--Congresses. WG300.3 C822 1978] RD598.C669 617'.412 79-10443

Softcover reprint of the hardcover 1st edition 1979

Printing: Beltz Offsetdruck, Hemsbach/Bergstraße
Bookbinding: J. Schäffer OHG, Grünstadt

2127/3140-543210

Preface

On the occasion of the inauguration of the Department of Heart Surgery at the Rehabilitation Center in Bad Krozingen, we held under the auspices of the European Society of Cardiology an International Symposium on March 17 to 18, 1978 with the topic:

"Coronary Heart Surgery - a Rehabilitation Measure"

This book contains the papers given at that time.
The editors of this book, together with the other members of the scientific committee - H. Denolin from Brussels, Ch. Hahn from Geneva, and F. Loogen from Düsseldorf - aimed at selecting controversial topics as well as speakers representing different viewpoints. Thus avoiding portrayal of an image of a world of coronary bypass surgery in which all problems have found a solution. In keeping with the topic of the meeting, special emphasis was drawn to the long-term functional results of aortocoronary bypass surgery; symptomatic improvement being, in most patients, significant enough and lasting for at least some years, thus allowing the patients to return to work. However, a combination of social, economic, and psychological factors may hamper optimal rehabilitation, as can be seen from some of the following papers. The incorporation of heart surgery into a rehabilitation center - being the motif of this symposium - may hopefully stimulate a global approach to cardiac rehabilitation which includes surgical, medical, psychological, vocational, and social rehabilitation measures.

Bad Krozingen, January 1979

H. Roskamm
M. Schmuziger

Table of Contents

Contributors

L'Abbate, Antonio, Dott., Fisiologia Clinica, Via Savi, 8, 56100 Pisa, Italy

Amende, I., Dr. med., Med. Hochschule Hannover, Abt. für Kardiologie, Postfach 61 01 80, 3000 Hannover, FRG

Benesch, L., Dr. med., Universität Düsseldorf, Medizinische Klinik B, 4000 Düsseldorf, FRG

Bleese, N., Priv. Doz., Universitätskrankenhaus, Abt. für Thoraxchirurgie, Martinistraße 52, 2000 Hamburg, FRG

Blümchen, G., Prof. Dr., Klinik Roderbirken, 5653 Leichlingen, FRG

Botvinick, E., M.D., University of California, Division of Cardiology, San Francisco, Cal. 94143, U.S.A.

Bregman, D., Asst. Prof., College of Physicians and Surgeons, Columbia University, 630 West 168th Street, New York N.Y., 10032, U.S.A.

Bussmann, W.D., Priv. Doz., Johann-Wolfgang-Goethe-Universität, Abt. für Kardiologie, Theodor-Stern-Kai 7, 6000 Frankfurt/Main, FRG

Clark, R.E., Ass. Prof., Washington University, School of Medicine, Division of Cardiology, St. Louis, Mo. 63111, U.S.A.

Cherrier, F., Prof., Hôpital de Brabois, Route de Neufchateau, 54400 Vandoeuvre-Les-Nancy, France

Cohn, L.H., M.D., Harvard Medical School, Department of Surgery, Boston, Mass. 02115, U.S.A.

David, P., M.D., Institute de Cardiologie de Montreal, 5000 Est, Rue Bélanger, Montreal, Que, HIT IC8, Canada

Dubost, Ch., Prof., Hôpital Broussais, Dept. Chir. Cardiovasc., 96, rue Didot, 75674 Paris, France

Ellestad, M.H., M.D., Memorial Hospital Medical Center, 2801 Atlantic Avenue, Long Beach, Cal. 90801, U.S.A.

Flemma, R.J., M.D., Cardiovascular Surgery Associates, 9800 West Bluemound Road, Milwaukee, Wis. 53226, U.S.A.

Frick, M.H., Dr. med., Cardiovascular Laboratory, University Central Hospital, Haartmaninkatu 4, 00290 Helsinki 29, Finland

Hall, R.J., M.D., Texas Heart Institute, P.O. Box 20269, Houston, Texas 77025, U.S.A.

Hempelmann, G., Prof. Dr., Abt. Anaesthesie, Universitätsklinik, Klinikstraße 37, 6300 Gießen, FRG

Holmgren, A., M.D., Karolinska Sjukhuset, 10401 Stockholm, Sweden

Huysman, H.A., Prof. Dr., St. Antonius Ziekenhuis, Chirurgsiche Afdeling, Utrecht, The Netherlands

Jehle, J., Dr. med., Universität Düsseldorf, 1. Med. Klinik, Moorenstraße 5, 4000 Düsseldorf, FRG

Johnson, W.D., M.D., Heart Surgery Association, 3112 West Highland Blvd., Milwaukee, Wis. 53208, U.S.A.

Kaltenbach, M., Prof. Dr., Johann-Wolfgang-Goethe-Universität, Abt. für Kardiologie, Theodor-Stern-Kai 7, 6000 Frankfurt/Main, FRG

Karp, R.B., M.D., University of Alabama, Thoracic Cardiovascular Dept., Birmingham, Ala., U.S.A.

Keon, W.J., M.D., University of Ottawa, Ottawa Civic Hospital, 1053 Carling Ave., Ottawa, Ont. K1Y4E9, Canada

Killip, Th., M.D., Evanston Hospital, 2650 Ridge Avenue, Evanston, Ill. 60201, U.S.A.

Klein, H., Dr. med., Universitätsklinik Düsseldorf, I. Med. Klinik, 4000 Düsseldorf, FRG

Lichtlen, P., Prof. Dr., Medizinische Hochschule Hannover, Abt. für Innere Medizin - Kardiologie, Postfach 61 01 80, 3000 Hannover, FRG

Lister, J.W., M.D., 1680 Michigan Avenue, Miami Beach, Fla. 33139, U.S.A.

Loeb, H., Prof., Veterans Administration Hospital, Section of Cardiology, Hines, Ill., 60141, U.S.A.

Mathes, P., Priv. Doz. Dr., Techn. Universität München, 1. Med. Klinik und Poliklinik, Ismaninger Straße 22, 8000 München 80, FRG

Mathieu, P., Prof., Hôpital de Brabois, Route de Neufchateau, 54500 Vandoeuvre-Les-Nancy, France

Neuhaus, K.H., Dr. med., Kliniken der Universität Göttingen, Med. Klinik und Poliklinik, Robert-Koch-Str. 40, 3400 Göttingen, FRG

Ochsner, J.L., Prof., Ochsner Clinic, Dept. of Surgery, 1516 Jefferson Highway, New Orleans, La. 70121, U.S.A.

Pachinger, O., Dr. med., Kardiologische Universitätsklinik Wien, Garnisongasse 13, 1097 Wien, Austria

Rivera, R., Prof., Clinica Privada, Dept. of Cardiovascular Surgery, Maiquez 9, Madrid, Spain

Schmuziger, M., Dr. med., Benedikt Kreutz Rehabilitationszentrum, 7812 Bad Krozingen, FRG

Selzer, A., Ass. Prof., Pacific Medical Center, Division of Cardiology, Clay at Buchanan Street, San Francisco, Cal. 94120, U.S.A.

Serruys, P.W., Dr. med., Academisch Ziekenhuis Rotterdam, Dr. Molewaterplein 40, Rotterdam 3002, The Netherlands

Sonnenblick, E.H., Prof., Albert Einstein College of Medicine, Division of Cardiology, 1300 Morris Park Avenue, Bronx, N.Y., 10461, U.S.A.

Stolte, M., Dr. med., Universität Erlangen, Pathologisches Institut, 8520 Erlangen, FRG

Stürzenhofecker, P., Dr., Benedikt Kreutz Rehabilitationszentrum, 7812 Bad Krozingen, FRG

Suter, P.M., Dr., Hôpital Cantonal, Dept. d'Anesthesiologie, 1211 Geneve, Switzerland

Tarhan, S., M.D., Mayo Clinic, Dept. of Anesthesiology, Rochester, Minn. 55901, U.S.A.

Urschel, H.C., M.D., Baylor Medical Plaza, 3600 Gaston Avenue, Dallas, Tex. 75245, U.S.A.

Varnauskaus, E., Prof. Dr., Med. Clinic 1, Dept. of Cardiology, Sahlgrenska Hospital, S 413 45 Göteborg, Sweden

Walter, P., Prof. Dr., Justus-Liebig-Universität, Abt. f. Kardiovaskuläre Chirurgie, 6300 Giessen, FRG

1. Controversial Points in Selection of Patients for Surgery

Changing Medical and Surgical Therapy in Coronary Artery Disease - Need for Prospective Studies

Th. Killip

Following the pioneering efforts of Favalaro, reported in 1968, it quickly became apparent that the aortocoronary bypass graft was the first surgical procedure to reliably and reproducibly increase coronary blood flow in patients with coronary artery disease. Coronary artery disease is generally a mechanical problem. In most patients the large external arteries proximal to the intramyocardial branches are blocked. Hence the success of bypass.

With increasing experience, the operative mortality for coronary bypass rapidly fell to a very acceptable 1% - 2% for good risk patients. In the United States the coronary bypass operation was enthusiastically applied in the large number of cardiovascular centers which had been busy performing valve replacement via open heart surgery in a dwindling population of patients with acquired valvular heart disease. Thus, it is estimated that in 1977 more than 70,000 coronary bypass operations were performed and perhaps 250,000 patients underwent coronary angiography in the United States, a country with a population of about 220 million. Coronary bypass and its attendant diagnosis and treatment has become a major growth industry in the United States costing currently about $1 billion annually.

Traditionally, new surgical procedures are evaluated by comparison with previous experience, and coronary bypass has been no exception. Comparative trials for surgical treatments have been uncommon. One could point, however, to the work of the Boston Liver Group which in a pioneering study evaluated the portal-caval shunt [1]. This prospective randomized study demonstrated some long-term good for patients surviving the procedure, but found short-term carnage. Operative mortality was unacceptably high due to continued hemorrhage or progressive liver failure. When the long-term salvage and the short-term mortality of the surgical group were balanced against the results of continued medical therapy in randomly selected patients, it was found that neither treatment had the advantage. These results had immediate impact on the medical and surgical management of gastrointestinal hemorrhage due to portal hypertension with bleeding varices.

That randomization should be applied to the development of new surgical procedures, however, is difficult to accept for many, and the traditional evaluation of surgical procedures by testimonial reports continues. When the physician, or the patient, must choose between the traditional and conservative medical treatment or a new, promising and "radical" surgical procedure, confusion abounds and serious differences of opinion arise. Thus, it is with the coronary bypass procedure.

Evaluation of new therapy requires a thorough understanding of the natural history of the disease being treated and a comparison of the new treatment with other forms of therapy. Although patients with significant but asymptomatic coronary artery disease are being recognized with increasing frequency, coronary artery surgery is generally applied to the patient with symptoms due to angina pectoris. It is the symptoms which bring the patient to the attention of the physician and permit the clinical diagnosis of coronary artery disease. This clinical impression is often evaluated by coronary angiography.

It is pertinent to ask whether the prognosis of coronary artery disease is well understood, and whether medical treatment is standardized and relatively unchanging. It is our thesis that during the past 10 years when effective surgery for coronary artery disease became widely accepted medical treatment was rapidly improving after having been static for many decades.

In 1925 Paul Dudley White began a study of 500 patients with angina pectoris whom he followed for the next 25 years, by which time they had all died. This series was subsequently reported by Richards, Bland, and White in 1956 who recorded an average annual mortality of 4% [2]. Subsequently two other major studies on longevity in angina pectoris revealed essentially the same results. Kannell and co-authors reporting the Framingham, Massachusetts study with a 14 year follow-up, found an annual mortality of 4% in individuals with angina pectoris [3]. Somewhat later Frank and co-authors described an annual average mortality of 4% in males with angina pectoris from New York City [4]. Frank was able to stratify risk according to other attributes. Thus, the low risk group, with normal blood pressure and normal resting electrocardiogram had an annual mortality of 1.9% compared to the mortality in the control population of 1.1%. A high risk group with hypertension and abnormal electrocardiogram had an annual mortality of about 9%.

Thus, three major American studies, separated by almost 50 years, reached essentially the same conclusion: In patients with symptomatic angina pectoris under medical treatment the annual mortality was approximately 4% per year. These observations suggested that the effectiveness of medical therapy, at least in the United States, had not changed much in more than a half a century.

In the past 10 years, however, the medical treatment of angina pectoris has become more aggressive and almost certainly more effective. The concept of identifying risk factors thought to increase the hazard of myocardial infarction or sudden death in patients with coronary artery disease is widely accepted and practiced. The influence of smoking, obesity, hypertension, lack of regular exercise, Type A personality, soft water, elevated serum cholesterol, and elevated triglycerides as well as many other factors to increase the risk of a symptomatic coronary event is well accepted. Physicians recommend therapy to alleviate these risks in cooperative patients and presumably this is having some effect.

The death rate from cardiovascular disease in the United States has been falling steadily since about 1960, and possibly even before. There is great dispute as to the cause of this decline; there can be no dispute about the fact that the death rate from myocardial infarction is continuing to decrease in my country.

During the past 10 years there have been significant changes in the medical treatment of patients with angina pectoris. Highly effective and relatively safe antihypertensive agents have become available. Massive educational programs have reached both the physician and the public pointing to the importance of detection and treatment of hypertension. When an average hypertensive patient encounters an average medical professional in the United States the hypertension is vigorously treated. This is especially true in the patient with angina pectoris. Although data clearly demonstrating the decline in mortality due to sudden death and myocardial infarction in well-treated hypertensives are not available, it is hard to believe that hypertension is good for the patient with coronary artery disease or that, conversely, adequate treatment is bad.

Epidemiologists in the western hemisphere have focused heavily on the adverse risk of smoking in the patient with coronary arters disease. In the United States there has been a significant decline in the incidence of smoking in middle-aged men. Less than 10% of physicians smoke, and the vast majority work hard and effectively to persuade patients at risk for coronary artery disease to stop smoking. It appears that smoking is additive but not causative since the risk of infarction declines rapidly after cessation of the habit to about the level found in the nonsmoker. Wilhelmsson and co-authors showed a significant decrease in incidence of reinfarction and cardiac death in a group of patients who stopped smoking after their first infarction compared with those who did not [5].

A major advance in the therapy of cardiovascular disorders has been the introduction of beta blockers. Beta blockers are now widely administered to patients with symptomatic coronary artery disease and to some patients with known coronary atherosclerosis and no ischemic symptoms. Recent reports suggest that these agents reduce the risk of sudden death and myocardial infarction in patients treated after a first infarct. Thus, Wilhelmsson and co-authors showed that alprenolol significantly reduced the incidence of sudden death in patients treated following a first infarction in comparison with placebo [6]. Similarly the study by the British Medical Research Council on the effect of practolol after acute myocardial infarction with an average follow-up of 14 months showed a significant reduction in nonfatal myocardial infarction and death due to cardiac disease in patients taking the drug compared to a randomized group receiving placebo [7]. A study on the effect of propranolol is just getting underway in the United States.

There is currently great interest in the influence of platelet aggregability on the genesis of coronary atherosclerosis. It has been known for some time in pigs with genetically induced von Willebrand's disease that spontaneous or induced atherosclerosis is much retarded [8]. As known, platelet aggregation is disturbed in von Willebrand's disease due to a missing plasma factor. A preliminary study by the National Institutes of Health (United States) coronary drug project suggested, but did not prove, that daily ingestion of aspirin might reduce the frequency of a second myocardial infarction. A major study is underway at the present time to test this thesis in the United States. A recent report described a 50% reduction in the incidence of sudden death in patients taking an agent sulfinpyrazone originally introduced for the treatment of gout but also now known to reduce platelet aggregability [9].

After much debate and a predominantly negative attitude which lasted many years, it is now recognized that longacting vasodilators produce measurable blood levels of nitrates, and improved exercise tolerance in patients with ischemic heart disease several hours after ingestion. Vasodilator therapy with a variety of agents is now vigorously promulgated by many cardiac groups not only to unload the overworked ventricle, but also to reduce ischemic manifestations.

Thus, the past 10 - 15 years have seen two important revolutions in the management of coronary artery disease: The introduction of an effective surgical procedure, namely coronary artery bypass; and rapid changes in medical therapy which appear to be favorably altering the outlook of the patient with ischemic heart disease. Medical treatment is clearly far more effective currently than it has been in the past. As a further index of the importance of improved medical therapy, it is interesting to note that in at least three major randomized trials comparing medical and surgical treatment in coronary artery disease, the medical mortality has proved to be far less than expected when the protocols were written, despite the fact that the protocols were developed by recognized experts after thorough surveys of the available medical literature.

It is apparent, then, that the influence of coronary artery surgery on the incidence of sudden death, myocardial infarction, and longevity cannot be determined by a comparison with accounts drawn from the literature or recent experience in a given clinic. When medical therapy is rapidly changing, the use of historical controls can be misleading. As Byar, Simon, and Friedewald and others have argued, clinical trials designed to evaluate which if any of two forms of therapy is more effective, require the concurrent use of a control population selected at random from the patients available for treatment [10]. Control and treatment groups must be identical in all aspects that can be currently measured. The method of randomization should be designed to eliminate all possible sources of bias. Randomization must be done properly to eliminate bias in the allocation of subjects to treatment groups, balance the prognostic factors, both known and unknown, and guarantee the validity of statistical tests.

In designing a study, it is important to determine what sample size is sufficient to reliably demonstrate a difference in mortality in the two treatment groups that would be clinically important. A difference between medical and surgical mortality in coronary artery disease of less than 25% - 30% (5% - 6% per year) after 5 years of study would probably not be clinically useful. It can readily be demonstrated that a study designed to detect this minimum difference would require several hundreds of patients to be valid.

"The concept that the first sick patient to receive a new drug, procedure, or operation should be randomized stems from recognition of the pernicious influence of pilot trials and postponing or eliminating a definitive therapeutic trial." [11] As Chalmers has pointed out there are three possible results from an uncontrolled pilot trial: apparent striking improvement, evidence of worthlessness, or no conclusive results. If the new procedure looks promising, often the early investigators become so convinced of its value that they come to believe that randomization is unethical. Or, as an alternative, the initial favorable results are reported with the comment at the end of the paper that the trial was, of course, uncontrolled and that a controlled trial should be carried out (by somebody else)[11].

The ethics of randomized studies have been well summarized by Chalmers [12]. As he has written, if the clinician knows or has good reason to believe that a new therapy (A) is better than another therapy (B) he cannot participate in a comparative trial of therapy A versus therapy B. Ethically the clinician is obligated to give therapy A to each new patient with a need of one of these treatments. However, if the physician or his peers have genuine doubt as to which therapy is better, he should give each patient an equal chance to receive one or the other therapy. The physician must fully recognize

Table 1. Randomized studies of surgery of coronary artery disease

Type angina	Investigators	Location	Multicenter	Year	No. subjects	Outcome
Unstable	Bertolasi[13]	Buenos Aires	No	1974	97	Preliminary report: Surgical mortality 8%; medical 20%.
Unstable	Conti[14]	US National Institutes of Health	Yes	1972-1976	288	24-month followup: No difference mortality or myocardial infarction rate; "quality of life" improved surgically.
Unstable	Selden[15]	Portland,Oregon	No	1975	40	No significant differences mortality, 4 months.
Stable	Mathur[16]	Houston,Texas	No	1975	70	No significant differences mortality, 28 months.
Stable	Kloster[17]	Portland,Oregon	No	1975	100	No significant differences mortality, 36 months.
Stable	Murphy[18]	US Veterans Administration	Yes	1972-1974	596	36-month followup: No significant differences mortality.
Stable	Varnauskas[19]	European Cooperative Study	Yes	1974-1976	750	No reports.
Stable	Killip (Coordinator)	US National Institutes of Health, CASS	Yes	1975-1979	900-1,000	No reports.

that the new therapy might be worse than the old. Each new patient must have a fair chance of receiving either the new, and hopefully better, therapy, or the limited effects of the old therapy. There is a further important caveat, "The conduct and reporting of poorly designed and conducted research is potentially unethical".

It is my personal view that the effect of coronary artery bypass surgery on the incidence of myocardial infarction, death from cardiac events, and prognosis in patients with symptomatic coronary artery disease is not known and that therefore randomized studies comparing medical and surgical treatment are not only ethical but must be carried out.

In the accompanying table are listed the randomized studies which are known to us. In addition to the eight tabulated, one further study from Dallas, Texas has been reported in abstract form, but the numbers randomized are so small, less than 30, that it is unlikely that any conclusions regarding infarction rate or death can be reached (Table 1).

Comments Regarding Table 1
It is doubtful that the study reported by Bertolasi should be included in this compilation. The technique for randomization is not reported; it is not clear whether consecutive cases were studied, and the reported medical mortality is unusually high [13].

A preliminary report of study of unstable angina sponsored by the National Institutes of Health in the United States involving nine clinical centers has appeared [14].

The number of subjects enrolled in the three studies reported by Mathur [15], Kloster [16] and Selden [17] will probably be too small to give any of these projects sufficient statistical power to demonstrate differences in survival, rate of myocardial infarction, or ventricular function between the medical and surgical groups. Mathur reported important observations in exercise tolerance. After 28 months there was significant improvement in exercise tolerance in both medical ($P < 0.001$) and surgical ($P < 0.001$) groups. However, the increase in exercise tolerance in the surgical group was significantly greater than in the medical patients ($P < 0.05$).

Data from the European Cooperative Study involving 13 institutions have not yet appeared. Prof. Varnauskas of Göteborg, Sweden is the coordinator. The Veterans Administration project involving 13 hospitals will be discussed by Dr. Loeb and others, including the special circumstances of left main stem disease [18].

A major study currently underway in the United States, and sponsored by the National Institutes of Health, is the Coronary Artery Surgery Study (CASS). The CASS protocol is quite similar to that of the European Cooperative Study. Sixteen different institutions in the United States are cooperating in this project. CASS consists of two parts, a *Registry* and a *Randomized Study*.

The *registry* is comprised of all consecutive patients at the cooperating institutions undergoing angiography because of a diagnosis of ischemic heart disease. Considerable clinical and objective information is recorded from each patient on multipage data forms, and entered by an "intelligent" computer terminal at each site into a central data bank in the Coordinating Center at the University of Washington in Seattle. Particular attention is paid to the analysis of objective data obtained from the angiocardiogram and also from the electrocardiogram. All electrocardiograms are now being read at a central site. Each angiocardiogram is analyzed at the individual site according to rigid protocol and data form. Ventriculographic data, including ejection fraction and wall motion, are determined in a standard manner. The quality of the angiogram is central to the study, and a special subcommittee has developed standard procedures for imaging and processing of the photographic film. This has led to a uniform high technical quality of the angiography. Furthermore, there are elaborate quality control measures concerned with interpretation of the coronary arteriogram.

Patients selected for *randomization* meet rigid criteria. The principle of informed consent is closely followed. Randomization is performed upon request by telephone call at the Coordinating Center. We believe that every possible element of bias has been eliminated. An important group of patients also being followed closely are those who met the criteria for randomization but chose not to follow this course. There are about twice as many patients in this group as have been randomized, and their baseline characteristics and clinical descriptors are generally similar to those who are randomized.

To date, as of 13 March 1978, 554 patients have been randomized, and the registry contains approximately 18,500 individuals. Intake for the study will continue until 30 June 1979, or until the accumulation of 1,000 randomized patients, whichever is achieved first.

Randomization is accomplished for three groups of patients:

1) Angina pectoris, less than severe, with normal ventricular function
2) Angina pectoris, less than severe, with abnormal ventricular function
3) Asymptomatic individuals following acute myocardial infarction

A major purpose of the registry is to accumulate sufficient data on a sufficiently large number of patients so that multiple studies can be initiated on small subgroups. At the present time these "spinoff" studies include analysis of the complications of angiography; results of exercise testing in men and women correlated with angiographic findings; perioperative infarction rate; influence of operative techniques on outcome; observer variation in angiographic interpretation; and many others.

The ongoing results, including surgical mortality, and medical and surgical outcome of the *randomized* study, are reviewed at regular intervals by a Police Board appointed by the National Institutes of Health, made up of prominent clinical investigators who are not connected directly with the study. The Police Board has the power at any time to modify or halt intake of randomized patients if preliminary analysis of data reveals trends that would require a major change in the study or adverse results. No data regarding the major goals of the study, namely, differences in survival between medical and surgical treatment, the rate of myocardial infarction during the follow-up period, or alterations in the "quality of life" will be revealed until intake of subjects for randomization has been completed.

References

1. Garceau, A.J., Donaldson, R.M. (Jr.), O'Hara, E.T., Callow, A., Muench, H., Chalmers, T.C.: Controlled trial of prophylactic portacaval shunt surgery. N. Engl. J. Med. *270*, 496 (1964)
2. Richards, D.W., Bland, E.F., White, P.D.: A complete twenty-five-year followup study of 456 patients with angina pectoris. J. Chron. Dis. *4*, 423-433 (1956)
3. Kannell, W.B., Feinleib, M.: Natural history of angina pectoris in the Framingham study. Prognosis and survival. Am. J. Cardiol. *29*, 154-163 (1972)
4. Frank, C.W., Weinblatt, E., Shapiro, S.: Angina pectoris in men. Circulation *47*, 509-517 (1973)
5. Wilhelmsson, C., Elmfeldt, D., Vedin, J.A., Tibblin, G., Wilhelmsen, L.: Smoking and myocardial infarction. Lancet *1*, 1975/I, 415
6. Wilhelmsson, C., Wilhelmsen, L., Vedin, J.A., Tibblin, G., Werkö, L.: Reduction of sudden deaths after myocardial infarction by treatment with alprenolol. Lancet *2*, 1974/I, 1157
7. A Multicentre International Study Report: Improvement in prognosis of myocardial infarction by long-term beta-adrenoreceptor blockade using practolol. Br. Med. J. *3*, 735 (1975)
8. Owen, C.A. (Jr.): Animal models of human diseases. Proc. Mayo Clin. *53*, 193-194 (1978)
9. Anturane Reinfarction Trial Research Group: Sulfinpyrazone in the prevention of cardiac death after myocardial infarction. N. Engl. J. Med. *298*, 289-294 (1978)
10. Byar, D.P., Simon, R.M., Friedewald, W.T., Schlesselman, J.J., DeMets, D.L., Ellenberg, J.H., Gail, M.H., Ware, J.H.: Randomized clinical trials: Perspectives on some recent ideas. N. Engl. J. Med. *295*, 74-80 (1976)
11. Chalmers, T.C.: Randomization of the first patient. Med. Clin. North Am. *59*, 1035-1039 (1975)
12. Shaw, L.W., Chalmers, T.C.: Ethics in cooperative clinical trials. Ann. NY Acad. Sci. *169*, 487-495 (1970)
13. Bertolasi, C.A., Trongé, J.E., Carreño, C.A., Jalon, J., Vega, M.R.: Unstable angina: prospective and randomized study of its evolution, with and without surgery. Am. J. Cardiol. *33*, 201 (1974)
14. Conti, C.R., Gilbert, J.B., Hodges, M., Hutter, A.M., Kaplan, E., Newell, J., Resnekov, L., Rosati, R., Ross, R.S., Russell, R.O., Schroeder, J.S., Wolk, M.: Unstable angina pectoris: Randomized study of surgical versus medical therapy: National cooperative unstable angina pectoris study group. Am. J. Cardiol. *35*, 129 (1975)
15. Selden, R., Neill, W.A., Ritzmann, L.W., Okies, J.E., Anderson, R.P.: Medical versus surgical therapy for acute coronary insufficiency: A randomized study. N. Engl. J. Med. *293*, 1329-1333 (1975)
16. Mathur, V.S., Guinn, G.A., Anastassiades, L.C., Chahine, R.A., Korompai, F.L., Montero, A.C., Luchi, R.J.: Surgical treatment for stable angina pectoris: Prospective randomized study. N. Engl. J. Med. *292*, 709-713 (1975)
17. Kloster, F., Kremkau, L., Rahimtoola, S., Griswold, H., Ritzmann, L., Neill, W., Starr, A.: Prospective randomized study of coronary bypass surgery for chronic stable angina. Circulation *52*[Suppl. 2], 90 (1975)
18. Murphy, M.L., Hultgren, H.N., Detre, K., Thomsen, J., Takaro, T., and participants of the Veterans Administration Cooperative Study: Treatment of chronic stable angina. A preliminary report of survival data of the randomized Veterans Administration study. N. Engl. J. Med. *297*, 621-627 (1977)
19. Varnauskas, E.: Need for Coronary Bypass Surgery in Europe. In: Coronary Heart Surgery — A Rehabilitation Measure. Roskamm, H., Schmuziger, M. (eds.), Berlin Heidelberg New York: Springer 1979

A Critical Review of the Veterans Administrative Cooperative Study

H. Loeb

I feel honored to have been invited to address this symposium and to have the opportunity to visit your country.

My remarks will deal with the Veterans Administration Cooperative Study of Surgery for Coronary Arterial Disease. As I am sure you are aware, this study has generated a considerable amount of interest in the United States and abroad.

At the onset, I wish to emphasize that I have the highest respect for all of the individuals who planned, initiated, and directed this study. Although certain aspects of the study have come recently under criticism, some justified, some not, it must be remembered that this study was undertaken at a time when both the medical and surgical treatment of coronary disease was undergoing rapid development. As a participant in the study, I can attest to the many difficulties encountered in its day to day operation. There is no doubt in my mind however, that all of the participants in this study attempted, whenever humanly possible, to adhere to scientific methodology while avoiding any bias they might have had.

This morning, I will briefly summarize the study as a whole and then present data obtained from our own VA Hospital in Hines, Illinois. Finally, I will enumerate certain factors which I believe are important in relating the results of the VA study to the practice of cardiology in 1978.

The primary goal of the study was to determine whether coronary artery surgery influenced longevity in patients with stable angina pectoris. There were various criteria for patients being admitted into the study. Males with symptoms of chronic stable angina pectoris of at least 6 months duration and who had been treated medically for at least 3 months were screened. In addition to a history of angina an abnormal electrocardiogram either at rest or during exercise was required. Prior to being entered into the study, all patients underwent cardiac catheterization. Patients with significant obstruction of one or more major coronary arteries, whose distal vessels were suitable for bypass surgery, and whose left ventricular function was not impaired sufficiently to preclude surgery, were asked to participate in the study. If the patient consented, he was then assigned by randomization to either medical or surgical therapy. Although follow-up has continued to the present and will continue for several additional years, preliminary results dealing with the influence of therapy on longevity have recently been published. The early experience from 1968-1972 included several patients who underwent internal mammary implantation rather than aortocoronary bypass. In addition, operative mortality during these early years was high in several hospitals. For these reasons, analysis of results deals only with patients entered into the study during the years 1972 through 1974. It soon became clear that patients with significant obstruction of the left main coronary artery who were treated surgically, had improved longevity, when compared to similar patients treated medically. Thus, our recent attention has been directed to those patients who did not have left main coronary artery obstruction.

During the period of 1972 through 1974, 596 patients from 13 participating hospitals with significant 1-, 2-, or 3-vessel disease and without left main coronary disease were admitted into the study and randomized to either medical therapy (310 patients) or surgical therapy (286 patients). According to the cumulative survival rates there has been to this date, no detectable significant difference between the medically randomized and surgically randomized groups. Similar analysis on subgroups according to number of coronary arteries with significant obstruction and degree of left ventricular impairment have also failed to show improved survival with either surgical or medical therapy. Of interest is the surprisingly benign course followed by the medically treated patients with an average survival of nearly 90% at 3 years.

Our own experience at Hines VA Hospital contrasts sharply with the results of the total series.

Our data includes 152 patients admitted into the study from 1968 through 1974, although the majority were entered after 1971. We have excluded 13 patients from our analysis; one patient because no significant coronary lesion was found upon review of the angiogram and three patients who underwent Vineberg procedures. Nine patients with significant left main disease were analyzed separately. No patient has been lost to follow-up. Of the 139 patients remaining, 72 were randomized to medical therapy and 67 to surgical therapy.

In order to see if the medical and surgical groups were comparable at the time of entrance into the study, several baseline characteristics were analyzed. The average age was 51.6 and 50.7 years in the medical and surgical groups, respectively. None of the characteristics listed which include: duration of angina, New York Heart Association class, history of infarction, hypertension, cardiac failure, or diabetes differed in incidence between the two groups. Likewise, the presence of obesity, hypertension, and cardiomegaly on chest x-ray was similar in the two groups. Of interest and unexplained, hypercholesterolemia was more prevalent in the medical group.

Hemodynamic characteristics at the time of initial catheterization were also similar in the two groups. It should be noted that few patients in either group had significant impairment of left ventricular function.

In order to better define the extent of coronary disease, we utilized a simple scoring system. Significant left main coronary obstruction, although not included in the present series, counted 4 (points) or 5 (points) for a dominant left system. Significant proximal lesions in the major 3 coronary vessels counted 2 points each and in the absence of significant proximal obstruction, lesions more distally counted a single point. The maximum number of points a patient could have was 6.

Utilizing this scoring system, it was shown that our medically and surgically randomized patients were similar with regard to the extent of coronary obstruction. Approximately 60% of the patients in each group had a point score of 4 or above.

In conclusion, the current status of the 139 patients is summarized. Of the 72 patients randomized to medical therapy, 55 have remained in the medical group. There have been 19 deaths in these 55 patients. The other 17 medically randomized patients have subsequently undergone aortocoronary bypass surgery usually because of severe anginal symptoms not controlled with drugs. There have been three deaths in this group.

Of the 67 patients randomized to surgical therapy, 63 underwent operation. To date, there have been 8 deaths in this group. Four of the patients randomized to surgical therapy were not operated and one of these four patients has died.

Because a significant number of patients did not adhere to the therapy as originally assigned, we analyzed our data three different ways, but the results were not markedly influenced by type of analysis used.

Comparing the two groups according to original randomization, the medical mortality of 31% is significantly higher than the surgical mortality of 13%. Similarly, the 34% mortality in the patients treated medically is significantly higher than the 14% mortality in the patients treated surgically. Finally, when the 17 patients randomized to medical treatment, but treated surgically, and the four patients randomized to surgery, but treated medically, are removed from analysis, the medical mortality still is significantly higher than the mortality in the surgical group.

We do not know why our results differ from those of the larger Cooperative Study, however, it is apparent that the major difference is reflected in the higher mortality of our medical patients since the longevity of our surgical patients was similar to that of the entire study group.

Although the difference between our results and those of the other cooperating hospitals may simply be a statistical phenomenon occurring by chance, we admittedly, and I think justifiably, are influenced primarily by our own experience when choosing therapy for our patients.

Finally, it must be remembered that the VA study data was obtained during the years 1972 through 1974. Extrapolation of data from this period to 1978 and beyond must take into consideration the following questions:

1. Can an operative mortality significantly below the 5.6% of the VA cooperative study be achieved today?
2. Is the extent of revascularization more than 4-6 years ago and how might this alter surgical results?
3. Can graft patency rates above 69% at 1 year be expected today?
4. How do patients who crossed over from medical to surgical therapy alter the results of the VA study?
5. Are there major changes in medical therapy which now alter the natural history of patients with coronary artery disease?

I am sure many of these questions will be dealt with during this symposium.

The Effect of Coronary Bypass on Longevity - a Nonrandomized Study

L. H. Cohn and J. J. Collins

The coronary bypass operation has been shown to alleviate angina [1,2], increase exercise capacity [3,4], reverse myocardial ischemia [5,6], and improve the quality of life for most patients undergoing the operation [7,8]. After 10 years of coronary revascularization the effect of coronary bypass on prolongation of life of patients undergoing this operation is still controversial. This study analyzes consecutive patients operated upon at the Peter Bent Brigham Hospital, Boston, Massachusetts from July, 1970, to January, 1977, to evaluate the effect of coronary bypass on life expectancy.

Clinical Material

Table 1. Indications for coronary artery bypass

1) Angina pectoris
    - Chronic stable
    - Unstable
    - Prinzmetal
    - Chronic global ischemia
2) Acute Myocardial Infarction
3) Ancillary
    - Valve replacement
    - Sequelae of AMI
4) "Asymptomatic"
    - + EET
    - Prior AMI
    - Multiple risk factors

Table 1 lists our indications for coronary artery bypass. Only patients undergoing coronary bypass for stable (699) or unstable (127) angina consecutively operated upon were utilized for analysis. Patients with congestive heart failure or cardiogenic shock or who underwent concomitant valve replacement were not included. There were 704 men and 122 women ranging in age from 23-78, with a mean age of 55 years. Included were 129 (15%) patients with left main coronary stenosis; 80 had stable angina and 49 had unstable angina (Table 2).

Table 2.

	#	# Left main	Op death	Late death
Chronic angina	699	80	12(1.7%)	24(3.4%)
Unstable angina	127	49	5(4.0%)	5(4.0%)
	826	129(15%)	17(2.0%)	29(3.5%)

Three or more coronary branches were significantly obstructed (> 70%) in 478 patients; 260 had two vessels obstructed and 88 patients had one vessel obstructed. Ejection fraction under 0.40 (normal = 0.50) was found in 62 patients (7.5%). Follow-up for all patients was by personal examination or written questionnaire. Survival data was calculated by the life actuarial table method [9].

Operative Methods

Operative techniques include cardiopulmonary bypass, hemodilution to a hematocrit of 20%-25%, intrathoracic cannulations utilizing a single right atrial cannula, and an ascending aortic perfusion cannula, running venocoronary anastomoses with 6-0 Prolene sutures and running aortovenous anastomoses with 5-0 Prolene. Since the patients were operated upon over a seven year period, there has been variation in myocardial protection techniques but at present, two main techniques are used: (1) intermittent ischemia with crossclamping of the aorta for periods of 5-10 min with reperfusion periods from 3-5 min or (2) continuous ischemia with profound local cardiac hypothermia and hyperkalemic cardioplegia. The cardioplegic solution consists of dextrose, 5%/0.2% NS, 30 mEq KCl/liter, and bicarbonate to make the solution basic and hyperosmotic at 340 mosmol. Three ore more bypass grafts were performed in 259 patients, 479 patients underwent two coronary bypass grafts, and 88 patients underwent one coronary bypass graft. Left ventricular venting was used in the earlier years of the study, but is generally not used now unless there is excessive bronchial return or aortic regurgitation.

Results

The summary of the operative results is shown in Table 2. There were 17 operative deaths; 12 occurred in the chronic angina group, 5 in the unstable angina group (4.0%), an overall mortality of 2.0% (17/826). Nine of the 17 operative deaths were patients with left main coronary stenosis. There were 29 late deaths from all causes; 24 occurred in the chronic angina group, yielding a late mortality of 3.4%, and 5 occurred in the unstable angina group, a late mortality of 4%; the overall late mortality was 29/826 (3.5%). The follow-up period was 12-72 months, with a mean of 30 months.

The results of the actuarially derived data from patients with one-, two-, and three-vessel coronary disease surgically treated have been compared to the 6-year survival results of the normal United States population, age matched, sex matched, and race matched compiled from the vital statistics of the United States Public Health Service [10]. In Table 3 the comparative data are summarized. Eighty-eight patients with one-vessel disease had a 6-year survival projected actuarially of 97.2%, versus a normal population survival of 92.4%; in two-vessel disease patients it was 89.6% versus 92.1% in the normal population; in the three-vessel disease group 86.4% versus 90.6%; an overall of 88.9% in 826 patients compared to a 91% survival of the 826 persons from the normal population. In 259 patients receiving three or more bypass grafts survival was 94.5% compared to 90.5% in the normal population.

Table 3

# VD	# PTS	Projected 6-yr survival	6-yr Survival normal population[a]
1	88	97.2	92.4
2	260	89.6	92.1
3	478	86.4	90.6
3[b]	259	94.5	90.5
Total	826	88.9	91.0

[a]Age-, sex-, race matched.

[b]Patients with triple-vessel disease receiving three or more bypass grafts.

Discussion

These results show that patients undergoing coronary bypass surgery at the Peter Bent Brigham Hospital have a survival curve similar to that of an age-matched, sex-matched, and race-matched general population of the United States. Though this is not a controlled study it does lend credence to the fact that the life expectancy of patients with severe coronary obstructive disease with reasonable left ventricular function undergoing coronary bypass may become similar to the normal population. "Natural history" studies of angiogrammed patients [11-14] over a 22-92 month period have yearly attrition rates of 0.7%-3.6% for single-vessel disease, 6.6%-13% for two-vessel disease and 9.0%-15.0% for three-vessel coronary disease. Our previously reported surgical data [15] and that of others [16-19] showed statistically significant differences between these data. These studies have been criticized because they took place in the "pre-propranolol" period, though no prospective randomized study utilizing propranolol has ever shown prolongation of life. The recent prospective randomized study by the U.S. Veterans Hospital [20] attempted to evaluate long-term mortality. In a preliminary study these data showed that there was no significant difference between medical or surgical therapy. Operative mortality, however, was excessive (5.6%) for a group of patients who had the best possible prognosis, that is, those without unstable angina, left main coronary stenosis, recent infarction, diabetes, or hypertension; there was also a 17% crossover rate of patients from medical to surgical treatment, treated only as a "lost-to-followup" in the medical curve. We have compared our 3-year surgical survival to the Veterans Administration Hospital (VA) medical and surgical survival results at 3 years (Table 4); the results are significantly different despite inclusion of left main coronary stenosis and unstable angina, two high-risk categories excluded by the national VA study [20].

Table 4

	# PTS	36 months act. survival
PBBH Surg.	826	93%
VA Surg.	286	88% *
VA Med.	310	87% **

*P = 0.22 between PBBH.
**P = 0.009 between PBBH.

Summary

Eight-hundred and twenty-six consecutive patients undergoing coronary bypass surgery for unstable and stable angina including 129 patients with left main coronary stenosis at the Peter Bent Brigham Hospital underwent statistical analysis of their longevity. It was found that in one-, two-, and three-vessel disease the projected 6-year actuarial survival curves are similar to that of the normal age matched, sex matched, race matched American population. Surgical survival data from this study were also significantly improved over that of the VA medical and surgical series at 3 years. These data suggest that longevity is improved in patients following coronary bypass graft procedures.

References

1. Barbovak, J.J., Hughes, C.V., Anderson, A.J., Rimm, A.A.: Effect of aortocoronary bypass operation on factors precipitating angina. J. Thorac. Cardiovasc. Surg. *75*, 47 (1978)
2. Chatterjee, K., Matloff, J.M., Swan, H.V.C.: Improved angina threshold and coronary reserve following direct myocardial revascularization. Circulation *51*, 81 (1975)
3. Barry, W.H., Pfeifer, J.F., Lipton, M.J. et al: Effects of coronary artery bypass grafting on resting and exercise hemodynamics in patients with stable angina pectoris: a prospective randomized study. Am. J. Cardiol. *37*, 823 (1976)
4. Siegel, W., Lim, J.S., Proudfit, W.L., et al: The spectrum of exercise test and angiographic correlations in myocardial revascularization surgery. Circulation *51*, 156 (1975)
5. Cohn, L.H., Herman, M.V., Gorlin, R., Collins, J.J. (Jr.): Surgical treatment of aorto-coronary occlusion. J. Thorac. Cardiovasc. Surg. *64*, 503 (1972)
6. Favaloro, R.G., Effler, D.B., Cheanvechai, C., et al: Acute coronary insufficiency (Impending myocardial infarction and myocardial infarction): Surgical treatment by the saphenous vein graft technique. Am. J. Cardiol. *28*, 598 (1971)
7. Special correspondence: a debate on coronary bypass. N. Engl. J. Med. *297*, 1464-1470 (1977)
8. DeBakey, M.E., Lawrie, G.M.: Aorto-coronary artery bypass. JAMA *239*, 837 (1978)
9. Cutter, S.J., Ederer, F.: Maximum utilization of the life table method in analyzing survival. J. Chron. Dis. *8*, 699 (1958)
10. U.S. Bureau of the Census: Statistical abstract of the United States: Expectation of life and mortality rate by age, race and sex — 1974, 97th ed. pp. 61. Washington (D.C.) 1976
11. Friesinger, G.C., Page, E.E., Ross, R.S.: Prognostic significance of coronary arteriography. Trans. Assoc. Am. Physicians *83*, 78 (1970)
12. Humphries, J.O., Kuller, L., Ross, R.S., et al: Natural history of ischemic heart disease in relation to arteriographic findings: a 12-year study of 224 patients. Circulation *49*, 489 (1974)
13. Webster, J.S., Moberg, C., Rincon, G.: Natural history of severe proximal coronary artery disease as documented by coronary cine-angiography. Am. J. Cardiol. *33*, 195 (1974)
14. Oberman, A., Jones ,W.B., Riley, C.P., et al: Natural history of coronary artery disease. Bull. N.Y. Acad. Med. *48*, 1109 (1972)
15. Cohn, L.H., Boyden, C.M., Collins, J.J. (Jr.): Improved long-term survival after aorto-coronary bypass for advanced coronary disease. Am. J. Surg. *129*, 380 (1975)
16. Sheldon, W.C., Rincon, G., Pichard, A.D., et al: Surgical treatment of coronary artery disease: pure graft operations with study of 741 patients followed 3-7 years. Progr. Cardiovasc. Dis. *18*, 237 (1975)
17. Lawrie, G.M., Morris, G.C. (Jr.), Chapman, D.W., et al: Patterns of patency of 596 vein grafts up to seven years after aorto-coronary bypass. J. Thorac. Cardiovasc. Surg. *73*, 443 (1977)

18. Reul, G.J. (Jr.), Cooley, D.A., Sandeford, F.M., et al: Aorto-coronary artery bypass. Present indications and risk factors. Arch. Surg. *111*, 414 (1976)
19. Barnes, H.B., Mudd, A.G., Mark, A.L., et al: Patency of internal mammary coronary grafts. Circulation *54*, 70 (1976)
20. Murphy, M.L., Hultgren, H.N., Detre, K., et al: Treatment of chronic stable angina. A preliminary report of survival data of the randomized Veterans Administration Cooperative Study. N. Engl. J. Med. *297*, 621 (1977)
21. Takaro, T., Hultgren, H.N., Lipton, M.J., et al: The VA Cooperative randomized study of surgery for coronary arterial occlusive disease. II. Subgroup with significant left main lesions. Circulation *54*, 107 (1976)

The Effects of Aortocoronary Bypass Surgery on Life Expectancy - a Nonrandomized Study

R. J. Flemma

The purpose of this study is to compare survival in two closely matched groups of patients, one treated surgically, and the other being the VA Cooperative medically treated group. Both groups represent patients treated in the period 1972-1974, the surgical group being personally operated for coronary artery disease and the VA Cooperative medical treatment cohort reported by Read et al. [1] in the Journal of Thoracic and Cardiovascular Surgery in January of 1978. Utilizing the demographic and angiographic criteria published by the VA Cooperative study, we withdrew from the data bank computer of the Milwaukee Cardiovascular Data Registry a closely matched cohort of surgical patients and compared survival.

Patient Groups

The group, consisting of 229 patients, on whom we had extensive preoperative, operative, and postoperative follow-up, were catheterized at St. Luke's Hospital. They were withdrawn from the computer registry to closely match those 310 medically treated patients presented by the VA Cooperative study. Tables 1 and 2 show the demographic and angiographic criteria which were utilized to as closely resemble the VA Cooperative patients as possible. No patients with significant left main coronary disease or ventricular aneurysms were included. The patients were 68 years of age or less. We did not exclude hypertensive patients or those with unstable angina.

The VA Cooperative study rejected generalized poor left ventricular function as we also did. The VA Cooperative study rejected patients "for marked elevation of LVEDP", yet, this number was not explicitly defined. We included patients with an LVEDP of 25 or less, excluding those patients with an LVEDP greater than 25. A large left ventricle, although a reason for exclusion in the VA Cooperative study was not then, or now, excluded from surgical intervention. The VA also excluded patients with a poor ejection fraction, although not clearly defined by number. We did not routinely measure ejection fractions in

Table 1. Demographic characteristics of the two groups to be compared. 1972-1974

VA Coop (Medical Rx)	Personal (Surgical)
No left main	No left main
Stable angina	Unstable + Stable
No hypertensives	Hypertensives
No aneurysm	No aneurysm
Age <68	Age <68)

Table 2. Comparative characteristics of LV function between the two groups compared. 1972-1974

VA Coop (Medical)	Personal (Surgical)
Rejection	*Rejection*
Generalized poor LV function	Generalized poor LV function
Marked elevation of LVEDP?	LVEDP >25
Large LV	Not routine at that time
Poor EF	
Abnormal LV defined as	
1) EF <45% or	One or more walls
2) one or more segments akinetic, hypokinetic dyskinetic or	akinetic
3) LVEDP >14 mmHg	

1972-1974 and still do not use this parameter alone as an exclusion to surgery. This parameter has many vagaries and must be done in two different projections in a stable hemodynamic condition to be valid. The definition of "abnormal" left ventricular function by the VA Cooperative study used a high lower limit of 45% for the ejection fraction, and a low upper limit of normal of 14 mmHg for the left ventricular end-diastolic pressure. Any one of these so-called "abnormal values" or one or more segments akinetic, hypokinetic, or dyskinetic lead to the label of abnormal ventricle. Our cardiologists used a definition of abnormal as one or more segments of left ventricle having akinesis, hypokinesis, or dyskinesis. We also included patients with an LVEDP of 25 or less as surgical candidates. We, therefore, feel that these groups of patients are similar in demographic characteristics, as well as, in ventricular function. Although we feel that we were more "liberal" in including patients with poor left ventricular function as judged by LVEDP and the inclusion of unstable angina patients, these groups were remarkably similar. Comparison could only be improved by utilizing randomization. There is no attempt to compare our surgical results with the VA surgical results, but it is important to note that approximately 17% of patients in the VA medical group "crossed over" to surgical therapy. We also had a 99% follow-up on our patients. Operative mortality is included in all curves.

Results

Figure 1 presents the gross survival curves of the 229 surgically treated patients compared with 310 patients treated medically in the VA Cooperative study. The difference in survival becomes readily apparent in 2 years. There was an operative mortality of 0.4% or 1 in 229 patients. The VA study had only a 4-year follow-up, while we had a 5-year follow-up in the overall group with a nearly similar number of patients followed up to 4 years.

To look further into subsets, we compared patients with three vessel disease. The VA cumulative survival for all patients with three vessel disease was 73%, while the surgical survival was 93%. This difference in survival was readily apparent by 1 year and points out the fact that a low operative mortality is necessary to detect a difference in 1 year (Fig. 2).

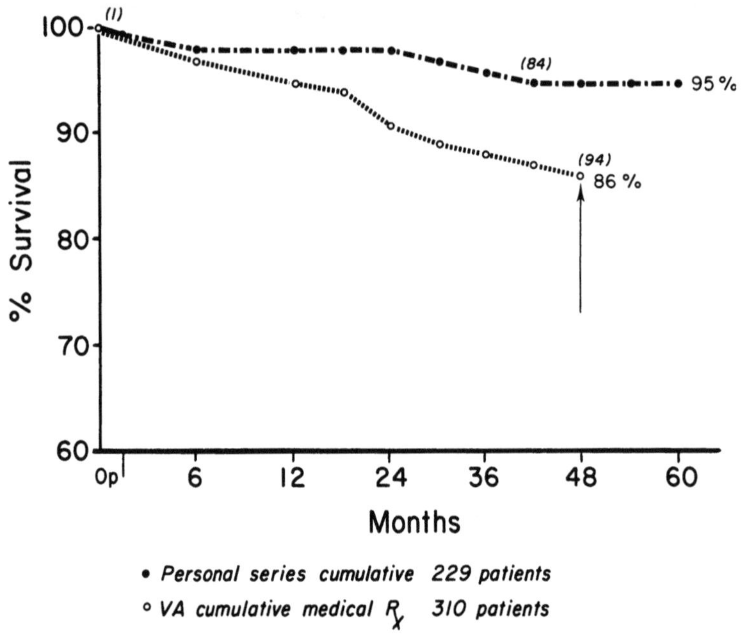

Fig. 1. The cumulative survival curve in 229 surgically treated patients compared with the cumulative VA medical therapy group of 310 patients. There was one operative death of the 229 patients

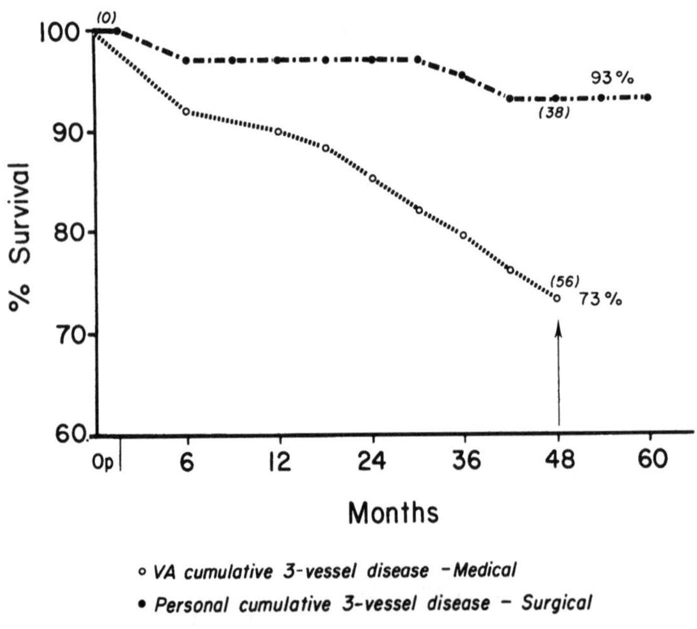

Fig. 2. Life table depicting survival in *all* patients with three-vessel disease. There is a 20% difference in survival at 4 years. There was no operative mortality in the 109 patient cohort and the difference in survival becomes apparent at 1 year

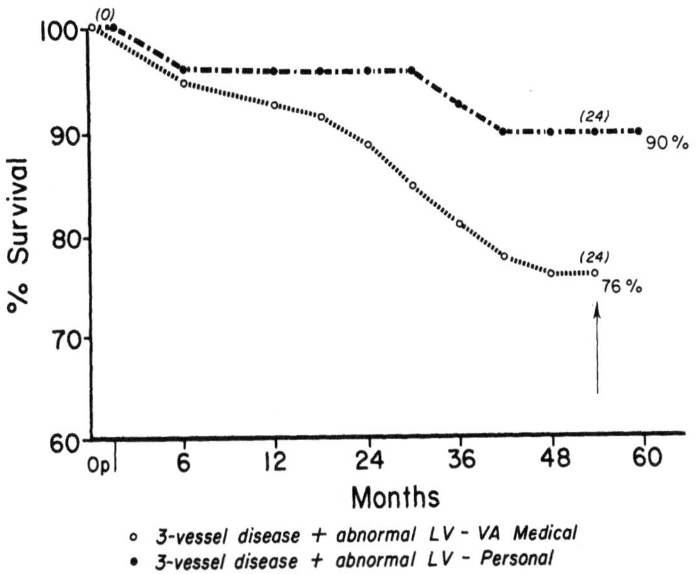

Fig. 3. This life table shows survival in the subset of patients with three-vessel disease and abnormal LV function with 54-month-survival tables

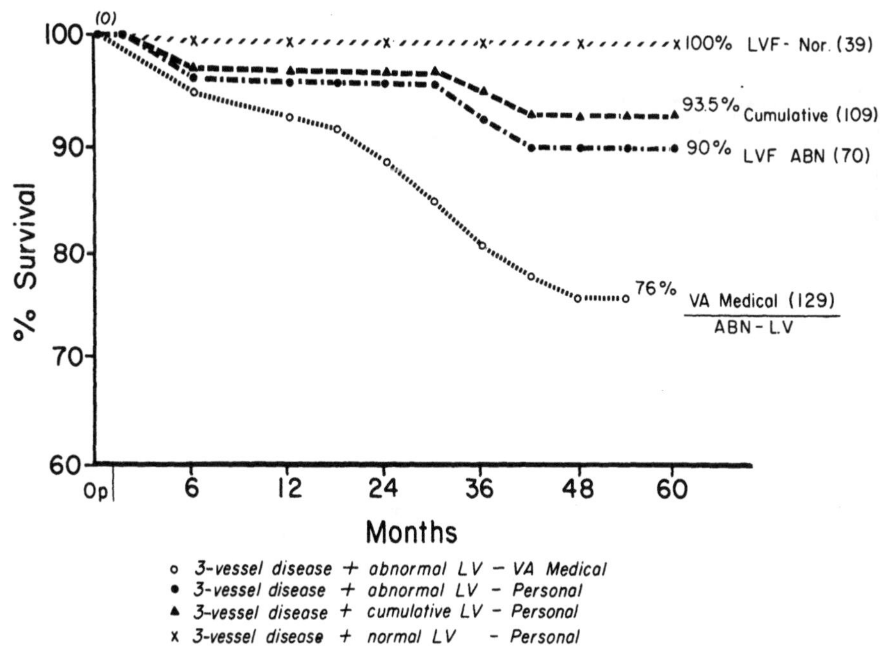

Fig. 4. This table has four groups. All surgically treated patients with three-vessel disease and normal LV are survivors. This is different than those with three-vessel disease and abnormal LV (LVF-ABN). All surgically treated groups demonstrate better survival curves than the medical treated cohort. The *best* curve was used for medically treated three-vessel disease to make this comparison

Figure 3 breaks this subset down even further to show the difference between the subset that has three-vessel disease and an abnormal left ventricle. Of the surgically treated patients in this group 90% are alive 5 years following operation and 76% of those treated medically are alive.

Figure 4 demonstrates that all patients in the subset with three-vessel disease and a normal left ventricle are alive 5 years post-operatively. This compares favorably with the VA medically treated group. The VA does not show what their survival is in this group. Figure 4 also shows that the three-vessel disease cumulative and abnormal left ventricular function group have markedly better survival than the 76% survival at 4.5 years for the abnormal LV group of the VA Cooperative study. It would appear from the VA Cooperative report that the three-vessel disease and abnormal LV did better than the three-vessel disease and normal LV since the cumulative (abnormal plus normal LV) patients had a lower 54 month survival than three-vessel disease and abnormal LV.

Figure 5 is a subset depicting survival in two-vessel disease showing that 95.6% of operated patients survive 5 years, while the VA Cooperative medically treated patients reveal an 87% 4-year survival. The number of patients in each group is similar. With single-vessel disease, we find no difference in survival at 4 years. The only surgical death occurred late and here one can only speculate on a difference in the quality of life which is not a subject of this discussion (Fig. 6). Figure 7 summarizes the curves, comparing the 4-year survival and annual attrition for each subset.

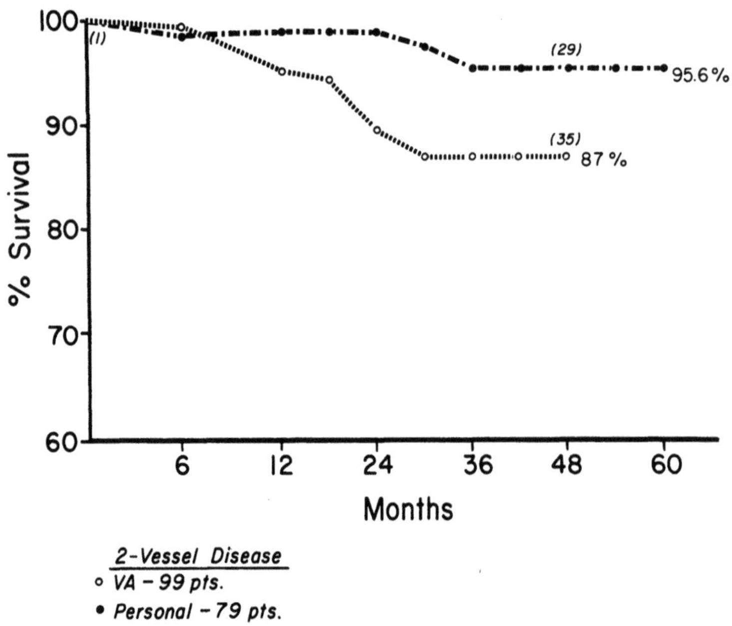

Fig. 5. Survival curve for two-vessel disease reveals a better curve for the surgical cohort than the medical, but the difference is not as striking as with three-vessel disease

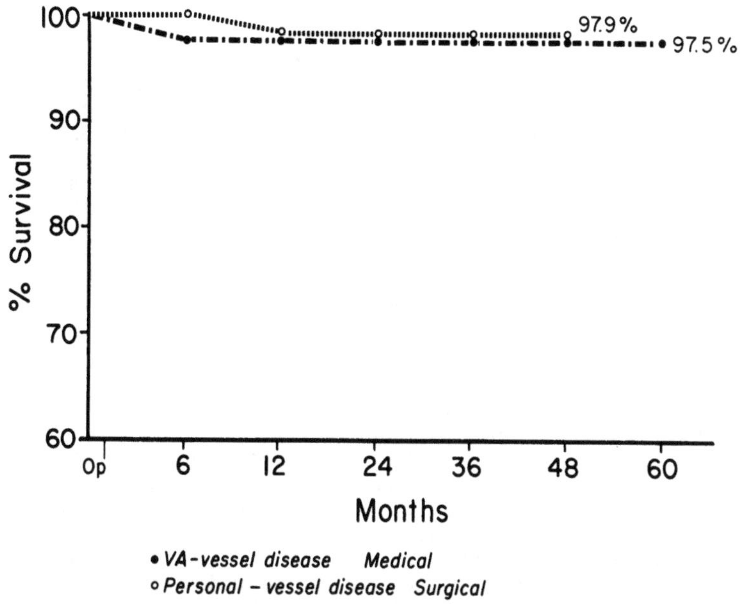

Fig. 6. No difference in survival curves noted in single-vessel disease. Both groups had one late death in a similar number of patients

SURVIVAL

	SURGERY			VA MEDICAL		
		4 yr	annual attrition		4 yr	annual attrition
OVERALL	229 pts	95 %	1.25 %	310 pts	86 %	3.5 %
3-VESSEL	109 pts			189 pts		
Cumulative	109 pts	93.5 %	1.6 %	189 pts	73 %	7 %
Abnormal LV	70 pts	90.0 %	2.5 %	129 pts	76 %	6 %
Normal LV	39 pts	100 %	0.0		?	?
2-Vessel	79 pts	95.6 %	1.1 %	99 pts	87 %	3.2 %
1-Vessel		97.5 %	0.3 %	45 pts	97.9 %	0.3 %

Fig. 7. This table summarizes the curves and shows that overall, and with three-vessel disease regardless of LV function, that the surgical cohort showed better survival and a much lower average annual attrition

Discussion

The ideal method for comparing two treatments of a problem is unquestionably a random study, but they must both represent the optimal currently available therapy. It was felt that the VA Cooperative study had some major defects. The surgical section had too high an operative mortality (5.8%) and too high a percentage of patients with all grafts closed (12%). We felt that the medically treated cohort represented the best results ever reported, but we agree this was more representative of medical therapy in the 1970s than the reports from the 1960s [2]. It did have a 17% crossover to surgical therapy that could have influenced their results, in having those patients with the worst angina cross to surgical therapy and thus, the most favorable group for medical therapy remained in the Medical Survival Tables. Nevertheless, we attempted to derive from our 1972-1974 experience those patients who compared closest with those described in the VA Cooperative group. Our surgically treated cohort was representative of our total experience as far as operative mortality was concerned. The operative mortality of all coronary bypass surgery for the years 1972-1974 was less than 2%.

In all subsets except single-vessel disease, survival was enhanced in the surgical therapy cohort. Left main coronary disease is acknowledged to have a better survival with surgical therapy and this study would suggest that triple-vessel disease with a normal or abnormal left ventricular function has increased survival with surgical therapy. A closer look at Fig. 4 further shows that survival in the presence of three-vessel disease is additionally enhanced by surgical intervention if the LV is still normal, and would prejudice one to a more aggressive surgical approach before LV damage has occurred. Either of these surgical subsets has a markedly better 4-year survival than medical therapy for the cumulative or abnormal LV, and triple-vessel disease, 73% and 76% respectively. Double-vessel disease treated by surgery shows a better, but less striking difference in favor of surgery. There is no question that a true randomized study would be the best method for comparing survival in the two groups of patients.

This study might be subject to criticism only in regards to comparability of left ventricular function, since in the medical therapy in the VA Cooperative study 68% of patients had abnormal left ventricular function. This difference may be more apparent than real, because we feel that the criteria the VA Cooperative study used to define abnormal were extremely liberal by using an LVEDP of 14 and an ejection fraction less than 45%. We included patients with an LVEDP up to 25 mmHg in our surgical group. We feel that the ventriculogram is the single most reliable determinant of ventricular function and our abnormal ventricular function occurred in 55% of patients and by ventriculographic criteria 68% of the VA group were abnormal. The percentages of patients with one-, two-, or three-vessel disease were very close, and any differences removed by comparing them in subsets, where the group numbers are comparable between the VA Cooperative study and this surgical series. We cannot compare directly three-vessel disease and normal LV function because the VA Cooperative study did not report the survival curve. These data would support an aggressive surgical approach to three-vessel coronary disease regardless of LV function within the boundaries of the population described.

Summary

Utilizing the VA Cooperative study criteria we have obtained from the Milwaukee Cardiovascular Data Registry one surgeon's experience with a similar cohort of 229 patients with coronary artery disease in 1972-1974 and followed 99% of these patients to date. They were compared to the VA Cooperative study medically treated group of 310 patients. The results of this comparison suggest: (1) that three-vessel disease and normal, and three-vessel disease and abnormal ventricular function had better survival with surgical intervention than when treated medically; (2) that two-vessel disease had a better survival with surgical therapy, 95.6% versus 87% at 4 years, but this is a less striking difference than seen with triple-vessel disease; and (3) that there is no difference in survival with single-vessel disease with coronary artery disease between medical and surgical therapy, and to recommend operation in this situation, it remains for us to prove a better quality of life and preservation of ventricular function. A randomized study that compares current optimal results of medical and surgical therapy would be desirable.

We would like to thank the Milwaukee Cardiovascular Data Registry for retrieval of the information, Mr. Jacob Assa, Coordinator.
We would like to thank the Cardiologists, Jack Manley, M.D., Howard Zeft, M.D., James King, M.D., John Walker, M.D., Henry Gale, M.D., Frank Cummins, M.D., Bernard Staller, M.D., H. David Friedberg, M.D., Richard Silberman, M.D., and Massoud Maleki, M.D. who entered all the preoperative data into the Data Registry and have followed these patients for many years.

References

1. Read, R.C., Murphy, M.L., Hultgren, H.N., Takaro, T.: Survival of men treated for chronic stable angina pectoris. J. Thorac. Cardiovasc. Surg. *75*, 1 (1978)
2. Webster, J.S., Moberg, C., Rincon, G.: Natural history of severe proximal coronary artery disease as documented by coronary cineangiography. Am. J. Cardiol. *33*, 195 (1974)

Does Coronary Bypass Surgery Prolong Life Expectancy?

R. J. Hall, D. A. Cooley, E. Garcia, V. S. Mathur, and C. M. de Castro, Jr.

While relief of disabling angina following coronary artery bypass (CAB) generally has been accepted, the influence of CAB upon long-term survival has remained controversial. Comparison of survival data of nonrandomized surgical series with "noncurrent" historic medical controls [1] has been criticized frequently, most recently by Braunwald [2]. In addition, the results of two recent multicenter cooperative studies of patients with unstable angina (NHLI)[3] and stable angina (VAH)[4], who were randomly assigned to medical or surgical therapy, show no difference in long-term survival.

From 1968 through 1976 at our Institute, 9,364 patients (Table 1) underwent direct revascularization of an ischemic myocardium with autologous saphenous vein grafts. Among these, 8,017 underwent CAB alone and 1,347, some other concomitant cardiac procedure [5]. In the 8,017 patients who underwent CAB alone, early mortality was 3.98%, while in the entire series, early mortality was 5.2%. During 1976, early mortality in patients who underwent CAB alone declined to 2.2% (52 deaths among 2,383 patients). The 5-year actuarial survival (Fig. 1) among these patients is 87.7%.

During this period, 846 patients from one cardiology section who underwent CAB alone came under my personal supervision and that of my colleagues and form the basis of this report [6]. Excluded from operation were patients with diffuse distal vessel disease that would have precluded satisfactory bypass, patients with notably impaired ventricular function but no angina, patients with lesser grades of occlusive disease according to angiography, and patients whose major occluded vessels were distributed to scarred areas discernable on angiography. The clinical profiles and early and long-term survival of these patients are detailed and compared with patients in the two multicenter random studies [3,4,7].

Of our patients 66% were 50 years or older (average, 53 years) (Table 2); 88% were males; 82% had angina, functional classes III or IV (NYHA); and 17% had unstable angina. Previous myocardial infarctions

Table 1. All cases of coronary artery bypass 1968 through 1976, Texas Heart Institute

Total patients	9,364
Coronary bypass alone	8,017
with aneurysm or valve surgery	1,347
Early mortality - bypass alone	3.98%
- all patients	5.2%
Early mortality - bypass alone (1976)	2.2%

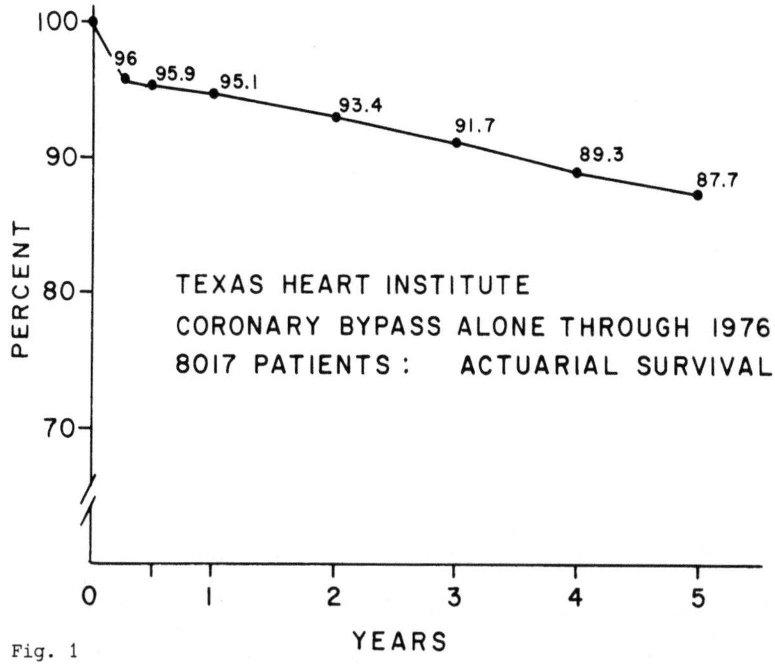

Fig. 1

Table 2

	THI Surgical	VAH[4] Random stable	NHLI[3] Random unstable
Males	88%	100%	-
Age ≥50	66%	-	59%
Average age	53 Yr	51 Yr	-
Angina FC II	15%	95% (FC II + FC III)	-
Angina FC III	63%		-
Angina FC IV	19%	-	-
Unstable	17%	None	100%

Table 3

	THI Surgical	VAH[4] Random stable	NHLI[3] Random unstable
Previous MI (total 846)	70%	62%	
Previous MI (unstable angina - 143 pts)	70%	-	31%
< 1 Month before CAB	3.2%		None
1-2 Months before CAB	3.5%	None	Within 3 months
2-6 Months before CAB	14.9%		
Hypertension	34%	29%	-
Diabetes mellitus	12%	12.5%	-

Table 4

	THI Surgical	VAH[4] Random stable	NHLI[3] Random unstable
Based upon reduction of luminal diameter of -	75%	50%	70%
Single vessel involvement	14%	16%	27%
Double vessel involvement	36%	34%	39%
Triple vessel involvement	50%	50%	33%
Main left coronary artery	8%	None	None
with stable angina	7.7%	-	-
with unstable angina	10%	-	-
Ejection fraction <0.45	18%	26%	23%

(Table 3) occurred in 70% in both the total group and the subset of 143 patients with unstable angina. Infarctions had occurred within 1 month of CAB in 3.2%, between 1 and 2 months in 3.5% and between 2 and 6 months in 14.9% (within 6 months in 21.6%). Hypertension was present in 34%, and diabetes mellitus in 12%. Based upon a 75% reduction in luminal diameter (Table 4), 14% had single major coronary artery occlusive disease (CAOD); 36% double CAOD; and 50% triple CAOD, indicating more extensive coronary artery disease than in either the VAH or NHLI series. Of the patients 8% (68) had involvement of the left main coronary artery, an exclusion in both random studies. Main left coronary disease was present in 7.7% of the patients with stable angina and 10% of those with unstable angina. The ejection fraction was reduced (less than 0.60) in 48% and was below 0.45 in 18%.

Single bypass (Table 5) was performed in 8%, double in 39%, triple in 45% and four or more bypasses in 8% of the patients, producing an average of 2.53 bypasses per patient. This compares to a greater frequency of single and double bypasses (79%) in the VAH series for an average of 1.9 bypasses per patient. Comparable data for the NHLI series are not available. The ratio of bypasses to major vessels involved, an index of completeness of revascularization, was 1.08, compared to 0.87 in the VAH study. The early mortality (30 day) was 2.96% (Table 6) for the total series studied; and was 3.4% during the years 1972-1974, the period of the two random studies. Early

Table 5

	THI Surgical	VAH[4] Random stable	NHLI[3] Random unstable
Single CAB	8%	28%	-
Double CAB	39%	51%	-
Triple CAB	45%	21%	-
Four or more CAB	8%	None	-
Bypasses per patient	2.53	1.9	-
Average major vessels involved per patient	2.34	2.18	
Ratio CAB/vessels involved	1.08	0.87	-

Table 6

	THI Surgical	VAH[4] Random stable	NHLI[3] Random unstable
Early mortality (846 pts)	2.96%	-	-
Years 1972-1974	3.4%	5.6%	5.0%
Male	2.6%	5.6%	-
Female	5.7%	-	-
Left main CAB (68 pts)	1.5%	-	-
Unstable angina (143 pts)	3.5%	-	5.0%

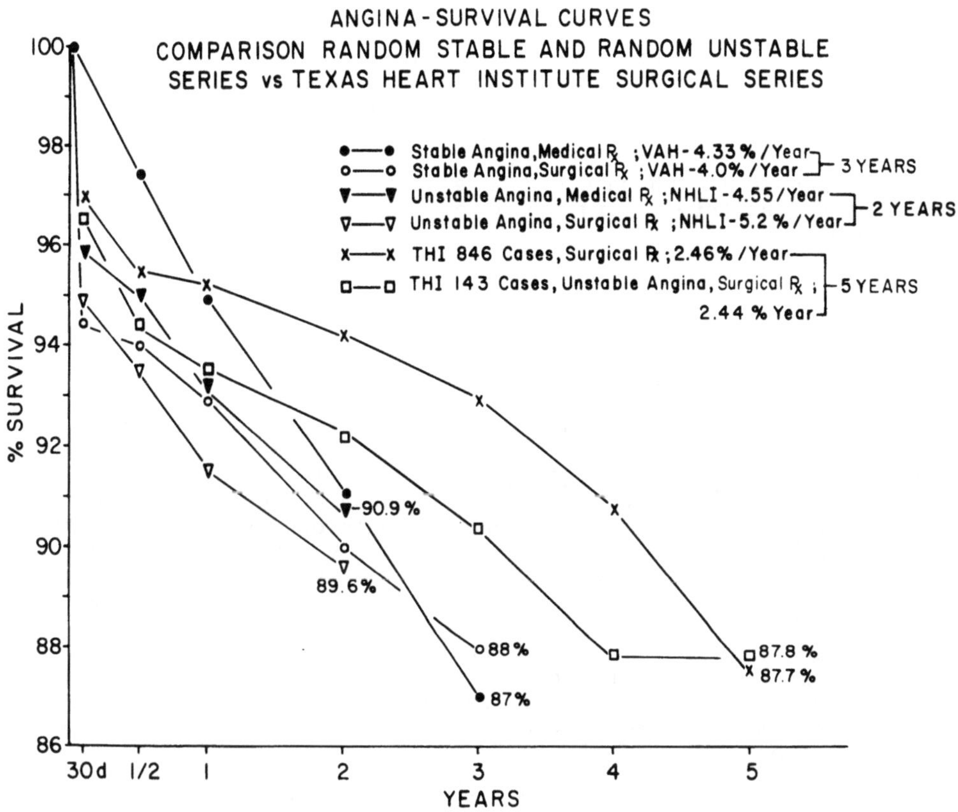

Fig. 2

mortality in males was 2.6%, while females experienced a 5.7% early mortality, a feature we have noted throughout our experience with CAB [8]. Early mortality in patients with left main coronary disease was 1.5% and in those with unstable angina, 3.5%.

The 5-year actuarial survival [9] of patients in this series (Fig. 2) is 87.7% yielding an average attrition, including early mortality, of 2.46% per year. The annual attrition of survivors of the first month is 1.9% per year. The 5-year survival for patients with unstable angina and for those with left main CAOD is 87.7% and 85.2%, respectively. In comparison (Table 7), the 5-year survival of Bruschke's historical "noncurrent" medically treated patients [1] is 64.4% (7.12%

Table 7

	THI Surgical	Bruschke[1] Clev. Cl. medical	VAH[4] Randomized Medical		NHLI[3] Randomized Medical	
			Medical	Surgical	Medical	Surgical
5-Yr survival	87.7%*	64.4%	-	-	-	-
Average yearly attrition	2.46%	7.12%	4.33%	-	4.55%	-
"Projected" 5-yr survival	-	-	78.3%*	83.7%	77.3%*	81.5%

(*P = 0.005)

per year average attrition); while in the two multicenter studies, the patients randomized to "current" medical treatment experienced an average annual attrition of 4.33% per year with stable angina [4] and 4.55% per year with unstable angina [3]. The "projected" 5-year survival in the latter two medically treated series is 78.3% and 77.3%, respectively (which would be statistically different from the Texas Heart Institute's surgical 5-year survival of 87.7% at the 0.005 level).

Discussion

The surgical experience at the Texas Heart Institute is composed of a consecutive series of patients with serious symptomatic and anatomic ischemic heart disease. Indicators of severity of disease were present in our patients with equal or greater frequency than in the populations comprising either of the two multicenter random treatment studies. Involvement of the left main coronary artery, excluded in the random studies, was present in 8% of the patients. Females, who experience more than double the early mortality [6] of males, were not present in the VAH study. Women made up 12% of our population. Identified exclusions in both random studies tend to develop a series of patients for randomization who have fewer traits of serious coronary artery disease. This bias toward less severe disease is further enhanced in the multicenter studies by exclusions, before randomization, of a subset of patients at "physician or patient preference" [10]. Slightly over one-quarter of the VAH patients eligible for randomization [11] were excluded: 8% by death, 38% unwilling to enter the study, and 48% for "other" but unspecified reasons. This could be construed, unless proved otherwise, as a diversion of patients with more severe disease to nonrandomized surgical treatment.

Further bias of the actuarial attrition of the medically randomized patients results from crossover of patients to surgical treatment during follow-up. Such patients comprised 16% of the medically randomized VAH patients [4] and 33% of the NHLI patients [12]. Dropping these patients from follow-up at the time of crossover may further improve the long-term results of medical treatment actuarially. When these exclusions of patients with more serious and prognostically unfavorable features are considered, medical therapy might not be an "approach better than previously reported" [3], and despite the current use of beta blockers, may be little, if at all, better than the medical statistics detailed by Bruschke [1]. In light of these observations, we should assess the immediate and long-term results of effective revascularization of the ischemic myocardium by means of coronary artery bypass grafting. In our institute and many other surgical centers, the immediate and long-term results are better than those reported in either multicenter random study. Of greater importance is the fact that the long-term survival after CAB is better than that of less critically diseased patients who were randomly assigned to current medical treatment. These differences, if projected to 5 years, are statistically significant.

It is evident that effective myocardial revascularization in patients with more severe coronary artery disease prolongs life at the 5-year point when compared with current medical management.

References

1. Bruschke, A.V.G., Proudfit, W.L., et al: Progress study of 590 consecutive nonsurgical cases of coronary disease followed 5-9 years. Circulation *47*, 1147-1153 (1973)
2. Braunwald, E.: Coronary-artery surgery at the crossroads. N. Engl. J. Med. *297*, 661-663 (1977)
3. National Cooperative Study Group of National Heart, Lung and Blood Institute: Medical approach better than previously reported. In: Acute unstable angina. Clinical Trends in Cardiology *6*, 1-3 (1977)
4. Murphy, M.L., Hultgren, H.N., Detre, K., et al: Treatment of chronic stable angina: A preliminary report of survival data of the randomized Veterans Administration Cooperative Study. N. Engl. J. Med. *297*, 621-626 (1977)
5. Cooley, D.A., Wukasch, D.C., Bruno, F., et al: Direct myocardial revascularization: Experience with 9,364 operations. Thorax *33*, 411-417 (1978)
6. Hall, R.J., Garcia, E., Mathur, V.S., et al: Factors influencing early and late survival after aortocoronary artery bypass: A preliminary report. Cardiovasc. Dis., Bull. Texas Heart Inst. *4*, 120-128 (1977)
7. Russel, R.O., Moraski, R.E., Kouchoukos, N., et al: Unstable angina pectoris: National Cooperative Study Group to compare medical and surgical therapy. I. Report of protocol and patient population. Am. J. Cardiol. *37*, 896-902 (1976)
8. Wukasch, D.C., Hall, R.J., Cooley, D.A., et al: Surgical versus medical treatment of coronary artery disease: Long-term survival. Vasc. Surg. *10*, 300-314 (1976)
9. Cutler, S.J., Ederer, F.: Maximum utilization of the life table method in analyzing survival. J. Chronic. Dis. *8*, 699 (1958)
10. Scheidt, S.S.: Unstable angina: Medical management or surgery? Editorial and comment. Cardiovasc. Med. *2*, 541-543 (1977)
11. Detre, K., Hultgren, H., Takaro, T.: Veterans Administration Cooperative Study for coronary arterial occlusive disease. III. Methods and baseline characteristics, including experience with medical treatment. Am. J. Cardiol. *40*, 212-225 (1977)
12. Hutter, A.M., Russel, R.O., Resnekov, L., et al: Unstable angina pectoris: National randomized study of survival vs medical therapy: Results in 1, 2, and 3 vessel disease. Circulation *5556* [suppl. 3], 60 (1977)

Are There Indications for Surgery in Asymptomatic Patients?

A. Selzer

In every form of treatment, be it medical or surgical, it is necessary to evaluate the risk-benefit relationship. The performance of aortocoronary bypass operation in patients who are free from symptoms, apparently in good health, requires a particularly careful analysis of factors involved because the operation is primarily of prophylactic nature, that is, aimed at prevention of future problems. Justification for the performance of a major heart operation in an apparently well subject rests upon four assumptions:

1) Stenotic lesions in coronary arteries are inevitably and rapidly progressive.
2) As a corollary of the previous statement, patients with significant stenotic lesions are always at the high risk of acute myocardial infarction or sudden death.
3) Bypass operations successfully and reliably protect the patient from these disastrous events.
4) Clinical symptoms are unreliable as guidelines to myocardial ischemia.

Thus, the answer to the question posed in the title depends on the analysis of these four assumptions: if they are correct then the operation is fully justifiable at all times provided a significant stenosis in the coronary artery is found. If incorrect, the operation should never be performed.

Starting with the first assumption it is true that plaques in the coronary arteries start as small lesions and gradually increase, encroaching upon the lumen and eventually producing complete occlusion of the artery. However, it should be emphasized that:

1) The rate of growth is quite variable.
2) Complete occlusion may develop abruptly, such as the result of subintimal hemorrhage, or rupture of atheromatous plaque, or of thrombosis, regardless of how small or how large the stenotic lesion.
3) Many plaques become burned out, that is, replaced by fibrosis and then remain stable and nonprogressive [1].

As a consequence, a single coronary arteriogram does not permit prediction of the future course of coronary disease.

In regards to the second assumption, while high degree of stenosis suggests a possibility of a future myocardial infarction or sudden death, collateral circulation may partly or completely compensate the reduction or cessation of coronary flow and thus avert the catastrophe. It is recognized that coronary arteriography cannot reliably estimate the available volume of collateral circulation [2].

The third assumption is probably the most controversial. It is tempting to accept the hypothesis that sizable artificial collateral blood supply to a stenosed coronary artery protects the appropriate portion of the heart from temporary or permanent ischemia, especially since the operative mortality in skillful surgical hands can be very low indeed. Yet it is necessary to review the overall risk of bypass surgery, that is, to add to the operative mortality the risk of interoperative myocardial infarction, the risk of diffuse myocardial damage resulting from the cardiopulmonary bypass, the risk of closure of the bypass graft, and the risk of rapid progression of the lesion in the bypassed arteries proximal to the anastomosis [3]. In terms of benefit there is general agreement that relief of symptoms and of other manifestations of ischemia is excellent, often dramatic. Furthermore, there is strong implication, perhaps not yet positive proof, that in significant lesions of the left main coronary trunk life is prolonged by the aortocoronary bypass operation [4]. Otherwise the suggestion that aortocoronary bypass surgery is effective in prolonging life and preventing myocardial infarction has no factual basis. There are suggested statistics but mainly in nonrandomized series in which comparison of the two groups lacks statistical validity. The two principal randomized series [4,5], in spite of some faults pointed out by many investigators, are still the best means of comparison that we possess and they show no difference between medical and surgical cases for the entire group of patients included in the studies. It should be emphasized that the widely used medical reference series' (dividing the material into one-vessel, two-vessel, three-vessel) are strongly biased toward unfavorable results and should not be used in comparing them with surgical results [6]. It can now be stated that two published [7,8] and several unpublished independent studies point to the fact that the deciding factor in prognosis is not the number of coronary vessels involved but the state of the myocardium. Thus, three-vessel disease carries the poorest prognosis because it is most likely to produce a damaged myocardium with a low ejection fraction.

The fourth assumption is based on observation concerning the frequency of sudden cardiac death as the initial manifestation in patients later found to have advanced coronary disease. Furthermore, acute myocardial infarction frequently develops in patients who had no previous clinical manifestation of coronary disease. Finally, there are many examples of electrocardiographic evidence of ischemia occurring spontaneously or in response to exercise without concomitant pain. However, the only point to be made is that myocardial ischemia *can* occur without pain or pain equivalent. How often this occurs is not known and one can muster good arguments in favor of this being rare. First, most clinicians recognize that statistics regarding unheralded sudden death are unreliable. Careful questioning of survivors frequently brings out the facts that the deceased suffered from "bursitis," "indigestion," "neuralgia" - all of which unquestionably represents unrecognized anginal pain. Furthermore, sudden death is undoubtedly a common manifestation of sudden increment of luminal stenosis, such as subintimal hemorrhage or thrombosis developing in patients who in spite of coronary disease did not previously have ischemia, therefore had no cause for symptoms. Finally, it is clear that painless ischemia during stress testing can be observed only in a small minority of patients.

From the preceding discussion it is clear that the four assumptions are not entirely correct. The first one - inevitable progression, and the second - inevitable development of myocardial infarction and sudden cardiac death - are clearly incorrect. The third postulate -

protective value of bypass operation - is unproven and probably incorrect except for a subset of patients with left coronary artery trunk lesions. The fourth - unreliability of symptoms - is true only for a small minority of cases.

Without these principal arguments the case in favor of considering coronary artery disease as a purely hydraulic problem becomes very weak. One can answer the question posed in the title, by stating that in general aortocoronary bypass surgery has, as a rule, no place when applied to asymptomatic patients. However, there are undoubtedly small subsets where consideration needs to be given to such patients as being exceptions to the above rule. Here I would place first severe obstructive lesion estimated at at least 75% of luminal stenosis in the left main trunk in patients who have no arteriographic evidence of large collateral circulation from the right coronary artery. Secondly, I would put in these categories patients with critical coronary lesions in any of the other branches in whom truly severe ischemia (ST segment elevation or segmental depression greater than 3 mm) is demonstrated without symptoms, particularly if a life-threatening arrhythmia, such as ventricular tachycardia or ventricular fibrillation, is triggered by the ischemia.

This discussion would not be complete without making a few comments about means of discovering coronary artery disease in asymptomatic subjects. In the light of the previous considerations regarding operations in such patients I am opposed to a broad case finding effort using coronary arteriography. I know that in some institutions a large number of asymptomatic subjects are being studied by means of coronary arteriography because of the mere presence of coronary risk factors, or following recovery from an eventful and uncomplicated myocardial infarction, or because of a mere presence of a mildly positive stress test. I see no justification for this approach. There is even serious reservation in my mind whether stress testing should be included in a routine examination of asymptomatic patients except in those who have had a myocardial infarction in the past or in whom there is other suggestive evidence that they may have coronary artery disease. If results of stress testing are used for indications for coronary arteriography then only those patients who show an unusually severe ischemic response or who show life-threatening arrhythmias with exercise should be further followed by arteriography.

In summary, aortocoronary bypass operation in asymptomatic patients is based on the assumptions which are in part or in their entirety incorrect and so not justify the performance of a prophylactic operation. The small subset of coronary disease in which prophylaxis may be justified on the basis of present knowledge is a severe lesion of the main left coronary trunk. It should be emphasized that the overwhelming majority of patients with this lesion has significant symptoms. The rare occurrence of asymptomatic main left disease does not justify a broad case finding search by means of coronary arteriography.

References

1. Vlodaver, Z., Edwards, J.E.: Pathology of coronary atherosclerosis. Prog. Cardiovasc. Dis. *14*, 256 (1971)
2. McGregor, M.: The coronary collateral circulation: A significant compensatory mechanism or a functionless quirk of nature. Circulation *52*, 529 (1975)
3. Pasternak, R., Cohn, K., Selzer, A., Langston, M.F. (Jr.): Enhanced rate of

progression of coronary artery disease following aortocoronary saphenous vein bypass surgery. Am. J. Med. *58*, 166 (1975)
4. Murphy, M.L. Hultgren, H.N., Detre, K., Thomsen, J., Takaro, T., et al: Treatment of chronic stable angina. N. Engl. J. Med. *297*, 621 (1977)
5. Hutter, A.M., Russel, R.O. (Jr.), Resnekov, L., Wolk, M., Rosati, R.A., Conti, C.R., Becker, L., Biddle, T., Schroeder, J.S., Kaplan, E.M., Gilbert, J.P., Mock, M.B.: Unstable angina pectoris. National randomized study of surgical vs. medical therapy: Results in 1, 2 and 3 vessel disease. Circulation *55-56* [Suppl. III], 60 (1977) (Abs.)
6. Selzer, A., Cohn, K.: Asymptomatic coronary artery disease and coronary bypass surgery. Am. J. Cardiol. *39*, 614 (1977)
7. Vlietsra, R.D.E., Assad-Morell, J.L., Frye, R., Elveback, L.R., Connoly, D.C., Ritman, E.I., Pluth, J.R., Barnhorst, D.A., Danielson, G.K., Wallace, R.B.: Survival predictors in coronary artery disease. Medical and surgical comparisons. Mayo Clin. Proc. *52*, 85 (1977)
8. Gross, H., Vaid, A.K., Cohen, M.V.: Prognosis in patients rejected for coronary revascularization surgery. Am. J. Med. *64*, 9 (1978)

Factors to Prolong Survival in Patients with Coronary Artery Disease

R. B. Karp, N. T. Kouchoukos and J. W. Kirklin

Summary

Coronary artery bypass grafting generally relieves angina. Our studies have shown that survival of these angina patients treated surgically is superior at 3-5 years than in similar matched (but not randomized) patients treated medically. Factors associated with this improved survival are 1) low operative mortality; 0.9% in 757 patients for 1977, 1.5% for the total series, 2) a diminishing perioperative infarction rate, 1.6% for 1975, in light of evidence supporting an association between perioperative infarction and late postoperative death, 3) a significant improvement in late survival of angina patients with LV dysfunction operated on compared to those not operated, 4) a similarity in survival among operated patients whether they have two- or three-vessel or left main disease.
Other factors which are presumed to favorably influence postoperative survival are 1) complete revascularization, 2) improved intraoperative myocardial preservation, 3) late overall SVG patency rate (80%).
Comparing our surgical results with an age/sex/race-matched normal population suggests that survival is prolonged in patients having SV grafting and is nearly equal to that of normal populations.

This symposium is directed toward approaches for prolonging survival in patients with coronary artery disease. It has been adequately demonstrated that operation has a very significant effect to improve quality of life by relieving angina in the majority of patients.

Table 1. Symptomatic status in coronary artery disease randomized study[a]

Treatment group	Status >1 year after treatment					
	Asymptomatic		Improved		Same or worse	
	No.	%	No.	%	No.	%
CABPG (n = 32[b])	24	75%	7	22%	1	3%
Medical treatment (n = 30[b])	4	13%	19	63%	7	23%
	P for difference <0.0001				P for difference = 0.02	

[a]Mathur et al., NEJM 292:710, (April 3, 1975).
[b]Surviving patients.
CABPG = coronary artery bypass grafting

Table 1 is reproduced from a study by Mathur and Guinn [1] and elegantly demonstrates the difference in relief of symptoms of patients with stable angina randomized to either surgery or medical treatment. Of the surgical patients at 1 year 75% were asymptomatic whereas only 13% treated medically achieved asymptomatic status.

Naturally, then most large surgical series have included the majority of patients operated upon for symptoms. The University of Alabama in Birmingham group is no exception. In order to form conclusions as to the effect of surgery on survival of these patients we must begin with certain assumptions. Some are quite clear, for example, that angina as a manifestation of coronary artery disease predisposes to a discouraging life expectancy compared to a normal, age-matched population. This has been shown in the Framingham study [2]. A more difficult proposition to prove is that operation produces better survival in any group of coronary artery disease patients than comparable patients treated medically. The Veterans Administration cooperative study [3] has suggested to some that there is no greater effect of surgery to reduce mortality of coronary artery disease than medical treatment. It must be remembered that the VA study included only selected patients with stable angina and good left ventricular function. Approximately only an average of seven patients per year were operated in each of the participating hospitals and operative mortality was 5.6%. So comparison of treatment modalities must take into account these important factors having to do with experience of the surgical team, 30-day mortality, and, indeed, the whole question of heterogeneity of the diseased population.

Generally, age, race, and sex can be matched in large, otherwise heterogeneous populations. However, the degree of left ventricular damage must be assessed in a uniform manner and the symptomatic status of the patient precisely noted (Table 2). It is also curious that a 95% proximal left anterior descending stenosis plus disease of one or two diagonals has the same notation, that is single-vessel disease, as does a 60% mid-left anterior descending lesion. Thus, completeness of revascularization is a relative term. Despite some of the difficulties implicit in answering problems of survival posed by this multifaceted population we shall use some of the information obtained at our institution from operated patients to attempt to give insight into factors which prolong survival in these coronary artery patients.

Table 2. Problems in *evaluating surgical* versus *medical treatment* in coronary artery disease

Heterogeneity of the patient population
Age, race, sex
Number of stenosed branches of the coronary system
Degree of left ventricular damage
Other atherosclerotic risk factors
Heterogeneity of surgical techniques
Hospital mortality rates
Completeness of revascularization
Myocardial preservation
Long-term patency rates
Possible recent changes in results of medical treatment

February 9, 1978

Table 3. Thirty-day mortality rates for coronary artery bypass grafting

Year of operation	No. of pts.	Mortality No.	Mortality %
1970	29	4	13.8
1971	134	2	1.5
1972	163	5	3.1
1973	264	5	1.9
1974	434	5	1.2
1975	537	7	1.3
1976	739	11	1.5
1977	757	7	0.9
Totals	3057	46	1.5

Table 4. Primary coronary artery bypass grafting, UAB, 1977

Age (years)	No. of patients		Hospital deaths No.	Hospital deaths %
< 20	-		-	
20 < 30	3		-	0%
30 < 40	26		1	3.8%
40 < 50	157	0.4%* (0.2%-0.8%)	1	0.6%
50 < 60	361		1	0.3%
60 < 70	190		0	0%
70 < 80	19	20.0% (10.4%-33.4%)	4	21.1%
≥ 80	1		-	0%
Total	757		7	0.9%

*P for difference < 0.0001.
( ) 70% confidence limits.

Most would agree that saphenous vein bypass grafting relieves angina in about 80% of patients at 1 year and is associated with low operative mortality. At the University of Alabama, as surgical experience has increased, 30-day hospital mortality for saphenous vein grafting has decreased and come to be about 1.5% in 3057 patients. It is 0.9% in 757 patients operated in 1977 (Table 3).

Of interest, the distribution of patients treated surgically comprised 67% with unstable angina, and one-third of the total had had symptoms of congestive heart failure, and over one-half had a previous myocardial infarction.

The operative mortality for patients under 70 years of age in 1977 was 0.4% and in the 20 patients over 70 it was 20% (Table 4). The difference in mortality in the group of patients over 70 is statistically significant and perhaps has relevance to planning a cost effective and efficient rehabilitation program.

Over an 8 year period the number of distal anatomosis performed per patient has increased (Fig. 1). During this period mortality has shown no related increase and probably actually decreased. We do not

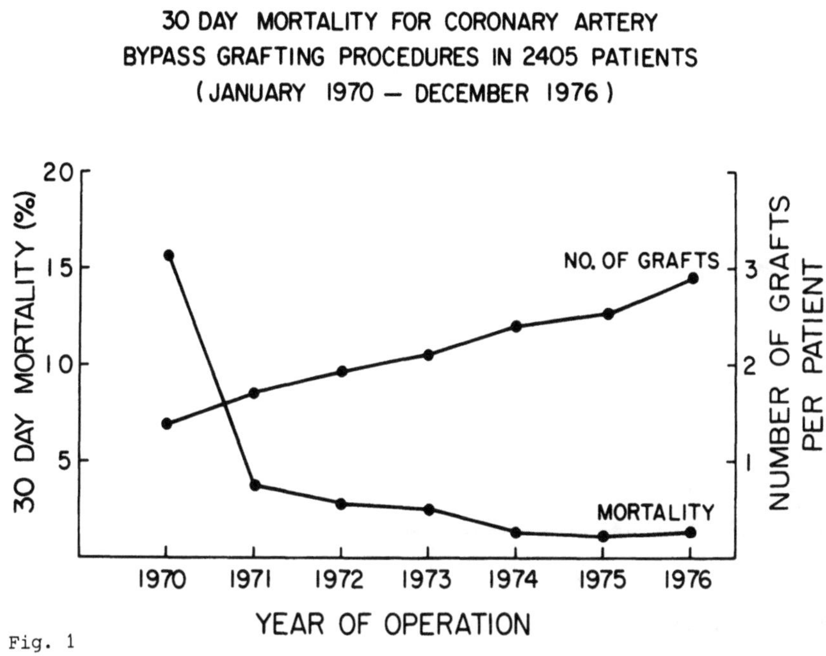

Fig. 1

Table 5. Primary coronary artery bypass grafting, UAB, 1977

No. of distal anastomoses	% of total patients	No. of patients		Hospital deaths No.	Hospital deaths %
1	5%	35		-	0%
2	32%	122	0.6%* (0.1%-2.2%)	1	0.8%
3		242		1	0.4%
4	47%	213	1.4%* (0.8%-2.4%)	2	0.9%
5		112		3	2.7%
6		22		-	0%
7		4		-	0%
Total		750		7	0.9%

*P for difference = 0.45 (0.75 with correction for continuity).
Chi-square test for trend of hospital deaths with increasing no. of anastomoses = 0.55.
( ) = 70% confidence limits.

know if a greater number of distal anastomoses improves long-term survival, or for that matter if any number greater than three, substantially increases the fraction of the patients free of angina. However, for 1977, 47% of patients had more than three distal anastomoses with no difference in surgical mortality (Table 5).

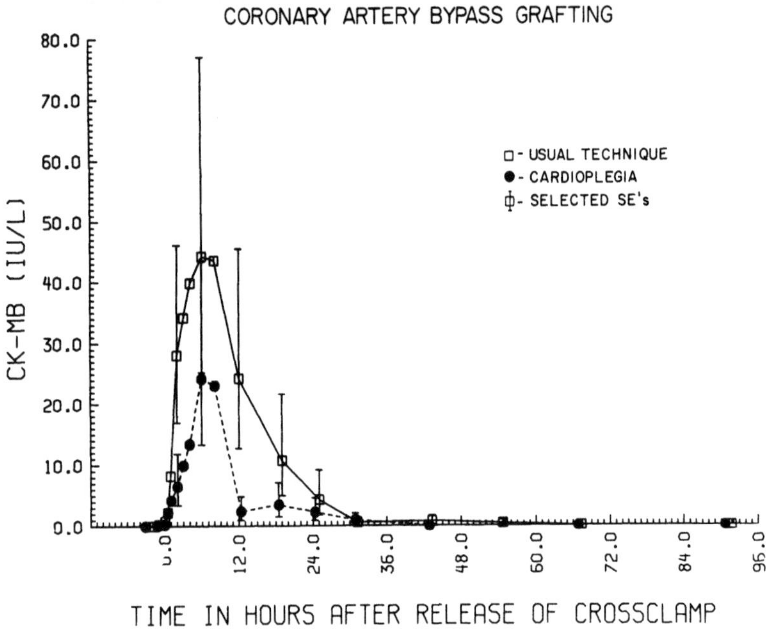

Fig. 2. Release of CK-MB in CABG patients using either hypothermic arrest or cardioplegic myocardial preservation [6]

The conduct of the coronary artery bypass operation is important to reducing surgical mortality and thus accentuating those positive factors leading to prolonged survival. Recently we have turned to cold potassium cardioplegic myocardial preservation with a single period of aortic crossclamping to do all distal anastomosis. CK-MB isoenzyme elaboration was diminished by this technique (Fig. 2).

In a randomized group of patients [4] evidence for electrocardiographic change occurring in the perioperative period was also less in the cardioplegia group compared to patients having hypothermic ischemic arrest. (ECG negative for change: 76% cardioplegia versus 47% hypothermia $P = 0.08$).

Perioperative infarction has decreased over the years and now is below 3% (Fig. 3). Measures to limit intraoperative myocardial damage are important as illustrated by the finding that late postoperative myocardial infarction occurred two and one-half times more frequently in patients having perioperative myocardial infarctions (Fig. 4). Additionally, survival was significantly decreased in those patients in whom there was electrocardiogram or enzyme evidence of intraoperative injury (Fig. 5).

As emphasized by others, graft patency is important to long-term relief of angina and probably also to long-term survival [5]. The VA cooperative study patients showed a 69% graft patency, not too different from UAB experience at that time (Fig. 6, Period I). There is, however, a statistically significant improvement in 1 year patency with time.

In our group, and as noted by Grondin [6], at second restudy there is little attrition in graft patency (Table 6). Of 55 patients with patent grafts 1 year postoperative 52 had continued patency at a second restudy.

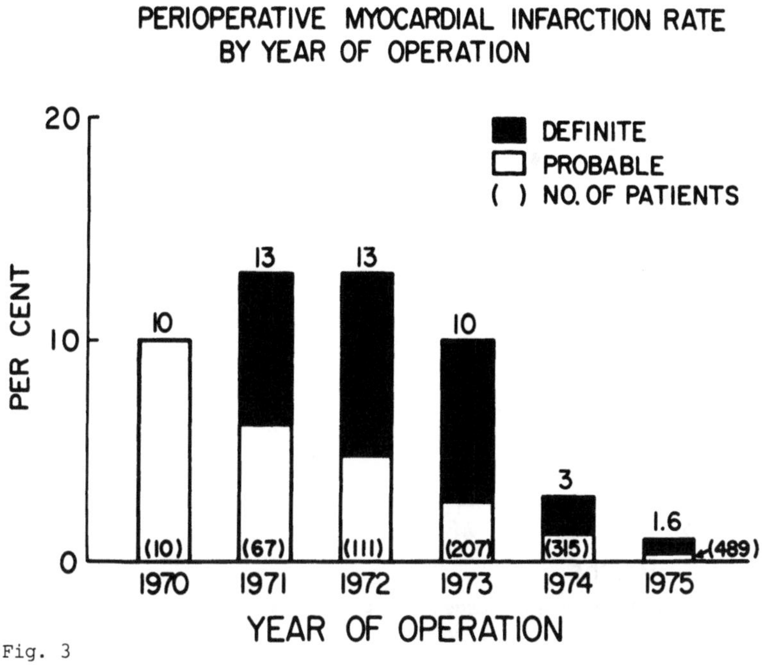

Fig. 3

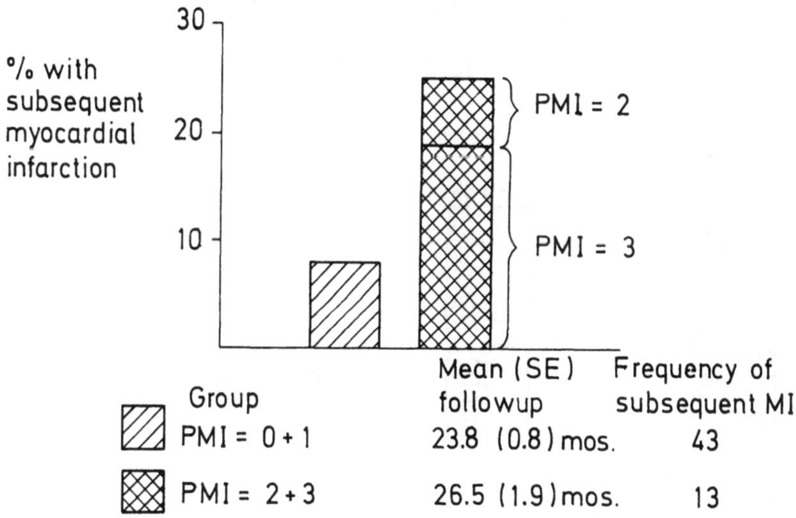

Fig. 4. Subsequent myocardial infarction in patients with and without perioperative myocardial infarction (PMI). 0 = no enzyme elevation, no EKG change; 1 = SGOT > 70 < 100; 2 = SGOT > 100 and EKG evidence of infarction

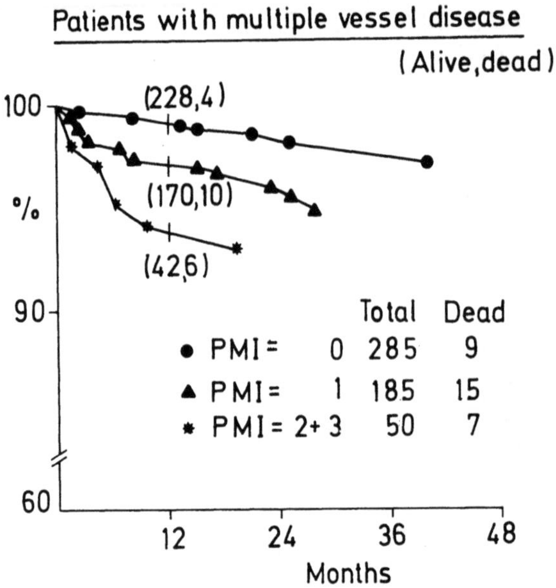

Fig. 5. Survival after coronary bypass surgery by perioperative myocardial infarction (PMI) class. (See Fig. 4 for key to PMI)

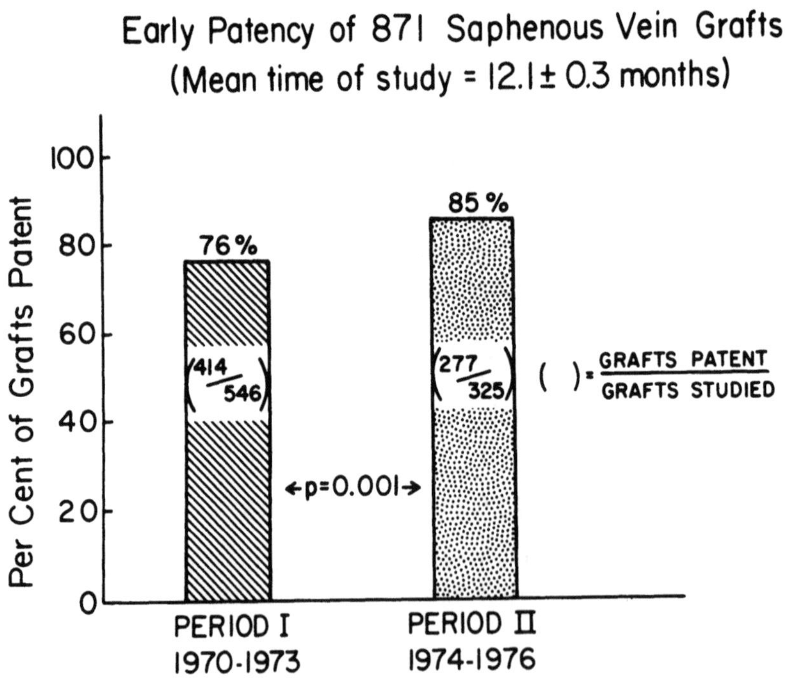

Fig. 6. Graft status 1 year after CABG

Table 6. Late patency of vein bypass grafts in 31 patients (Mean time of study = 37 ± 11 months)

System grafted	No. of grafts	Patency rates			
		One year		Late[a]	
		No.	%	No.	%
Right	25	23	92%	22	88%
Anterior descending	28	21	75%	19	68%
Circumflex	11	11	100%	11	100%
Totals	64	55	86%	52	81%

[a] Seventeen patients studies between three and five years after operation.

What now about survival of our own group of operated patients? When patients operated on with three-vessel disease are compared to patients considered surgical candidates but not operated on we found the following (Fig. 7):

At 36 months survival of matched but not randomized patients managed surgically was statistically better than patients considered candidates for operation but managed medically. Survival in patients treated medically who were not deemed candidates for surgery by unsuitable anatomy or depressed ventricular function was poor.

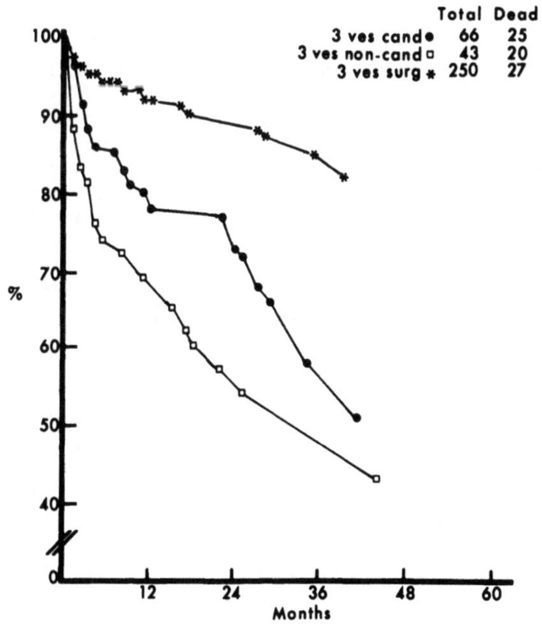

Fig. 7. Survival of candidates, non-candidates and total surgery with 3-vessel disease. Survival of surgical group compared to medically treated patients. "Non-candidates" are those patients medically treated who were considered by anatomy or left ventricular dysfunction not suitable for operation. Surgery has improved survival significantly ($P < 0.05$) at 36 months [1]

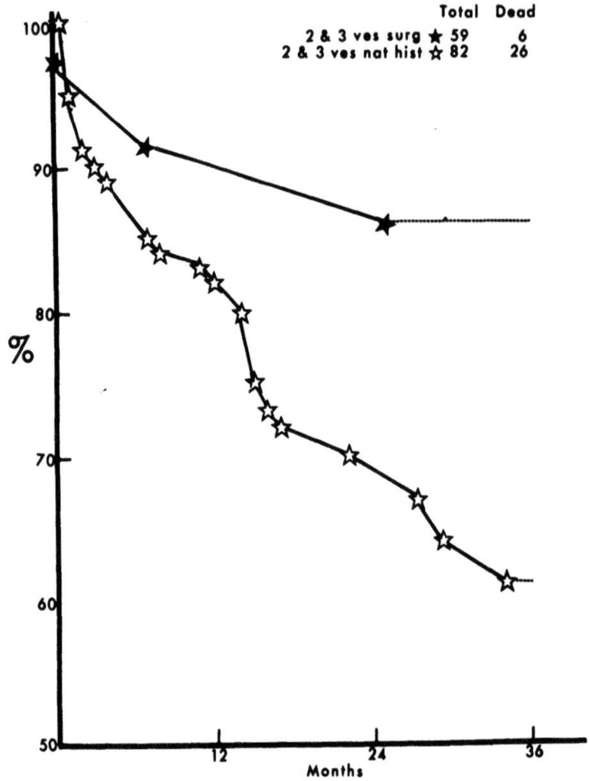

Fig. 8. Survival of surgery and natural history groups with multiple vessel disease, generalized hypokinesis and cardiomegaly. Survival of surgical group is significant ($P < 0.05$) at 24 months [1]

However, in our recent experience even patients with poor left ventricular function if operated upon sustain better long-term survival than similar patients treated medically (Fig. 8). Improved survival of the surgical group is significant at 24 months.

Following an example of Green [7], we and others [8] believe it useful to compare our treated groups of diseased patients (surgical group) to a normal group of age/sex/race-matched population.

An example is shown in Fig. 9 of patients with three-vessel disease treated medically at four institutions. The VA group is by far superior, but we believe it is constituted of patients with simply stable angina and good ventricular function. The medical cohorts of three other studies are shown with their survival at 4 years, all significantly less than a matched normal population.

Shown in Fig. 10 is the survival of University of Alabama surgical group for patients with three-vessel disease: Survival is only slightly less at 5 years than an age/sex/race-matched group of United States normals and is in this nonrandom comparison superior to VA cooperative study medical treatment.

In Table 7 we have data for survival at 5 years of all patients operated on with one-, two-, three-vessel, and left main disease at the University of Alabama. Two points emerge: Survival of triple vessel

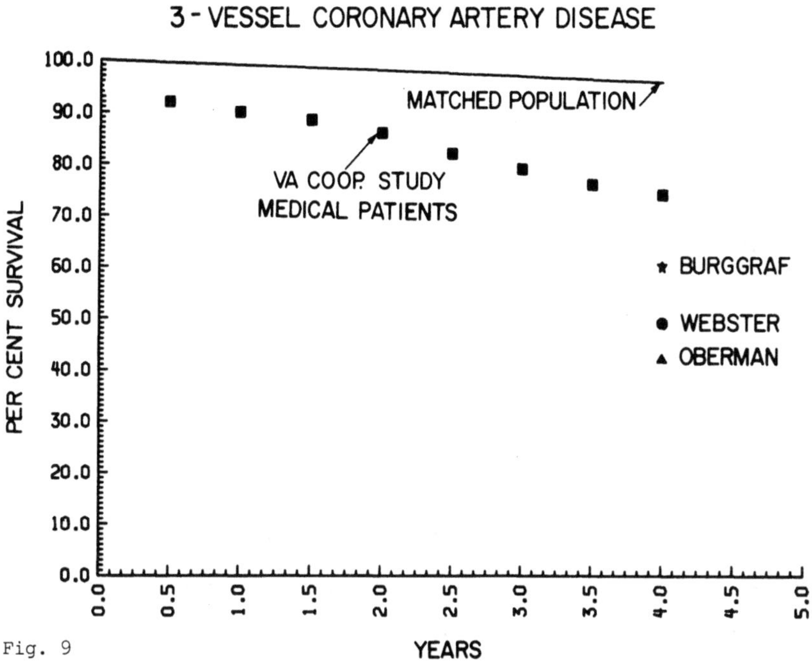

Fig. 9

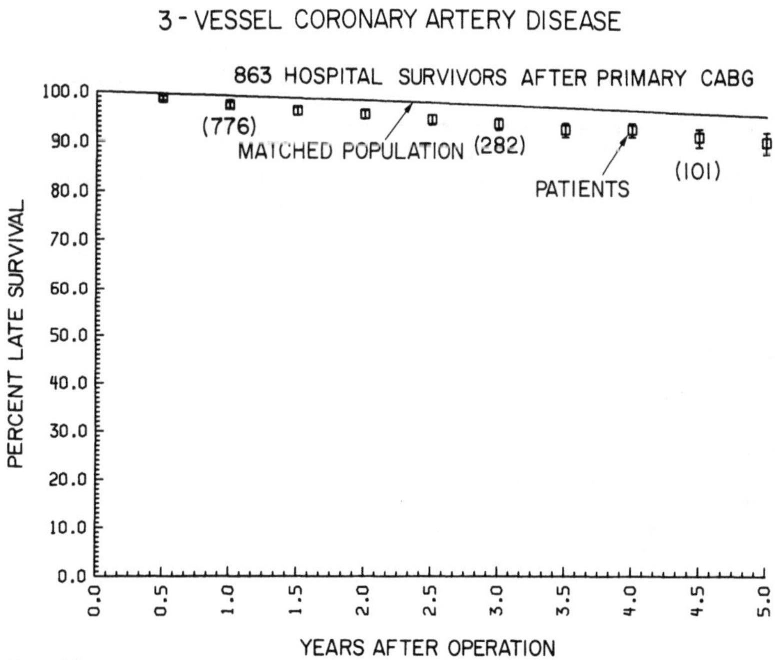

Fig. 10

disease at 5 years is only 7% less than that of a matched normal population; and surgery has converted the various differences in prognosis of two-, three-, left main vessel disease untreated, or treated medically to a uniform, similar survival among those anatomic categories.

Table 7. Comparison of survival of surgically treated coronary artery disease with matched population at 5 years

Category	Survival (Percent)		Significance level of difference
	Surgical treatment[a] (±SE)	Matched population	
1-Vessel	93.9±2.63	94.9	$P = 0.7$
2-Vessel	87.6±2.47[b]	95.0	$P = 0.003$
3-Vessel	88.9±1.89[b]	95.0	$P = 0.001$
Left main	86.7±3.90[b]	94.4	$P = 0.05$

[a]Hospital mortality assumed to be 0.9% for all categories.

[b]P for differences between these categories > 0.6 .

In summary, factors that influence survival in coronary artery disease are low surgical mortality and the consequent positive effect of surgery on life expectancy as contrasted to patients managed in other fashions.

References

1. Mathur, V.S., Guinn, G.A.: Prospective randomized study of coronary bypass surgery in stable angina: The first 100 patients. Circulation *51-52* [Suppl. I], 1-133 (1975)
2. Kannel, W.B., Feinleib, M.: Natural history of angina pectoris in the Framingham study. Am. J. Cardiol. *29*, 154 (1972)
3. Murphy, M.L., Hultgren, H.N., Petre, K., Thomsen, J., Takaro, T., participants of VA cooperative study: Treatment of chronic stable angina. N. Engl. J. Med. *297*, 621 (1977)
4. Conti, V.R., Blackstone, E.H., Digerness, S.R., Bertranou, E.G.: Cold cardioplegia versus hypothermia as myocardial protection: A randomized study in coronary artery bypass grafting. Presented at the American Association of Thoracic Surgeons. New Orleans (Louisiana), 9 May 1978
5. Herman, J., Corbara, F., Lesperance, J., Bourassa, M.G., Campeau, L.: Influence on late survival of graft status and degree of correction following aortocoronary bypass graft surgery. Am. J. Cardiol. *41*, 357 (1978)
6. Grondin, C.M., Lesperance, J., Bourassa, M.G., Pasternac, A., Campeau, L., Grondin, P.: Serial angiographic evaluation in 60 consecutive patients with aortocoronary artery vein grafts 2 weeks, 1 year, and 3 years after operation. J. Thorac. Cardiovasc. Surg. *67*, 1 (1974)
7. Green, et al.: Exhibit at the Meeting of the American Heart Association. Miami Beach (Florida), November 1977
8. DeBakey, M.E., Lawrie, G.: Aortocoronary bypass: Assessment after 13 years. JAMA *239*, 837 (1978)

Preinfarction Angina due to LAD Stenosis - a Surgical Follow-up

F. Cherrier, C. Pesch, J. L. Neimann, G. Braganti, and D. Souris

Preinfarction angina due to severe left anterior descending (LAD) stenosis must be differentiated [1,2] from different types of unstable angina because of the important mass of myocardial tissue being threatened. The possibility of clinical diagnosis and the seriousness of prognosis must be emphasized [3,4]. For these reasons, we believe that the preinfarctional angina syndrome requires surgery. In our study bypass grafting was always indicated except in patients with general or technical contraindications.

The aim of this nonrandomized study is the evaluation of surgery in the "syndrome de menace de l'interventriculaire antérieure." Other authors [5,6] have tried to duplicate this study after randomization [7]. This was not our goal; we only attempted in a group of patients who underwent surgery to assess results by means of perioperative mortality, functional and clinical results, rest and stress test, ECG, and angiographic controls.

Definition

The term "preinfarction angina due to LAD" stenosis must be strictly defined according to the following criteria:

- Increasing frequency and/or prolonged duration of spontaneous angina attacks (at rest) with onset of less than 3 months
- Transient evidence of myocardial ischemia such as T wave inversion or ST segment elevation on ECG recordings at least during chest pain and/or persistence after crisis
- Arteriographic LAD stenosis of at least 75%

Included are patients with isolated Prinzmetal attacks with stable LAD stenosis of at least 75%. Excluded are patients with immediate development toward myocardial infarction and previous anterior infarction.

Material

Sixty-five patients with a mean age of 51 years (range 33-67) were selected: 13 women and 52 men. Fifty-six patients were followed up for an average of 17.3 months (range 6-48 months). Forty-six patients had postoperative coronary arteriography after 8-12 months. Five patients had previous inferior myocardial infarction. The preinfarctional angina through LAD stenosis was the first symptom of coronary heart disease in 27 patients. Time interval between the onset of coronary heart disease and preinfarctional angina was less than 6 months in nearly 80% of our patients (Fig. 1). The delay between the onset of preinfarctional angina and coronarography was

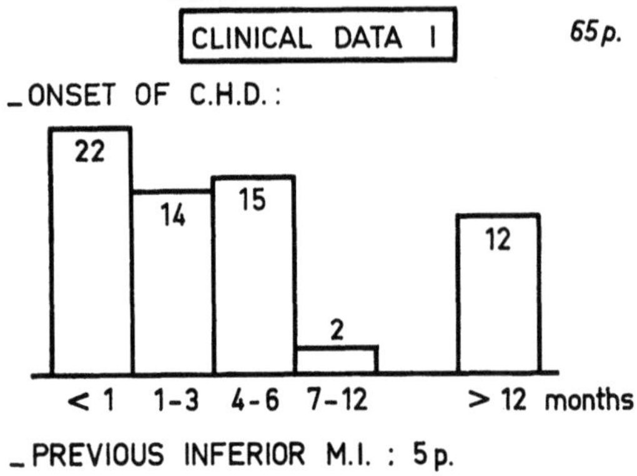

Fig. 1

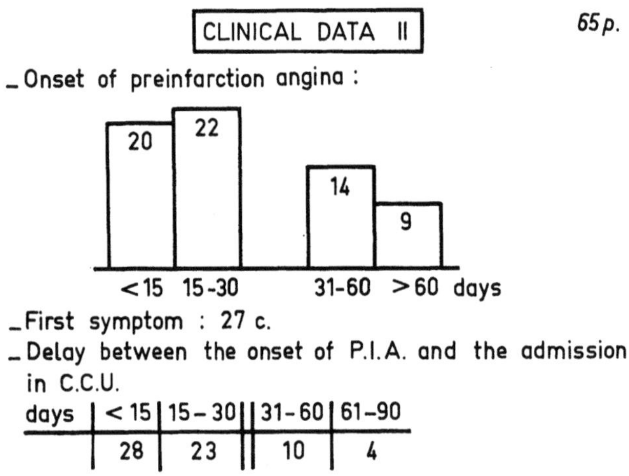

Fig. 2

less than 1 month in two-third of our patients (Fig. 2). The interval between the onset of preinfarctional angina and admission into coronary care unit was less than 15 days in 28 cases and 15-30 days in 23 cases; the remaining cases were admitted later (>30 days).

During anginal attacks, ECG recordings gave evidence of ischemic T-wave inversion in 26 patients, ST elevation with T-wave inversion in 35 patients, and a Prinzmetal pattern in 24 patients. Also ischemic ST depression was often indicated (14 cases), and ischemic Q waves occurred in 6 patients. In 36 patients ECG recordings always showed the same pattern during crises, whereas in 29 patients two to four different patterns were encountered. Severe disorders of cardiac rhythm, essentially ventricular tachycardia, occurred in 15 cases. Repolarization abnormalities remained in 44 patients after crisis.

Coronary angiography was performed in 55 patients during the unstable status. Ten patients underwent investigation after effective medical therapy. Twenty-nine patients had a normal left ventriculogram, 21 a mild hypokinesis, and 15 a severe one. A dyskinesis of the anterior wall was observed in only 11 patients. Thirty-nine patients had a normal ejection fraction (>0.55), 23 had a moderately impaired ejection fraction (0.40-0.55), and 3 a drastic one (<0.40).

Coronary angiograms showed one-vessel disease in 26 patients (40%), two-vessel disease in 22 cases, and three-vessel disease in 17 cases. Complete LAD obstruction was not present. The LAD stenosis ranged from 75% to 89% in 41 and from 90% to 98% in 24 patients. Thirty-eight stenoses were proximal; the remaining were situated between the first septal and the second diagonal arteries.
The delay between the onset of preinfarction angina and operation was variable. Surgery was performed immediately subsequent to coronary arteriography in 40 patients, 15 underwent bypass grafting 1-15 days after investigation, and in 10 patients this delay was more than 15 days. The mean graft/patient ratio was 1.2. Thirteen saphenous vein bypass grafts and 52 internal mammary artery anastomoses were performed on the LAD. Furthermore, 9 right coronary arteries and 6 circumflex arteries were bypassed. Revascularization was considered complete if ≥75% main coronary artery stenosis was bypassed. Revascularization was complete in 48 of our 65 patients.
There were four perioperative deaths[1] (6.1%): one by hemorrhagic complication and one by rupture of a right saphenous vein bypass graft with subsequent cardiac tamponnade. Two patients with a long history of coronary heart disease and previous inferior infarction died due to postoperative low output. Myocardial infarction developed in 9 patients (13.8%); 3 were of inferior and 6 of anterior location; 3 of these were severe.
Of 65 patients, 56 were followed up for 17.3 months (range 6-48 months): 4 patients died and 5 patients were lost to follow-up. Forthy-two patients (75%) were completely asymptomatic, 10 patients (17.9%) had a very mild angina, and 4 (7.1%) severe. No anterior infarction pattern was recorded after hospitalization discharge. The ECG was normal in 42 patients (75%), myocardial infarction was shown in 8 (14.3%), and an ischemic pattern in 6 patients (10.7%). Thirty-seven patients could perform a maximal stress test without an antianginal drug. The test was positive in 8 and negative in 29 cases. The patency rate of grafts evaluated in 46 patients was 91.3% (42/46). Thirty-four of 37 mammary artery anastomoses (91.9%) were patent, but only 30 were of good quality; the remaining showed narrowing. Therefore we had an excellent result in only 81.1% of our patients. Of 9 saphenous vein grafts 8 were patent (88.9%).

Comments

We must emphasize that preinfarctional angina has very precise criteria in our study. We eliminated "spontaneous" accelerated and prolonged anginal attacks caused by trigger effects, namely emotional factors. On the other hand, we choose patients with severe anterior ischemic ECG. This selection differed slightly from that of the national randomized study of A.C.C. (13), which could explain discrepancies.

The necessity for surgery in this group was emphasized by the recent onset of coronary heart disease, since the first symptoms appeared after less than 6 months in most cases. The frequency of one-vessel disease (40%), significantly higher than in stable angina (19% in our experience), also confirmed the necessity of surgery. This is also supported by other authors [8] and explains the low graft/patient ratio already described by Bonchek [9].

[1] At the Symposium of "Syndrome de menace" in Toulouse, (February 2, 1979) we presented 70 cases of *isolated* severe stenosis on LAD *without* perioperative mortality.

The high frequency of Prinzmetal ECG patterns either isolated or associated with other ischemic ST changes is noteworthy. The frequency of severe arrhythmias is correlated to this form of preinfarction angina.

The delay in performing coronary arteriography is explained first by insufficient information about this syndrome, second by not yet accomplished attempts of medical improvement in coronary care units.

The left ventricular function was often impaired, even after trinitroglycerine; in 11 patients mild to severe hypokinesis of the anterior wall was evident. The coronary angiogram was remarkable for the frequency of one-vessel disease and for the absence of complete LAD obstruction. LAD collateralization was mostly absent, and it is worth noting that we found it in only four cases (16%) with LAD stenosis greater than 90%. This type of lesion may perhaps explain the "crescendo" development of anginal attacks. We were dealing with a relatively privileged population that had not yet experienced infarction, but was sufficiently jeopardized to draw attention by clinical symptomatology. The coronary heart disease was limited enough to consider complete surgical revascularization and to provide a good future prognosis.

We must emphasize that in our overall experience of unstable angina five patients developed myocardial infarction between the 6th and 36th hour after coronary arteriography. We preferred to carry out this investigation before surgery since we were concerned about the risk of myocardial infarction or death during the interval in which patients await elective operation.

The operative death rate remained within a tolerable limit. The death of two of our patients resulted from hemorrhage. Our results were similar to those described by Bonchek: 5% [9], Geha: 2% [10], Wiles: 4.8% [12], and those usually encountered in unstable angina. Similar results were reported at the 7th European Congress of Cardiology [6]. In contrast to these results Russell [13] reported at a recent A.C.C. scientific session an perioperative mortality of 12% in preinfarction angina due to LAD stenosis.

The frequency of myocardial infarction in our group is noteworthy. However, only 3 of them were severe, the others were all of limited extent. It was likely that, when occurring in anteroseptal location, complete obstruction of the LAD proximal to the graft was responsible for collateral occlusion. These infarctions were regressive as shown by our followup study, since infarction pattern was evident in only 8 cases instead of 12 (old and perioperative infarctions included).

The functional results of our patients, who underwent surgery were excellent and were similar to those of other authors. Seventy-five percent of our patients were NYHA class I. Seven percent complained of severe angina. Stress tests revealed some discrepancies: Eight positive tests may be due to graft obstruction in 4 cases and in the 4 other cases to incomplete surgical revascularization. In contrast, in 2 of 29 negative stress tests the graft was completely occluded.

The patency rate of grafts was good and was similar to that of operated stable angina. The small number of patients in our group does not allow pertinent statistical comparison between saphenous vein bypass graft and internal mammary artery anastomosis. We would like to note that despite emergency surgery 52 mammary arteries could be dissected. The 13 remaining patients needed saphenous vein grafts because the internal mammary artery could not be adapted to a large distal LAD. In accordance with Geha [10], we prefer mammary artery anastomosis, provided the vessel is of perfect quality.

Conclusion

We prefer surgery for the "syndrome de menace sur l'I.V.A." when possible because anginal pain is quickly relieved, excellent functional results are obtained, and perioperative mortality is held within tolerable limits, especially in isolated stenosis on LAD.

We attempted to obtain rapid admission to the Coronary Care Unit for correct surveillance and medical treatment by rest, Heparin, Isosorbide Dinitrate, and beta blockers. Prinzmetal attacks were treated preferentially by Nifédipine or Amiodarone (but not by beta blockers which were less effective) [11]. Pre- and perioperative intraaortic balloon pumping was carried out in patients with severe arrhythmias, previous myocardial infarction, and depressed left ventricular function. If within 2 or 3 days no rapid improvement was observed and/or severe dysrhythmias persisted, immediate surgery was performed.

On the other hand, we preferred to postpone surgery for 1 month, if preinfarctional angina rapidly and persistently improved by medical therapy.

In all cases coronary arteriography immediately preceeds subsequent surgery.

We hope that this approach will permit a correct work status in most our patients.

References

1. Bruntz, J.F.: Les syndromes de menace d'infarctus. A propos de 81 cas. Nancy, Thesis 1976
2. Neimann, J.L., Cuilliere, M., Paquis, M., Mathieu, P., Cherrier, F.: Le syndrome de menace de l'I.V.A. Considérations diagnostiques et thérapeutiques. Arch. Mal. Coeur *68*, 1123-1132 (1975)
3. Gazes, P.C., Mobley, E.M., Faris, H.M., Duncan, R.C., Humphries, G.B.: Preinfarctional (unstable) angina. A prospective study. Ten year follow up. Prognostic significance of electric changes. Circulation *48*, 331-337 (1973)
4. Berk, G., Kaplitt, M., Padmanadbhab, V., Frantz, S., Morisson, J., Culotta, S.J.: Management of preinfarction angina. Evolution and comparison of medical and surgical therapy in 43 patients. J. Thorac. Cardiovasc. Surg. *71*, 110-117 (1976)
5. Kouchoukos, N.T., Oberman, A., Russell, R.O.: Surgical versus medical treatment of occlusive disease confined to the left anterior descending coronary artery. Am. J. Cardiol. *35*, 836-842 (1975)
6. Cherrier, F., Short, D.: Unstable angina what is it, what to do. 7th European Congress of Cardiology. Amsterdam, 1976. (Abs. I)
7. Russell, R.O., et al: Unstable angina pectoris: national cooperative study group to compare medical and surgical therapy. I. Report of protocol and patient population. Am. J. Cardiol. *37*, 896-902 (1976)
8. Tremblay, G., Cosette, R., Bonard, P., Proulx, A.: La coronarographie est-elle justifiée dans l'angine instable? Arch. Mal. Coeur. *68*, 1143-1148 (1975)
9. Bonchek, L.I., Rahimtoola, S.H., Anderson, R.P., Mc Anulty, J.A., Rosch, J., Bristow, J.D., Starq, A.: Late results following emergency saphenous vein bypass grafting for unstable angina. Circulation *50*, 972-977 (1974)

10. Geha, A.S., Baue, A.E., Krone, R.J., Kleiger, R.E., Oliver, G.C., Mc Cormick, J.R., Salimi, A.: Surgical treatment of unstable angina by sapenous vein and internal mammary artery bypass grafting. J. Thorac. Cardiovasc. Surg. *71*, 348-354 (1976)
11. Cherrier, F., Neimann, J.L., Groussin, P., Aliot, E., Cuilliere, M., Beissel, J.: Prinzmetal Angina: a study of 100 cases. 3rd Symposium on Coronary Heart Disease. Frankfurt/M. 1978, February 8-11. (Abs. 29)
12. Wiles, J.C., Peduzzi, P.N., Hammond, G.L., Cohen, L.S., Langou, R.A.: Pre-operative predictors of operative mortality for coronary bypass grafting in patients with unstable angina pectoris. Am. J. Cardiol. *39*, 939-943 (1977)
13. Russell, R.O., et al: Unstable angina pectoris national randomized study of surgical versus medical therapy: results in L.A.D. disease. Report of the 27th Annual Scientific Session of A.C.C., 8 March 1978

Aortocoronary Bypass Surgery in Patients with Organic Coronary Atherosclerosis Combined with Spasm

A. L'Abbate and A. Maseri

This presentation deals with the rationale and the indications of aortocoronary bypass surgery in patients with vasospastic angina on the basis of what is presently known on the pathogenesis of angina, rather than on the results of the treatment.

It is commonly recognized that transient ischemia may result from the discrepancy between supply and demand. The pathogenetic mechanism of exertional angina (angina for constant level of exercise or stable angina) is recognized to be *secondary* to the increase of myocardial oxygen demand not matched by an appropriate increase of flow because of the presence of an organic coronary stenosis not adequately compensated by collateral circulation. In this case the rational therapeutical approach appears to be the bypass of the stenosis, or alternatively, the reduction of myocardial demand.

On the other hand, transient myocardial ischemia, especially at rest, has also been reported to be related to a *primary* reduction of coronary blood flow rather than to an increase of oxygen demand. In this case the cause of the ischemia is a functional reduction of coronary blood supply that may occur both in presence or absence of severe coronary atherosclerosis. Thus, in this case, the presence of coronary stenosis is not the limiting factor in the genesis of the anginal attack. The demonstration of the existence of this type of angina derives from a series of convergent studies carried out in our institution which led to the following conclusions:

1) There is no increase of metabolic demand immediately before the onset of the attacks of angina at rest.
2) There is actually a decrease of coronary blood flow in a region of the myocardium.
3) Coronary spasm is responsible for the reduction of blood flow.

The first study was carried out in 22 patients with angina at rest by continuous hemodynamic monitoring for 10-24 h. Over 300 ischemic episodes were recorded on analog tape records. None of the episodes were preceded by an increase of the hemodynamic parameters controlling myocardial oxygen consumption [1,2] (Fig. 1). These findings confirm and extend previous reports [3,4] and are in agreement with recent observations [5]. It was interesting that in the same patients, as well as in different patients, with or without chest pain, episodes with ST segment elevation, ST depression, and pseudonormalization of T wave, were characterized by similar hemodynamic patterns.

Evidence for a primary reduction of coronary flow, in absence of an increase of oxygen demand, is suggested by preliminary studies in which we performed continuous monitoring of the coronary sinus oxygen saturation in patients with angina at rest, which show a consistent reduction of coronary sinus oxygen saturation preceding the onset of ECG changes by few seconds [6].

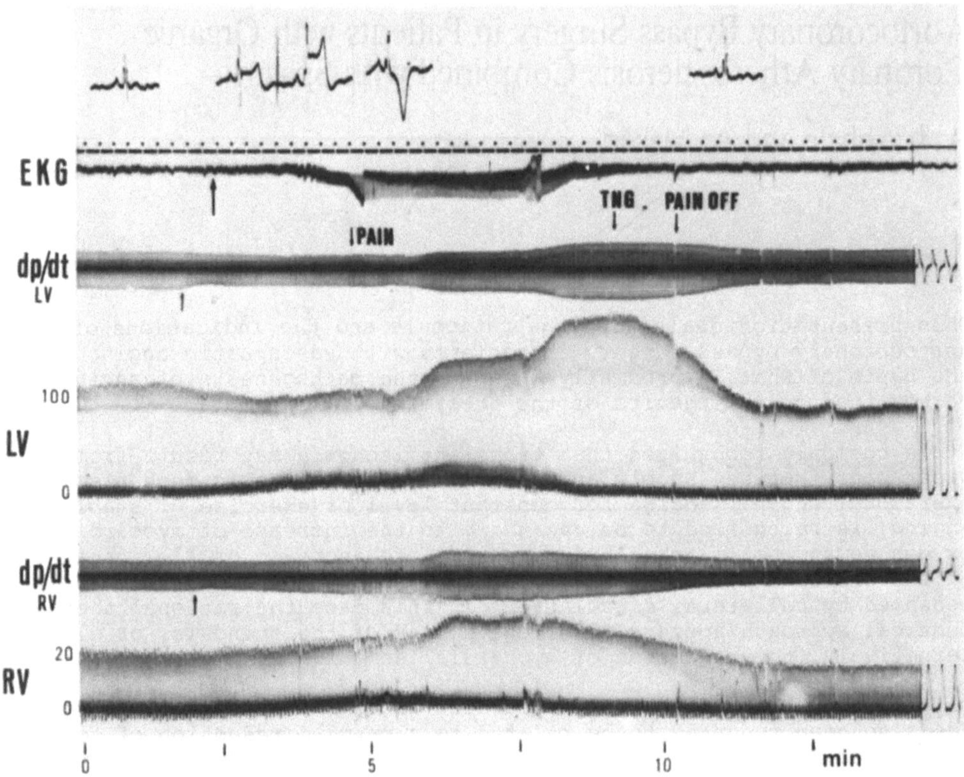

Fig. 1. Low speed playback of ECG lead 3, left and right ventricular pressure, showing the onset of an ischemic episode. Arrows indicate beginning of changes of various parameters as determined on high-speed tracings. High-speed ECG during various phases of the attack is superimposed at the top. The onset of ST segment elevation is not preceded by increase of pressures, but rather by reduction of peak relaxation dp/dt of LV and RV and peak contraction dp/dt of LV.
(From Maseri, A., et al.: Chest 68, 625, 1975)

A reduction of myocardial perfusion was also documented in 30 patients by ^{201}Tl scintigraphy. Tracer was injected during the attack and serial scintigrams obtained within 5-20 min. A massive transmural defect was present in cases with ST segment elevation [2] (Fig. 2) and in those with pseudonormalization of T wave. Episodes with ST segment depression showed a less massive defect with fuzzy limits suggestive of diffuse subendocardial ischemia [7].

In 44 patients coronary spasm was documented by coronary angiography performed during attacks occurring spontaneously or induced by ergonovine maleate [8] (Fig. 3). Table 1 summarizes the results of the angiographic study in 37 patients with anginal attacks characterized by ST segment elevation [9]. The extent of coronary atherosclerosis, the vessels involved by the spasm, and its morphological aspect are reported. In all seven patients who had only episodes with ST segment depression, a diffuse, severe atherosclerosis of the coronary arteries was present, and during the attack, a diffuse narrowing of several branches without complete obstruction or spasm of a small branch was observed [8,10].

Table 1. Location and extension of coronary vasospasm

	Normal vessels			1-Vessel disease			2-Vessel disease			3-Vessel disease		
	LAD	LCA	RCA	LAD	LCA	RCA	LAD	LCA	RCA	LAD	LCA	RCA
Occlusion without distal filling	X		*(X)	**(X)	()		X			()	()	X
				()	*(X)							
				()	X							
				(X)	X							
				X								
Occlusion with poor distal filling			X	()		()			***X	() ↔	()	X
						()	()			X		
							()					
							X					
Diffuse lumen reduction delayed filling			(X)	()			()			()		
				()			X			()		
				()			()			X		
							()					

X Spontaneous attack
() Ergonovine induced attack
(X) Spontaneous and ergonovine induced attacks
LAD = Left anterior descending coronary artery
LCA = Left circumflex coronary artery
RCA = Right coronary artery
* = the spasm was not occlusive following ergonovine maleate
** = the spasm was occlusive only following ergonovine maleate
*** = spontaneous spasm in RCA; in a second study, 3 months later spasm of first septal branch
↔ = spasm of the LAD and LCA simultaneously

The characteristics of the coronary vasospasm can be summarized as follows:

1) Although in patients with single-vessel disease, the spasm involved consistently the stenotic vessel, in those with double-or triple-vessel disease no correlation was found between the location and degree of coronary obstruction and location and extension of coronary spasm;
2) often the spasm involves a long segment of the vessel making questionable the indication for bypassing a diseased vessel which may go into spasm;
3) vasospastic angina can coexist with typical and severe effort angina. The myocardial region becoming ischemic during effort angina may not be the same as that becoming ischemic during vasospasm, suggesting that different segments of the coronary vasculature can be involved in the two conditions;
4) spasm may involve main branches as well as secondary branches.

On the basis of these observations the role of indiscriminate coronary bypass in patients with primary vasospastic angina appears questionable. Persistence of coronary spasm in patients who underwent heart denervation and autotransplantation [11] suggest the failure of the surgical approach in preventing coronary spasm.

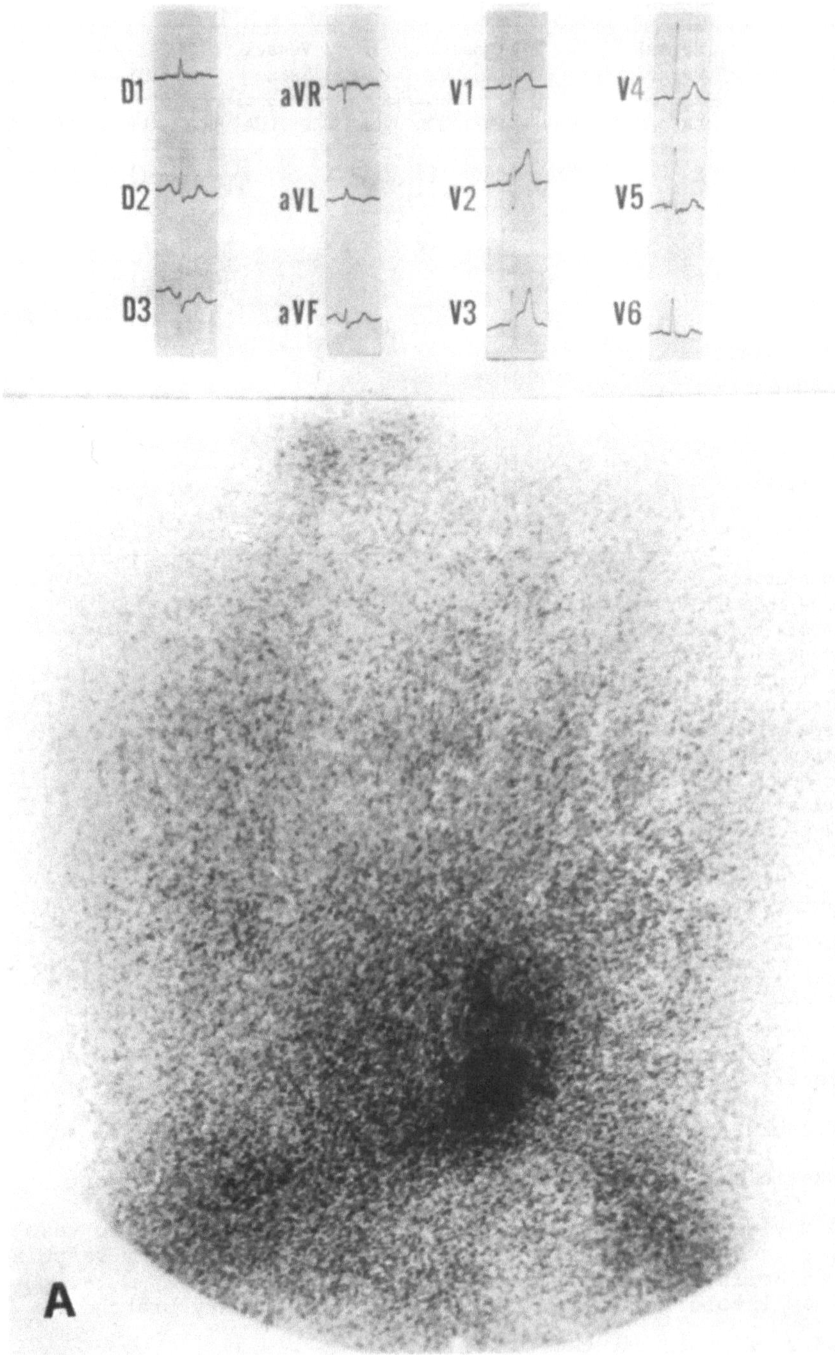

Fig. 2. LAO myocardial scintigrams obtained by ^{201}Tl injection during an ischemic episode characterized by ST segment elevation in the anterior leads (A) and one week later in absence of symptoms (B). A massive transmural perfusion defect of the anterior wall is present during the ischemic episode.
(From Maseri, A., et al.: Circulation 54, 280, 1976)

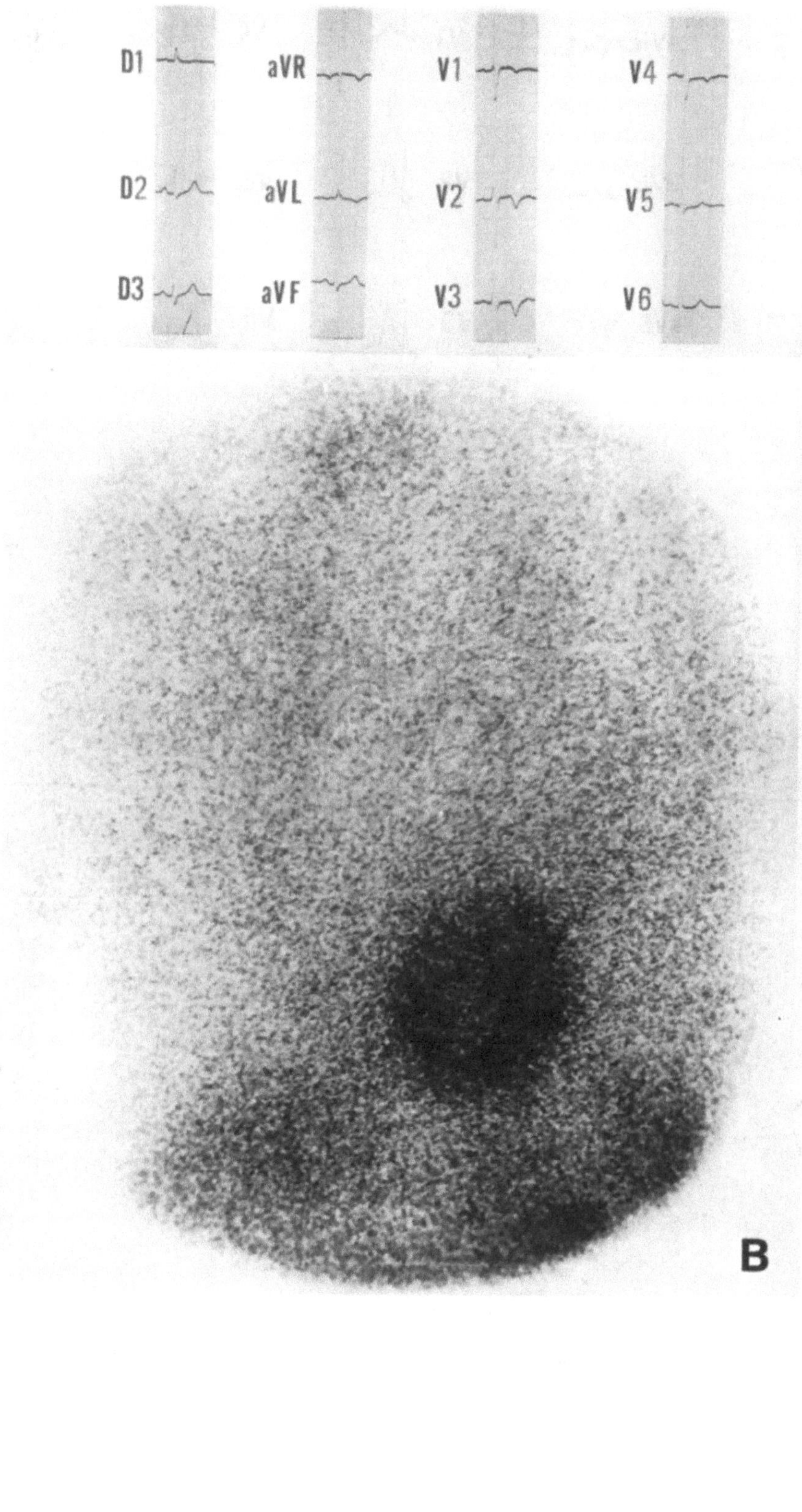
D1
aVR
V1
V4
D2
aVL
V2
V5
D3
aVF
V3
V6
B

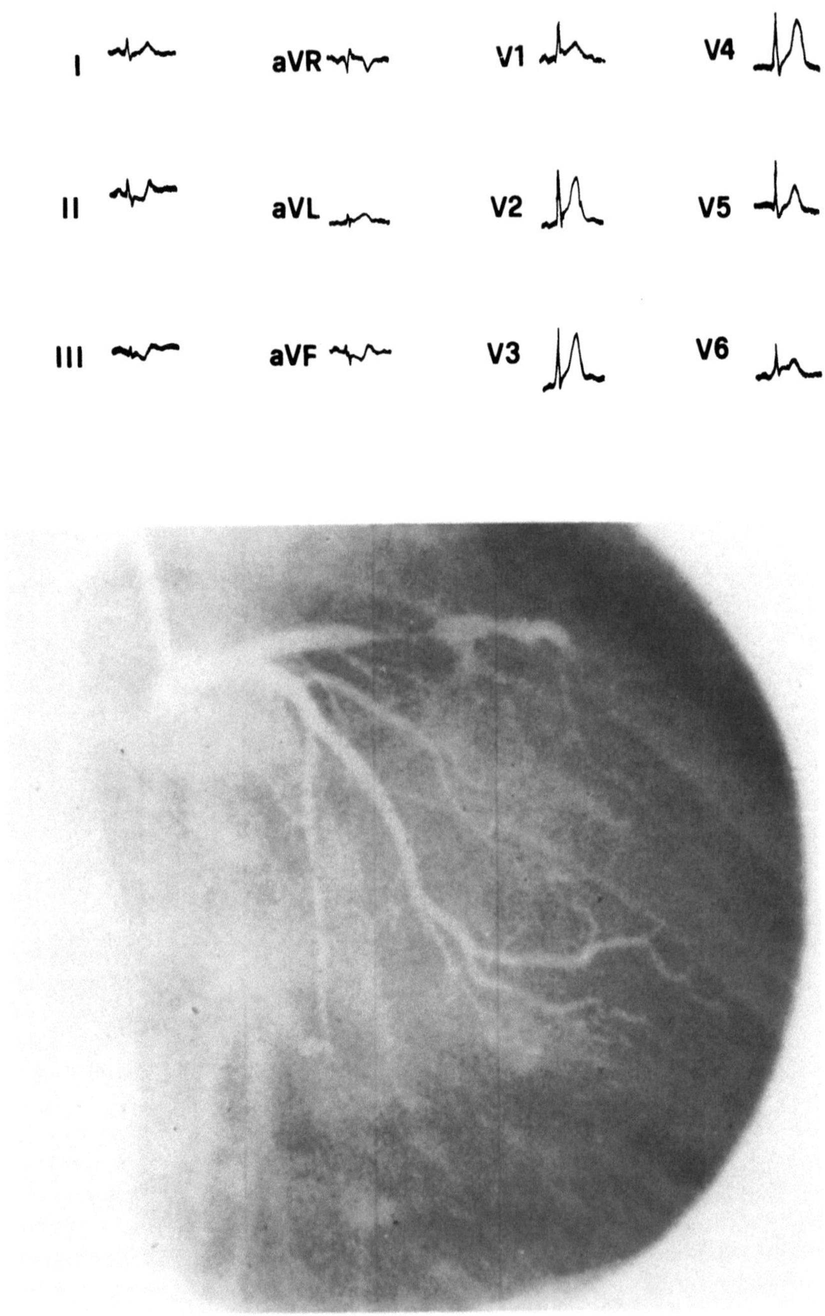

Fig. 3. RAO left coronary angiograms during a spontaneous anginal attack characterized by ST segment elevation on the precordial leads (*left*) and ist resolution (*right*). Complete occlusion of the LAD at the level of the distal stenosis is present during the attack

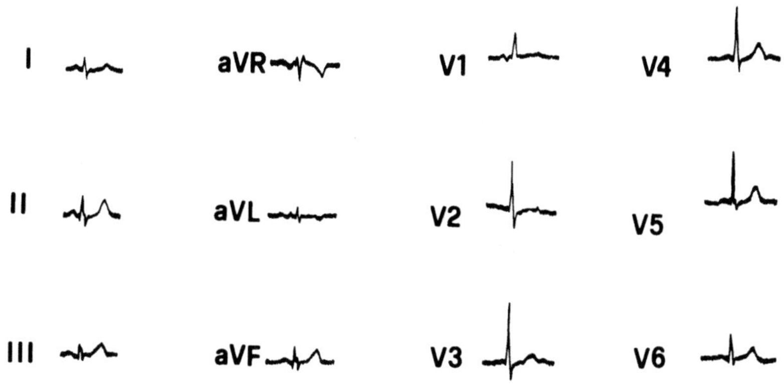
I
aVR
V1
V4
II
aVL
V2
V5
III
aVF
V3
V6

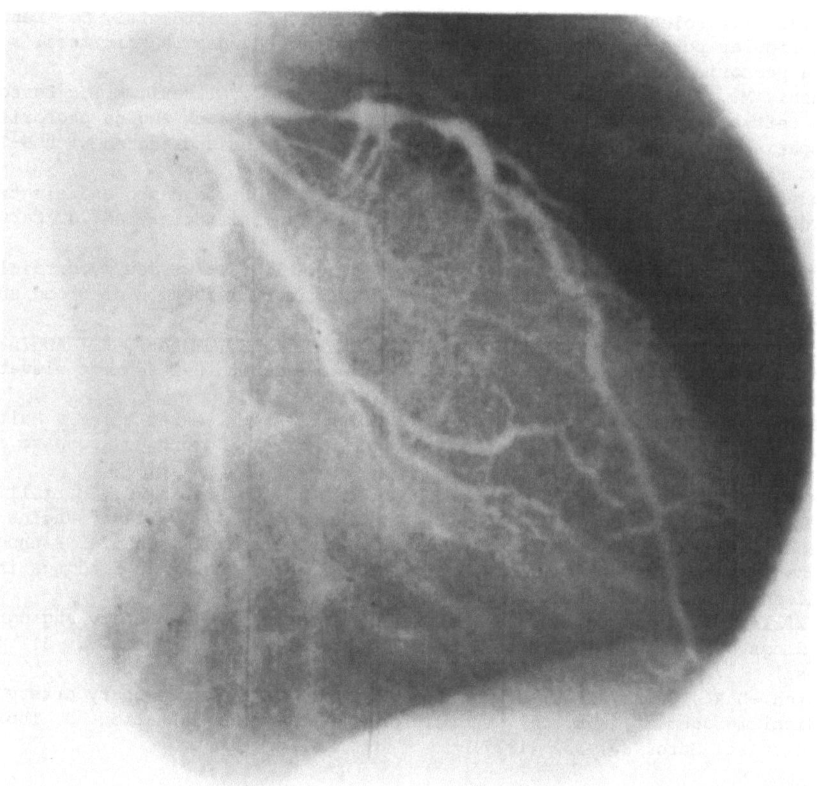

Thus, in our opinion, bypass should be reserved for those patients with vasospastic angina who have also exertional angina that, in spite of medical therapy, limits considerably their exercise tolerance; bypass should be used only when surgical intervention may be expected to improve life expectancy.

An accurate functional diagnostic characterization of the anginal patient should be the prerequisite for the evaluation of medical versus surgical treatment. Furthermore, the optimal medical treatment should be defined with regard to possible vasospastic components.

References

1. Maseri, A., Pesola, A., Mimmo, R., Chierchia, S., L'Abbate, A.: Pathogenetic mechanisms of angina at rest. Circulation [Suppl.] *51/52*, 89 (1975) (Abs.)
2. Maseri, A., Mimmo, R., Chierchia, S., Marchesi, C., Pesola, A., L'Abbate, A.: Coronary artery spasm as a cause of acute myocardial ischemia in man. Chest *68*, 625 (1975)
3. Guazzi, M., Polese, A., Fiorentini, C., Magrini, F., Bartorelli, C.: Left ventricular performance and related haemodynamic changes in Prinzmetal's angina pectoris. Br. Heart J. *33*, 84 (1971)
4. Guazzi, M., Polese, A., Fiorentini, C., Magrini, F., Olivari, M.T., Bartorelli, C.: Left and right heart haemodynamics during spontaneous angina pectoris. Comparison between angina with S-T segment depression and angina with S-T segment elevation. Br. Heart J. *37*, 401 (1975)
5. Figueras, J., Ganz, W., Singh, B.N., Swan, H.J.C.: Hemodynamic and electrocardiographic accompaniments of resting post-prandial angina. Am. J. Cardiol. (in press) (1978)
6. Chierchia, S., Maseri, A., Simonetti, I., Brunelli, C.: Oxygen myocardial extraction in angina at rest. Evidence of a primary reduction of blood supply. Circulation *56*, 135 (1977) (Abs.)
7. Parodi, O., Severi, S., Uthurralt, N., Solfanelli, S., Maseri, A.: Angina pectoris at rest: regional myocardial perfusion during S-T segment elevation or depression. Circulation *56*, 891 (1977)(Abs.)
8. Maseri, A., L'Abbate, A., Pesola, A., Ballestra, A.M., Marzilli, M., Maltinti, G., Severi, S., De Nes, M., Parodi, O., Biagini, A.: Coronary vasospasm in angina pectoris. Lancet *1977 I*, 713
9. Maseri, A., Severi, S., De Nes, M., L'Abbate, A., Chierchia, S., Marzilli, M., Ballestra, A.M., Parodi, O., Biagini, A., Distante, A.: "Variant" angina: one aspect of a continous spectrum of vasospastic myocardial ischemia. Pathogenic mechanisms, estimated incidence, clinical and coronarographic findings in 138 patients. Am J. Cardiol. *42*, 1019 (1978)
10. Marzilli, M., L'Abbate, A., Ballestra, A.M., Maseri, A.: Coronary angiographic findings during angina at rest with S-T depression. Circulation *56*, 312 (1977) (Abs.)
11. Clarch, D.A., Quint, R.A., Mitchell, R.L., Angell, W.W.: Coronary artery spasm Medical management, surgical denervation and autotransplantation. J. Thorac. Cardiovasc. Surg. *73*, 332 (1977)

Indications and Results of Emergency Coronary Revascularization

A. Deloche, Ph. Menasche, A. Carpentier, J. N. Fabiani, A. Piwnica, J. Relland, and Ch. Dubost

The operative indications in acute coronary insufficiency remain controversial. The long-term results of 191 patients after surgical treatment of acute coronary insufficiency are reported in this study operated on between 1970 and 1976 at the Clinic for Cardiovascular Surgery of the Broussais Hospital, Paris.

Clinical Material

Patients were classified into three groups:

Group I: Unstable Angina
The criteria of selection were:

- Angina of recent onset and increasing severity within the preceding 4 weeks
- Stable angina with a recent increase in severity within the preceding 4 weeks
- No response to medical treatment
- Transient electrocardiographic changes (myocardial ischemia) without the appearance of significant new Q waves or other electrocardiographic evidence of recent infarction
- Normal serum enzyme levels (LPH, SGPT, CPK).

This group consisted of 113 patients from 30-71 years of age (mean: 52 years). A preexisting myocardial infarction was present in 28 cases. The lesions documented by coronary arteriography are summarized in Table 1. The most frequent contractile disorder was hypokinesis, which was variable in degree, and most often limited to the ischemic areas.

The lesions were treated only by saphenous vein bypass grafts: 62 single grafts, 46 double grafts, and 5 triple grafts were performed.

Table 1. Unstable angina

Angiocardiography	
One-vessel	42
Multiple vessels	63
Left main	8
Abnormal ventricular contractility	62%
Operations	
Single bypass	62
Double bypass	46
Triple bypass	5

Group II: Prinzmetal Variant Angina
The criteria of selection were:

- Transient angina at rest
- Simultaneous EKG changes (elevation of ST segment without Q waves)
- Normal serum enzyme levels

This group consisted of 60 patients (52 male, 8 female) from 36-66 years of age (mean: 51 years). Twenty-one patients (35%) had been previously free of angina. A preexisting myocardial infarction was present in 13 cases.

Coronary arteriography showed a predominance of single-vessel disease. In 41 cases (68%) the left anterior descending artery was involved. Nine cases of arterial spasm were detected during angiography by the nitroglycerin test (Table 2). All patients underwent saphenous vein bypass grafting; 47 single grafts, 12 double grafts, and one triple graft were performed.

Group III
This group was comprised of 18 patients who underwent saphenous vein bypass grafting within the first 10 h following a myocardial infarction (14 cases), and patients with postinfarction angina, the so-called extending infarction.

Methods

Results were compiled in these three groups by clinical examination, electrocardiography, repeated coronary arteriography in 51 patients, and treadmill tests in 55 patients.

During the postoperative period 151 patients were followed for an average time of 2,5 years. We classified the results into three classes: *good*: absence of pain and normal activity without myocardial infarction, *fair*: residual angina, *poor*: severe angina, late infarction or death.

Results

Group I: Unstable Angina (Fig. 1a, b, and c).
The operative mortality was 8% and six patients died during the first 5 years (four from cardiac causes). At 5 years the survival rate was 84%. Theincidence of postoperative infarction was 12%. Late infarctions occurred in two cases, both in the areas of the grafts. Using

Table 2. Prinzmetal variant angina

Angiocardiography	
Single	41
Multiple	10
Spasm	9
Operation	
Single bypass	47
Multiple bypass	13

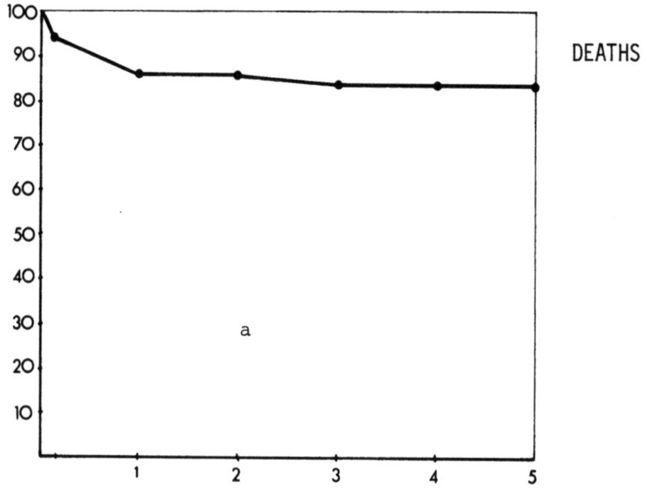

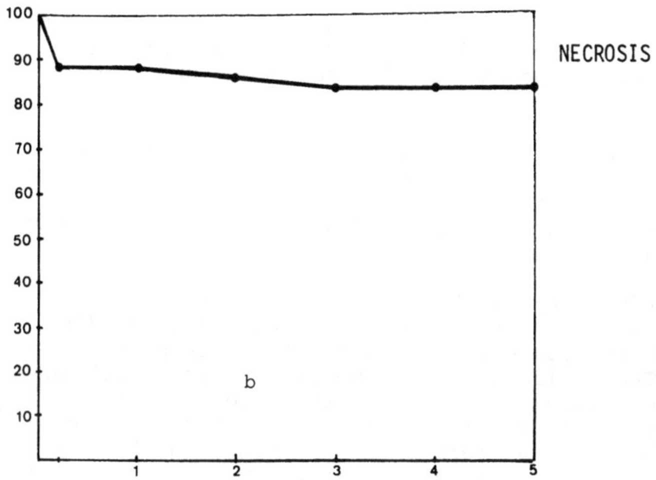

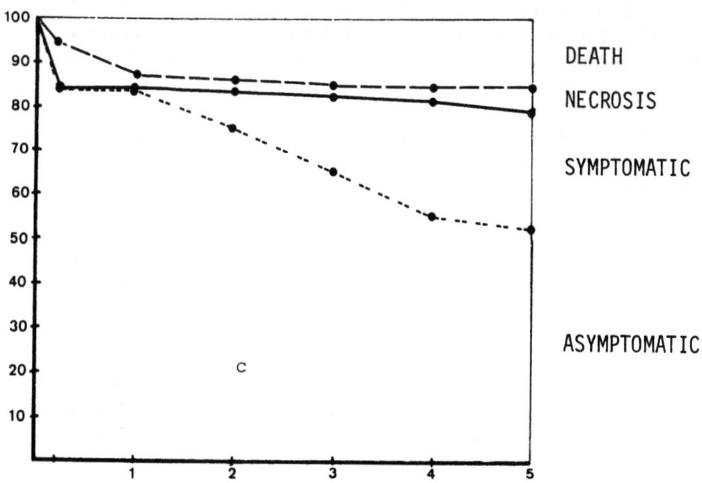

Fig. 1. *Group I*: unstable angina (113 patients). a) Actuarial survival curve: b) Actuarial curve of infarctions. c) Combined actuarial curves showing survival and infarction rates plus the proportion of patients with and without postoperative angina

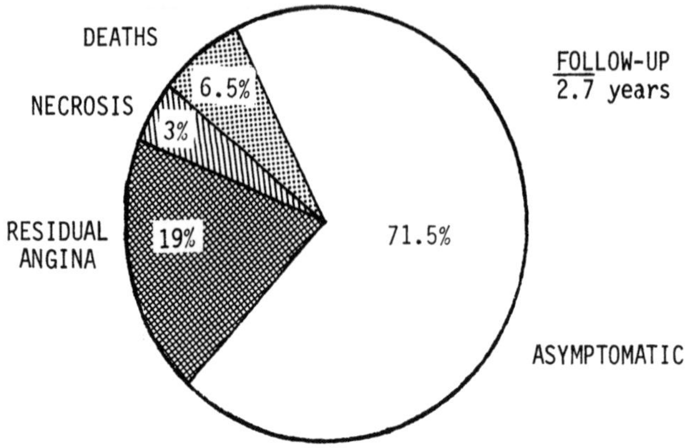

Fig. 2. *Group I*: unstable angina (113 patients). Long-term postoperative results of unstable angina

actuarial curves, the infarction rate was 15% at 5 years. 71,5% of the patients were free of angina and 19% had residual angina (Fig. 2). Re-operation was necessary in one patient for recurrent unstable angina.

Of the 86 patients followed, 47 had good results, 23 had fair results, and 16 had poor results. No correlation could be established between the clinical or anatomic findings and the quality of the long-term results. Nor did the results show any significant differences between the various types of angina, "de novo" or Crescendo angina.

Group II: Prinzmetal Variant Angina (Fig. 3a, b, and c).
The operative mortality was 3.3% and in addition, two patients died during the first year, both from cardiac causes. At 5 years, the survival rate was 91%. The incidence of postoperative myocardial infarction was 20%. Two additional infarctions were noted during the first 2 years. At 5 years, the overall incidence of infarction was 24%. Of the surviving patients 76% were free of angina, 14% had residual angina (Fig. 4). Re-operation was necessary in one patient for recurrent stenosis in the area of the graft.

Of the 43 patients followed, the long-term results were judged to be good in 31 cases, fair in seven cases, and poor in five cases. No correlation could be established between clinical and anatomic findings.

The Prinzmetal angina group caused by spasm had poor results. Of nine patients in this subgroup, we noted one operative death, three infarctions, and on postoperative angiography, two competitive flows and one occluded graft.

In groups I and II, 56 late angiograms were performed with a patency rate of 83% (Table 3). Treadmill tests were performed at 6 months in 55 patients; 33 were negative (60%) and 22 were positive (40%).

Group III: Infarction
In the group of four patients with impending extension of recent infarction, there was no operative mortality. The long-term results were good in one case and fair in the three others. In the group of

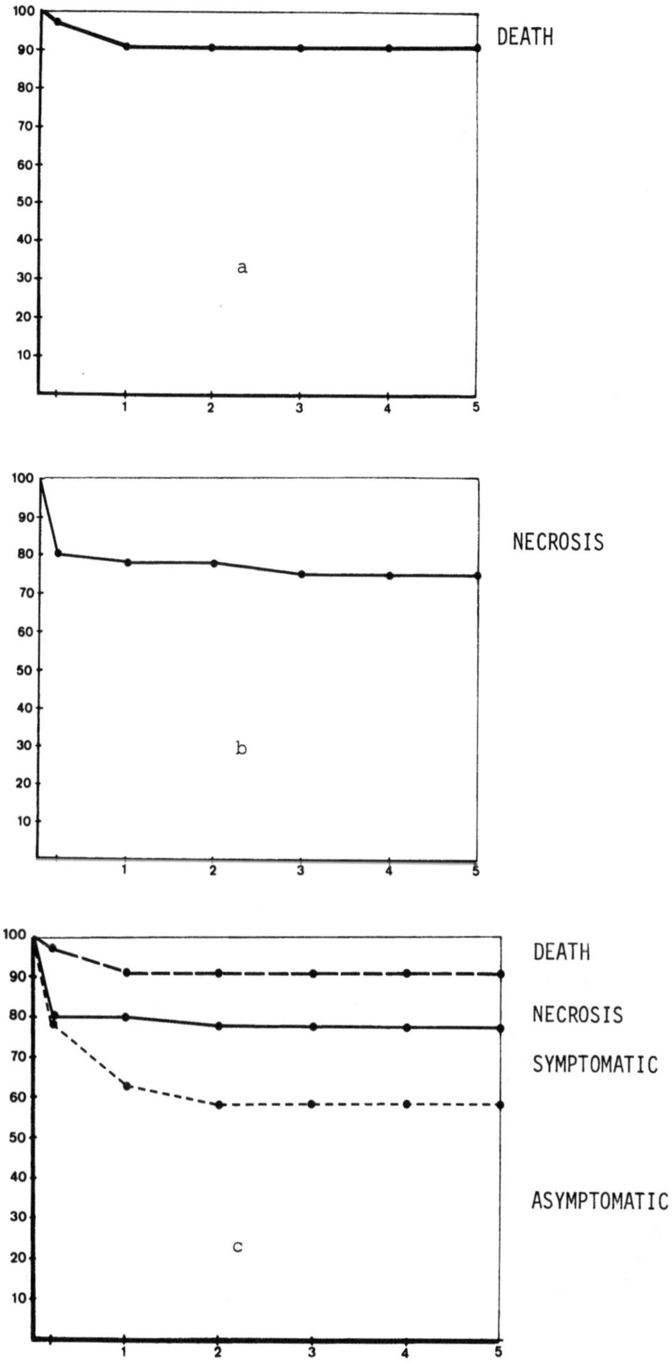

Fig. 3. *Group II*: Prinzmetal variant angina (60 patients). a) Actuarial survival curve. b) Actuarial curve of infarctions. c) Combined actuarial curves showing survival and infarction rates plus the proportion of patients with and without postoperative angina

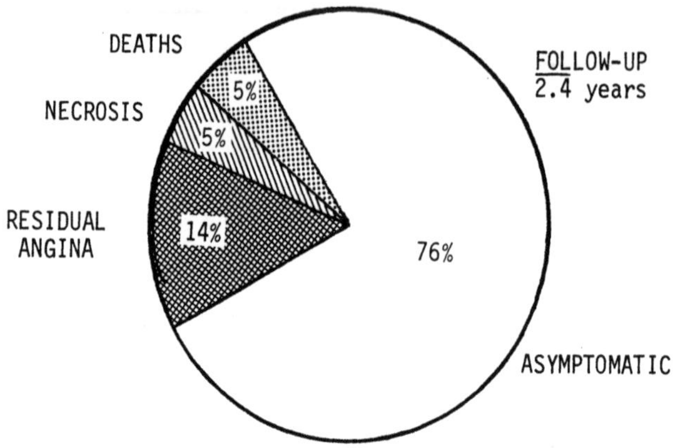

Fig. 4. *Group II*: Prinzmetal variant angina (60 patients). Long-term postoperative results of Prinzmetal angina

Table 3. Groups I and II

Stress EKG (55 patients)	Negative:	33
	Positive:	22
Angiocardiography (56 patients)		
Grafts	Patent:	47 (83%)
	Occluded:	9 (17%)
Ventricular contraction	Improvement:	21
	No change:	29

patients with myocardial infarction revascularized within the first 10 h, the operative mortality was 21%. Long-term results were fair in two patients, good in six, and in four good electrocardiographic and angiographic results were noted.

Conclusions

There was low operative mortality, in spite of the often critical condition of the patients. High incidence of intra-operative infarction, especially in the Prinzmetal group was most likely due to persistent spasm. Stable results were found following surgery up to 5 years. There was relief of angina in the majority of patients.

Our current indications for operation in acute coronary insufficiency are:

1) In the unstable angina group: angina unresponsive to medical treatment, stenosis of the left main coronary artery, irrespective of the response to medical treatment.

2) In the Prinzmetal angina group: patients with an organic lesion or a minor spasm, as demonstrated by the nitroglycerin test, and especially by the ergonovine maleate test during coronary angiography.
3) In the acute myocardial infarction group: patients with post-infarction angina (extending infarction) and the majority of patients undergoing intra-aortic balloon counter pulsation. The indications for acute revascularization of a recent myocardial infarction remain controversial.

Summary

Long-term results of surgical treatment of acute coronary insufficiency are reported in this study of 191 patients operated on between 1970 and 1976.

The patients were classified into three groups:

- *Group I*: Unstable angina (113 patients).
  In this group, the survival rate at 5 years was 84%. The overall rate of infarctions was 15%. 71,5% of the patients were free of angina.
- *Group II*: Prinzmetal variant angina (60 patients).
  In this group, the survival rate at 5 years was 91%. The overall rate of infarctions was 24%. 76% of the patients were asymptomatic.
- *Group III*: (18 patients).
  This group was comprised of patients who underwent acute revascularization of a myocardial infarction (14 patients) and patients with postinfraction angina (4 patients).

2. Controversial Points in Surgical Tactics and Techniques

Complete Revascularization, Including Moderate Stenosis?

H. A. Huysmans, F. E. E. Vermeulen, and A. V. G. Bruschke

When performing a coronary artery bypass operation, no surgeon will hesitate nowadays to include all branches with a stenosis of 70% or more in the revascularization procedure. However, when vessels with a moderate stenosis, i.e., around 50%, are present, some questions arise. A 50% stenosis is hemodynamically unimportant and it is improbable, that it will ever give rise to anginal complaints or myocardial infarction.
So placing a bypass graft on moderately stenosed vessels will only be done in view of the possible progression in the future, which might lead to the necessity of a second operation. In order to know whether or not such a procedure is justified, we will have to know what to expect from the development of moderate lesions in the natural history of coronary heart disease, as well as after coronary surgery. Secondly, we will have to know, whether the bypass grafts will stay patent for a longer time than it takes a moderate lesion to develop into a significant stenosis. It has been said, that bypass grafts on moderately stenosed vessels might have a lower patency rate, due to the fact, that there will be lower flows through the graft, because of a smaller demand in cases of moderate stenosis. Others however, have stated that graft patency is not related to flow rate through the bypass graft or to the diameter of the coronary artery, etc., but only to the surgical technique of the anastomosis.

In order to find some of the answers to the above questions, three groups of patients were studied. All had one or more moderate lesions in the proximal parts of graftable major coronary artery branches; they also had significant stenosis in other branches. Moderate stenosis was thought to be present when the lesion caused about 50% stenosis. In view of the interobserver differences in interpretation, lesions from the groups of 30%-50% and of 50%-70% were taken into account, but all were less than 60%. The first group consisted of patients who had coronary bypass surgery for significant lesions, and who had moderate lesions that were not bypassed. The second group had moderate lesions next to significant lesions and had no bypass surgery. The third group had bypass surgery for both significant and moderate lesions.
Most patients were recatheterized nonselectively as part of the follow-up study. Progression of a lesion was only considered to be present if there was at least 25% more stenosis; this was done in order to take care of the interpretation inaccuracies.

The first group consisted of 75 patients in whom 145 significant lesions were bypassed and who had 100 moderate lesions that were not treated surgically. A follow-up angiography was performed with a mean interval of 26 months after the operation (14-62 months). The development of the moderate lesions is shown in Fig. 1. Of the lesions 65% were unchanged, i.e., showed less than 25% increase of the stenosis; 22% of the moderate lesions had progressed to a significant stenosis of more than 70%. Of the 19 patients who together had 22

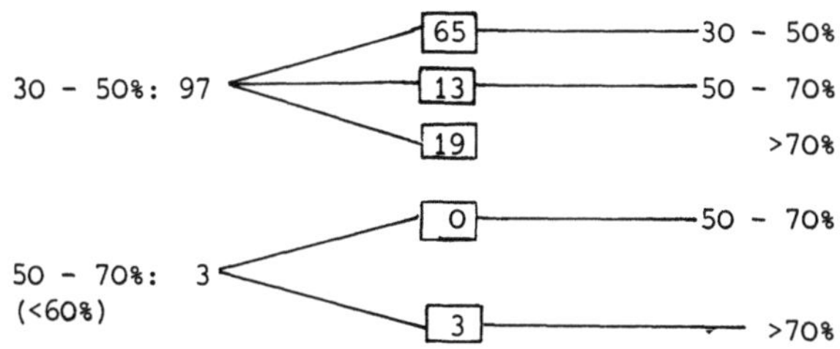

Fig. 1. Moderate stenosis: surgery for other coronary lesions

lesions that had progressed to more than 70% stenosis, eight were symptomatic with angina pectoris, which brought them into NYHA class II or III; in these patients the grafts to other coronary arteries were functioning well (with only 1 exception), so that symptoms were almost completely due to progression of the ungrafted moderate lesions. Time seems to be a factor in the development of progression; as shown in Table 1, relatively more significant stenoses and more symptomatic patients were found in the patients, who had their follow-up angiography more than 30 months postoperatively, as compared to those patients, who had their postoperative study after less than a 30 month interval. According to the figures from this small group of patients, 23% of the patients with ungrafted moderate lesions might become candidates for a reoperation as shortly as 2.5 years after coronary bypass procedures for their other lesions.

Table 1. Moderate stenosis: surgery for other coronary lesions

Followup	<30 months	>30 months
No. patients	49	26
Stenosis >70%	13	9
Angina pectoris	2	6

The same trends of development of progression seemed to be present in the second group, consisting of 88 patients, who were followed up in a natural history study. In this group 67 patients together had 100 moderate lesions in the proximal segments of the coronary artery system. These patients were treated medically and had a second angiography after a mean interval of 34 months (4-82 months). Of these lesions 23% progressed into significant lesions of more than 75% and 68% were unchanged (which means less than 25% increase of stenosis).

The influence of time was very marked here; many patients changed from one-vessel to two- or three-vessel disease by progression of the moderate lesions, as shown in Fig. 2. Other conclusions from the history study were that progression was essentially the same in the different branches of the coronary system, more pronounced in proximal segments, and more pronounced when more branches were primarily involved.

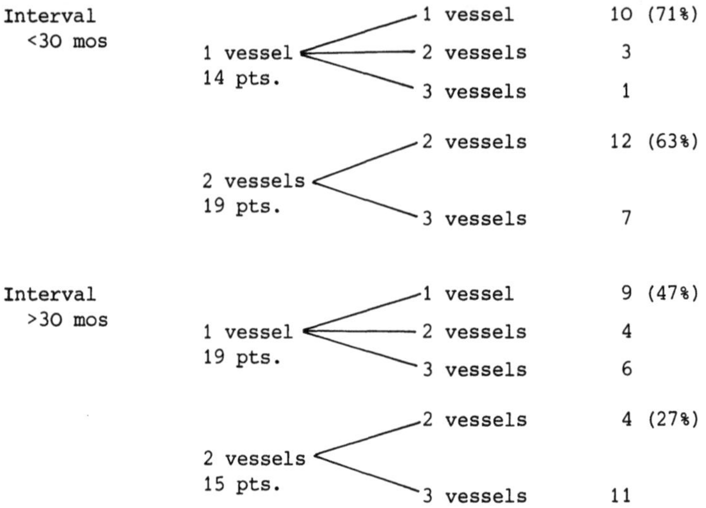

Fig. 2. Progression in one- and two-vessel disease. Natural case history

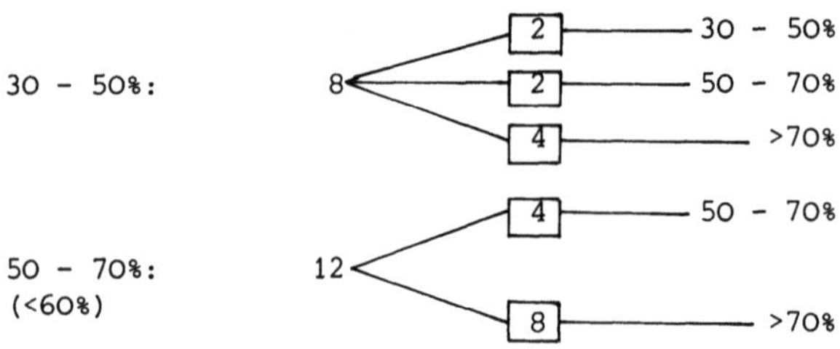

Fig. 3. Moderate stenosis: surgical therapy

The third group consisted of only 19 patients, in whom 20 moderate lesions were grafted as part of a revascularization procedure wherein 33 other significant stenoses were involved. The mean interval between operation and postoperative angiography was 21 months (18-42 months). As shown in Fig. 3 progression seemed to be stronger here; 60% of the moderate lesions had progressed into significant lesions of more than 70%, whereas only 30% were unchanged (progression less than 25%). Of the 20 bypass grafts 19 were patent at follow-up (95%), which seems satisfactory. In a larger group of patients with grafted moderate lesions, on whom an early follow-up angiography was performed, the patency rate of the bypass grafts was at least as good as in other grafted lesions.

Although the numbers of these studies are small, the results seem to indicate, that progression of moderate lesions can be considerable in a relatively short time. Progression of moderate lesions has been reported to be one of the reasons for reoperation after coronary artery bypass grafting. In view of the somewhat higher risk of reoperations and of the physical and psychological burden a second operation carries for the patient, it seems advisable to bypass also the moderate lesions whenever a revascularization procedure is performed. The additional bypass grafts do not seem to add a higher risk to the operation and the patency rate of such bypass grafts is satisfactory.

Is Revascularization Limited to Good Quality and High Caliber Vessels?

M. Schmuziger, H. Roskamm, P. Stürzenhofecker, Ch. Hahn, and M. Stolte

The occlusion of an aortocoronary bypass can occur either due to technical failure and/or poor surgical indication; the graft quality itself can of course also play a part (Fig. 1).

The more bypasses we perform on a single heart, the smaller will be the diameter of the coronary vessel, its length, and the myocardial area to be revascularized.

The questions we tried to answer in our first angiographic follow-up study in 203 patients operated from 1973-1975 and controlled routinely at a 1-year interval (Fig. 2) were:

- Should minor branches of the coronary tree be revascularized or not?
- Does the local and peripheral status of the coronary vessel play a major role in bypass occlusion?

The diameter of vessel was measured by means of preoperative angiography and the results were compared with indication of the operation report (Fig. 3).

The diameter of a totally occluded vessel is difficult, if not impossible to determine by preoperative angiography, due to the impaired filling. Therefore, we also considered the length of the vessel and obtained similar results (Fig. 4).

<u>Technical failures:</u>

- careless anastomosis (proximal and distal)
- incorrect length of bypass (kinking) } localization of revascularization
- incorrect conduction of bypass }
- torsion
- incorrect implantation of the bypass

<u>Indicational failures:</u>

- length of vessels } size of revascularized myocardial area
- diameter of vessels }
- quality of vessels
- revascularization of infarction areas

<u>Insufficient quality of material:</u>

- bad quality of bypass

Fig. 1. Possible reasons for bypass occlusion

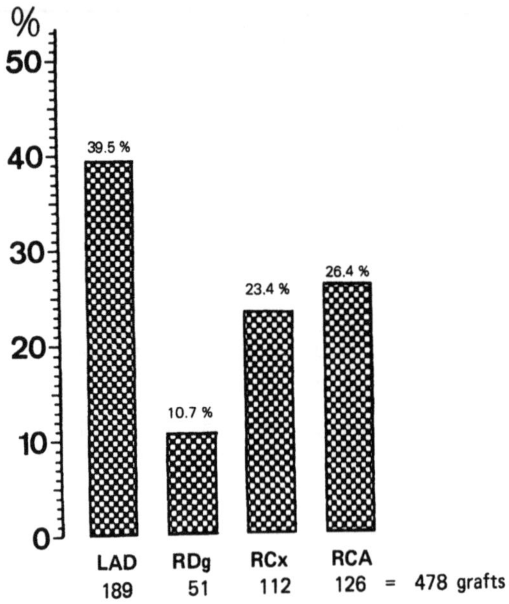

Fig. 2. 203 patients operated between 1973 and 1975 with 478 revascularizations (2.35 bypasses/ patient) had a routine control angiography 12 months postoperatively. The most common bypass was on the LAD, followed by that on the right coronary artery and the circumflexa

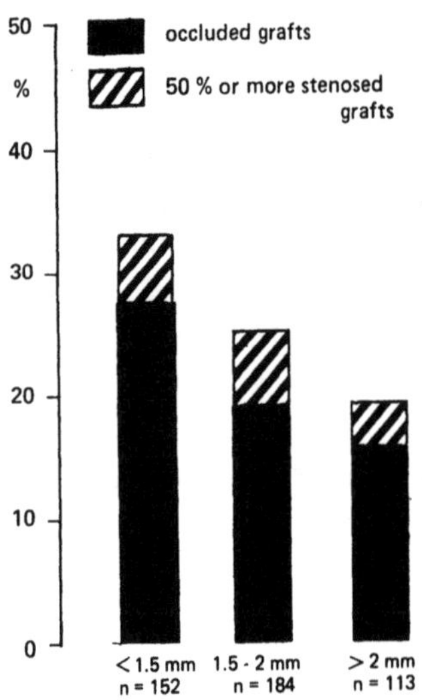

Fig. 3

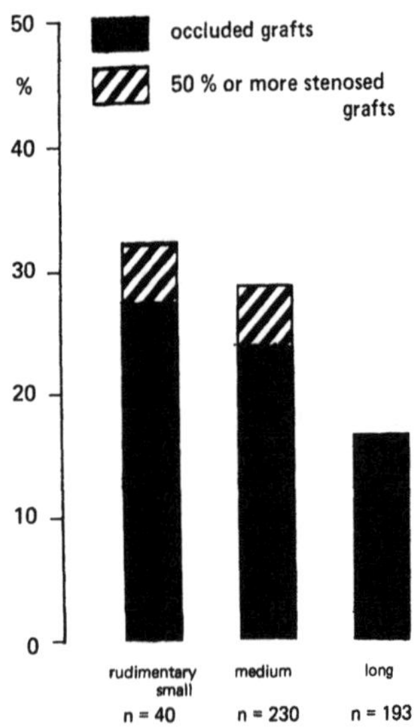

Fig. 4

Fig. 3. Relationship between diameter of the grafted vessels and graft occlusion (in 29 vessels preoperative estimates were not possible).
There is no doubt that occlusion rate in smaller grafted vessels is higher than in large ones

Fig. 4. Relation between length of the grafted vessel and occlusion rate (in 15 cases the length of the vessel could not be determined).
There is also a good correlation between length of the grafted vessel and graft occlusion: the longer the grafted vessel, the smaller the occlusion rate

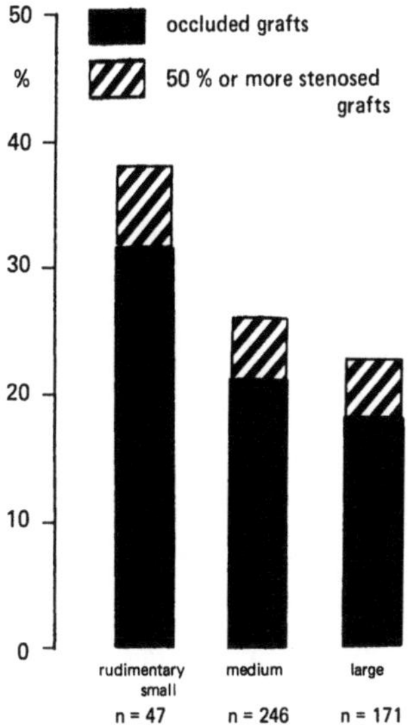

Fig. 5. Relationship between the estimated size of revascularized myocardial area and graft occlusion (in 14 cases this estimate was no longer possible). There is a high correlation between the preoperatively estimated size of the myocardial area and occlusion rate. It seems to us that this estimate is one of the most important criteria in the prediction of long-term results of revascularization

Length or diameter of a coronary vessel is not always proportional to the myocardial area to be revascularized. This mainly applies to the circumflexa-area. Therefore, we tried to find out if there is a correlation between the preoperatively estimated size of the myocardial area to be revascularized and the occlusion rate (Fig. 5).

In the beginning of aortocoronary bypass surgery we were dealing with patients who mostly had only proximal coronary lesions and good quality peripheral vessels. Today we operate more and more on patients with diffuse triple-vessel-disease. To avoid bad vessel quality in the anastomotic site, the tendency is to make distal anastomosis more and more on smaller, secondary coronary branches and to increase the number of bypasses.

To verify the validity of this attitude we checked the influence of local and peripheral vessel quality on graft occlusion (Figs. 6 and 7).

Based on the results of our study we have to conclude that the abovementioned tendency to make more bypasses on smaller peripheral coronary vessels in case of diffuse coronary triple-vessel-disease is not always justified.

Other questions are:

- Is it reasonable to revascularize infarcted areas?
- Does infarction increase the occlusion rate? (Fig. 8)

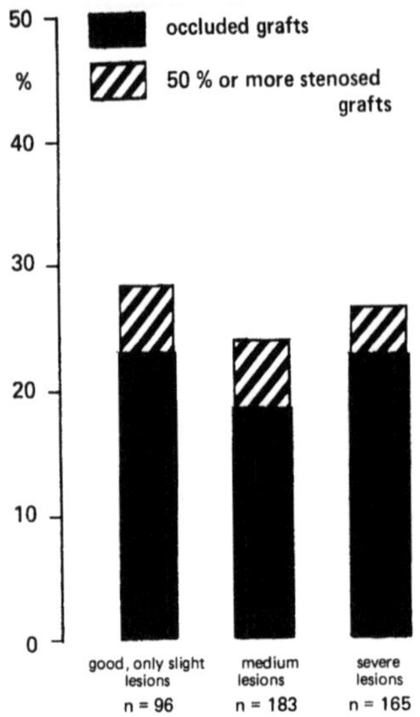

Fig. 6. Correlation between local vessel status and occlusion rate (in 34 cases local status could not be re-evaluated).
No direct influence of local vessel quality on graft occlusion could be found.
A prequisite must be that the grafted vessel at the anastomotic site is permeable and the anastomosis technically feasible

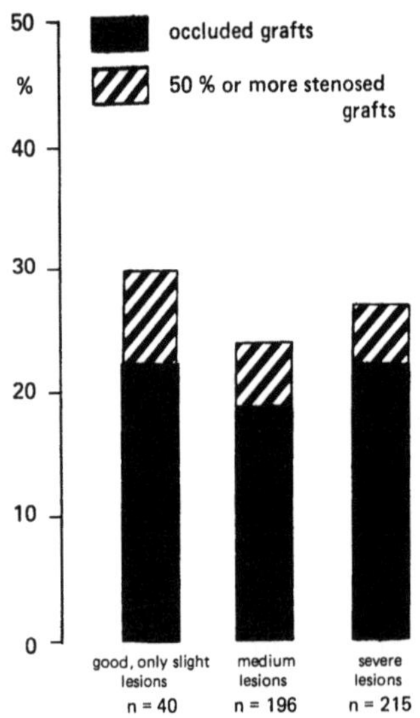

Fig. 7. Correlation of peripheral vessel quality and graft occlusion (in 27 cases peripheral status could not be determined anymore).
As for local quality the peripheral status of the grafted vessel does not influence the occlusion rate. Obviously, we are talking of vessels which pre- and perioperatively were considered graftable

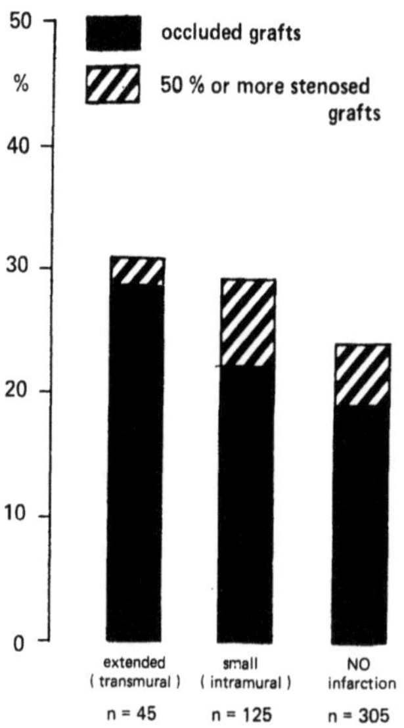

Fig. 8. Correlation between graft occlusion rate and size of infarction of the revascularized area (in 3 cases evaluation of infarction size was impossible). Revascularization of huge infarctions is not indicated because of the very high occlusion rate. On the other hand, whenever technically possible, we still revascularize small and medium size infarcted areas because patency rate is good. We believe, but cannot prove, that this kind of revascularization can be beneficial to still living myocardium

In Figs. 9 and 10 we analyze our newest results, 337 control coronary angiograms in the operation period 1973 - 1977.

The more bypasses per patient, the greater the number of occlusions or more than 50% stenosed grafts. However, when we consider the absolute and optimal patency rate per patient (bottom of Fig. 9), the best results, namely 2.51 patent bypasses per patient, are in the group of patients with 4. In the group with 5, results are not as good, only 2.17 bypasses were open per patient.

Total failure, i.e. all grafts occluded or more than 50% stenosed, occurred in 6.2% of all patients (6.8% of the patients who received 3 or more bypasses).

Total success, i.e. optimal patency of all anastomoses was obtained in 51.9% of all patients (in 36.1% of patients who received 3 or more bypasses).

39.8% of all patients had at least one optimal functioning graft.

80.5% of all patients with 3 and more bypasses had 2 and more, 49.3% even 3 and more optimally patent grafts.

Results of revascularization procedures with 5 bypasses are disappointing but note the small number of only 6 cases in these statistics.

Our present operative tactics are clearly influenced by these data: in triple-vessel-disease we do in most cases 3, if necessary 4 bypasses, seldom 5 or 6.

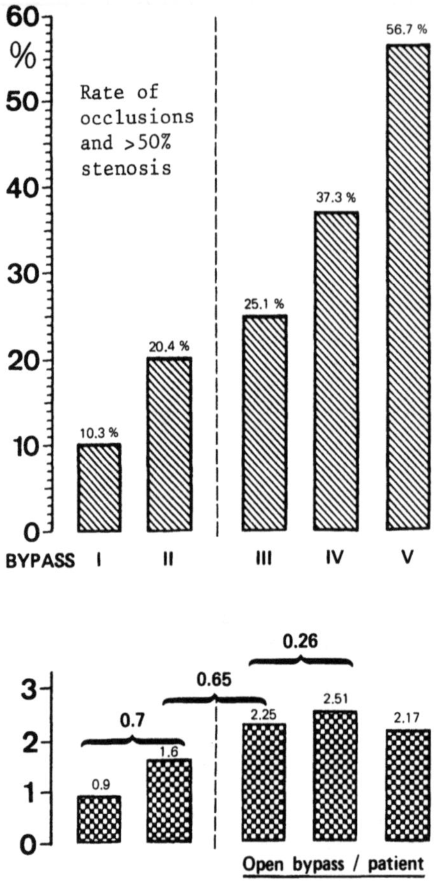

Fig. 9. Occluded and more than 50% stenosed grafts in relation to the number of bypasses made per patient

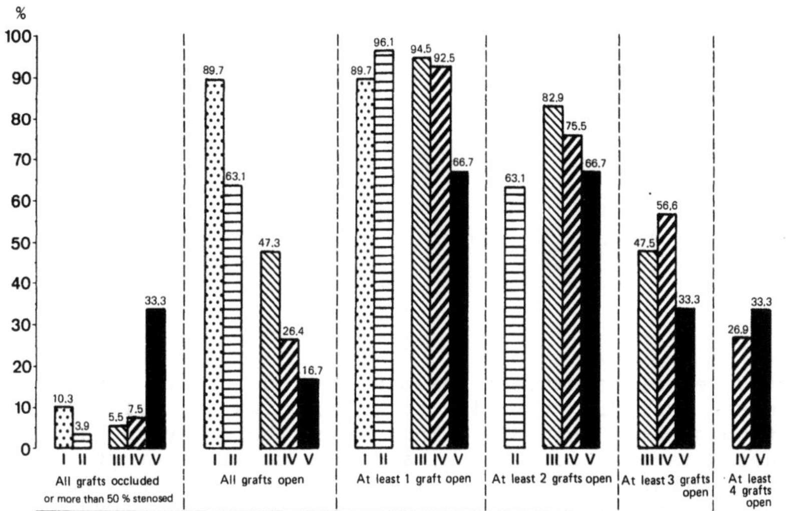

	All grafts occluded or more than 50 % stenosed	All grafts open	At least 1 graft open	At least 2 grafts open	At least 3 grafts open	At least 4 grafts open
of all revascularized patients	6.2 %	51.9 %	93.8 %	68.3 %	29.9 %	4.7 %
of patients with 3 and more revascularizations	6.8 %	36.1 %	93.1 %	80.5 %	49.3 %	7.8 %

Fig. 10. Summary of our results of 337 routine control coronary angiograms of patients operated from 1973-1977

We are convinced that the consideration of the above-mentioned data will ensure better long-term results.

On completion of the above analysis slightly different operative tactics and techniques were adopted which resulted in a significant decrease in the bypass occlusion rate. Patients who had been operated on during the first months of 1978 showed at 1-year-postoperative control coronary angiography an occlusion rate of 10% (16 of 161 grafts) and 5% of all grafts were more than 50% stenosed.

Diffuse Coronary Artery Disease; Is it a Contraindication for Surgery?

W. D. Johnson

Abstract

During the past 9 years, no patient has been denied surgery because of diffuse disease, providing ventricular function was satisfactory (ejection fraction greater than 30%). This means that many secondary coronary branches were used for bypass, and five to seven grafts were commonly inserted. Bypass grafts to smaller arteries have been carefully evaluated. Dilators in 0.5 mm increments are used to measure this size of the distal anastomosis in surgery. Graft patency has been correlated with the largest sized dilator which the coronary would accept. With 1.5 mm lumen, the patency has been 84%, only 3% less than the overall average. With 1 mm lumen, 67% of grafts have remained open. Flows are routinely measured at surgery and no significant change in patency occurs unless the flow is less than 20 cc/min. Even with less than 20 cc/min flow, 68% of grafts were later shown to be open. Long-term studies have shown no accelerated failure in the small vessel group. We have followed a group of patients operated on from 1970 through 1975 with normal ventricular function, but diffuse disease requiring four to eight grafts. Late mortality has been 0.86% per year, which is slightly less than the mortality rate of the general population for a comparable age group. While bypasses to multiple normal secondary branches are routinely performed, endarterectomy of any major artery is done when necessary. The perioperative infarct rate has been carefully monitored in all of our patients using standard EKG and also with pyrophosphate scan. Four percent of the patients developed new Q waves and 8% had positive pyrophosphate scans.

In summary, disease so diffuse as to contraindicate surgery is yet to be found in patients with reasonably good ventricular function. Similar results with small arteries have not been achieved by all centers, and it is recommended that all surgery be carefully evaluated and the results of each center should be used as the major criteria in the selection of further patients for surgery.

In 1968, when coronary bypass surgery was first introduced to our center, several studies were initiated to evaluate bypass grafts. Operative graft flow measurements were recorded and have been studied ever since that time. Recordings of the lumen size of grafted arteries were made. Postoperative cine studies were performed and pre- and postoperative bicycle ergometric studies were done. All of this, and more, plus late follow-up data have been continuously recorded in a computer based data registry system.

Early angiographic studies of single grafts rarely showed collaterals to other critically ischemic coronaries. Bicycle ergometric studies preoperatively consistently showed marked deterioration in left ventricular function under stress when critical coronary lesions were present. These same stress studies often showed little or no improvement postoperatively if one major area was left ischemic either by graft closure or by not grafting the artery. Full revascularization very quickly became the goal in order to maximally relieve ischemia and induce optimal improvement in function. Clinical experience quickly followed and it seemed apparent that relief of symptoms increased and perioperative infarction decreased when all major arteries were grafted. Operative graft flow into these smaller branches was, on the average, less than in larger arteries, but the grafts appeared to stay open. When necessary, endarterectomy was commonly done on the right, and rarely on the left system. Sufficiently small arteries were successfully bypassed so that by late 1969, too diffuse disease ceased to be a contraindication to surgery providing ventricular function was satisfactory. During the past 8 years, no patient with good function has been declined surgery because of too extensive coronary atherosclerosis.

Postoperative catheterization studies have not been done routinely and usually have been performed on patients suspected of having a closed graft or progression of disease. Despite that, correlations have been made between coronary lumen size and patency and between operative flow measurements and patency (Table 1 and 2). These studies have shown very satisfactory patency as long as operative flow exceeded 20 cc/min. Under 20 cc/min, two-thirds of grafts have remained open.

Patency related to lumen size has also been tabulated. Dilators in 0.5 mm increments are regularly inserted into the coronary lumen and the largest dilator admitted is recorded. Results show excellent patency down to the 1.5 mm size. Still, two-thirds of grafts are open when only a 1 mm probe can be inserted (Table 2).

Observing graft patency by these methods appeared to justify our attempts at grafting smaller, more peripheral arteries when obstructed proximally. Long-term studies relating time to patency have failed to show any evidence of accelerated closure in smaller arteries. Overall graft patency after 2 years (85%) is the same as graft patency under 6 months.

Table 1. Correlation between operative flow measurements and patency

Graft flow/ min	0-20 cc	21-40 cc	41-60 cc	61-80 cc	81-100 cc
Number of grafts studied	38	190	160	113	123
% Patency (1968 to July, 1975)	67%	93%	81%	90%	86%

Table 2. Correlation between coronary lumen size and patency

Lumen size	1 mm	1.5 mm	2.0 mm	2.5 mm	3.0 mm
Number of grafts studied	21	116	469	71	46
% Patency (1968 to July, 1975)	67%	84%	82%	92%	87%

Our experience with polygrafting (four or more grafts) to primary and secondary arteries was reviewed in 1976. From January, 1970, through June, 1975, 636 patients received this therapy. Of 495 patients with normal or moderate ventricular malfunction (severe malfunction in one wall only), surgical mortality was 3% (14 patients), and only one late death (0.2%) occurred during the entire period. One hundred forty-one patients had severe ventricular dysfunction (severe malfunction in two or more walls) and the surgical and total late mortality was 6% and 3%, respectively.

Complete relief of angina was reported by 75% versus 58% reported by the Milwaukee Cardiovascular Data Registry for comparable years. Five percent reported no improvement versus 11% for all patients from the registry.

Regardless of the number of major arteries involved, complete revascularization of all primary and secondary diseased arteries has been the goal in each operation. Results in recent years continue to show gradual improvement. Survival curves for patients operated from January, 1972 through June, 1976, show better results (Fig. 1). The number of grafts per patient steadily increased to over four per patient in 1976. Women, with generally smaller arteries, have done equally well. Five year survival in women with good ventricular function was equal to men at 98%. With poor ventricles, women actually have 6% better 5-year survival. As noted earlier, this series with good function includes all patients, most with diffuse three-vessel disease. No patient in this category of function has been denied surgery due to too diffuse disease.

Postoperative catheterization studies in patients with four or more grafts continue to show graft patency comparable to the overall experience. In the series reviewed in 1976, 58% had all grafts open and no patient had all grafts closed. Overall patency was 85%. In this group also, recatheterization was mostly on patients with symptoms, and it is expected that the results on asymptomatic patients may be better.

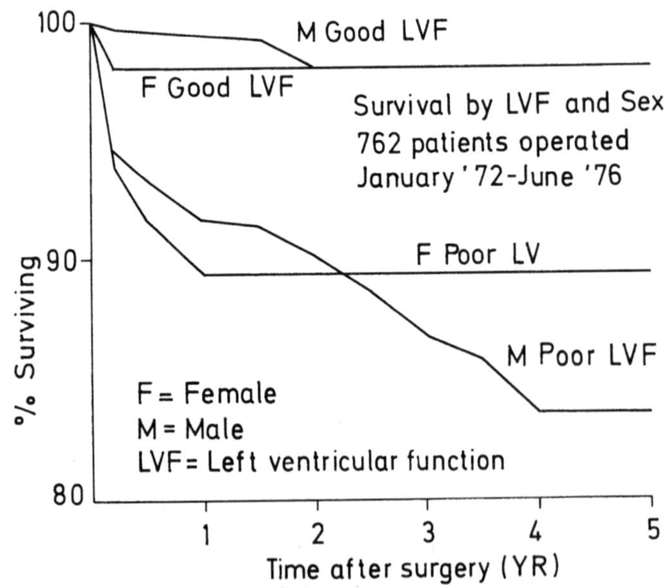

Fig. 1 Survival curves for patients operated from January, 1972 through June, 1976

Patients with poor contraction are often denied surgery. Despite their poor function, these patients obviously have some myocardium remaining which is usually in jeopardy of further damage. In these patients with limited reserve, it is perhaps even more important to graft all compromised branches. Considering patients with major malfunction in two or more walls, and generally with ejection fractions from 5%-40%, a great reduction in surgical and late mortality has been noted since 1971. Surgical mortality has dropped from 14% to under 8% and late mortality from 4.5% per year to 2%-4% per year. This is dramatically less than the medical mortality rate of 11% per year noted in unoperated patients with poor function from 1968-1971 [1].

Total revascularization can provide significant benefit to coronary patients in nearly all stages of ventricular function. It is clear that bypass grafts can only be inserted to preserve, and at times improve, myocardial function. Grafts do not alter scar, and best results are obtained when surgery is done prior to infarction. Since infarction (and death) can result from stenotic arteries, with or without symptoms, surgery is commonly done on the basis of anatomy alone. One thousand consecutive catheterizations in adults, at Mount Sinai Hospital (Milwaukee) in 1976-1977, were reviewed. Chronic to severe failure was not considered a contraindication to catheterization. Associated disease under control were not cause to avoid catheterization (diabetes, hypertension, chronic lung, and/or renal disease, etc). Of the 1000 catheterizations, six patients were rejected for surgery who were felt to have too severe ventricular dysfunction, plus too severe atherosclerosis.

This aggressive approach is based on our experience with total revascularization. This approach is clearly not recommended for all others. Bypassing small arteries could hardly be recommended when grafts to major vessels carry a 31% closure rate. Surgery for asymptomatic patients, similarly, could not be justified in that setting. When closure rates approach 40% in grafts with 30 cc/min flow, clearly this group should not accept patients for surgery with distal disease.

The major problem today is not who is a candidate for surgery, but rather, is in defining the ability of the surgeon in handling the different subsets of coronary patients. Some surgeons can and do handle small vessels with good results. For these surgeons, diffuse disease is rarely, if ever, a contraindication to surgery.

Reference

1. Manley, J.C., King, J.F., Zeft, H.J., Johnson, W.D.: The "bad" left ventricle. J. Thorac. Cardiovasc. Surg. *72*, 841-848 (1976)

Revascularization of Partially Infarcted Areas - Pathologist's Point of View

M. Stolte, H. Selz, U. Fiegl, and H. Müller

In cases with restricted function of the left ventricle due to myocardial infarctions, the results of coronary bypass surgery are clearly poorer than in the case of bypassing coronary stenoses that have not yet led to irreversible damage to the myocardium [1,11].

But are we justified in concluding from this that surgery is indicated only when the contractility of the left ventricular myocardium has been completely preserved? It certainly makes little sense to attempt to revascularize transmural scars. It does, however, become a problem to decide when areas of myocardium in the blood supply region behind coronary stenoses or occlusions are only partially infarcted. Is it worthwhile trying to protect remaining myocardium from progressive cicatrization in this region by creating a new blood supply? It is our aim to make a contribution to the solution of this problem from a pathologic-anatomic point of view.

Material and Method

One hundred sixty-five hearts of patients with clinically manifest coronary heart disease were subjected to postmortem angiographic and pathologic-anatomic examination.

The following methods were applied: coronary angiography using a mixture of gelatine and X-ray contrast medium [12], X-rays taken under image-intensifier control, fixation of the heart in 10% formalin under physiologic pressure, transversal sectioning in 1 cm thick slices, X-ray examination of the slices (Fig. 1), preparation and X-ray examination of the coronary arteries (Fig. 2), sequential sectioning of the coronary arteries in 2-3 mm steps, and macroscopic and histologic assessment of the degree of coronary stenosis and the state of the myocardium (stains: Hematoxylin and Elastica van Gieson).

Old and fresh myocardial infarctions were graded I: fine, disseminated subendocardial areas of infarction, grade II: interrelated, subendocardial infarctions, grade III: semitransmural infarctions and grade IV: transmural infarctions (Fig. 3). Grading of the size of the infarction with respect to the area supplied was diveded into small, medium and large.

Grading of the intercoronary anastomoses was done as follows: multiplication of the "intensity factor" (grade I, II, and III) of the individual anastomosis fields by an "evaluation factor" for the localization of these anastomoses (atria = 1, posterior wall = 3, AV node artery = 1, septal = 6, apical = 2, Ramus ventricularis dexter = 1, Ramus marginalis dexter = 1, intramyocardial = 2, graduation of the anastomosis into five groups).
In order to evaluate the intramyocardial vascularization in the infarction area the classifications: hypervascularization, normal vascularization, and devascularization grades I-IV, were used.

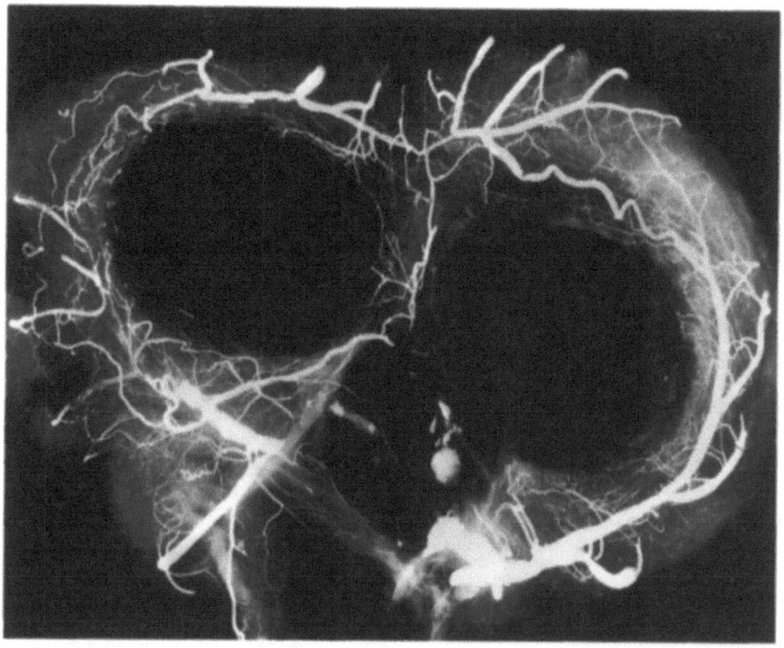

Fig. 1. X-ray of the first slice after transversal section: occlusion of the right coronary artery, intense anastomoses

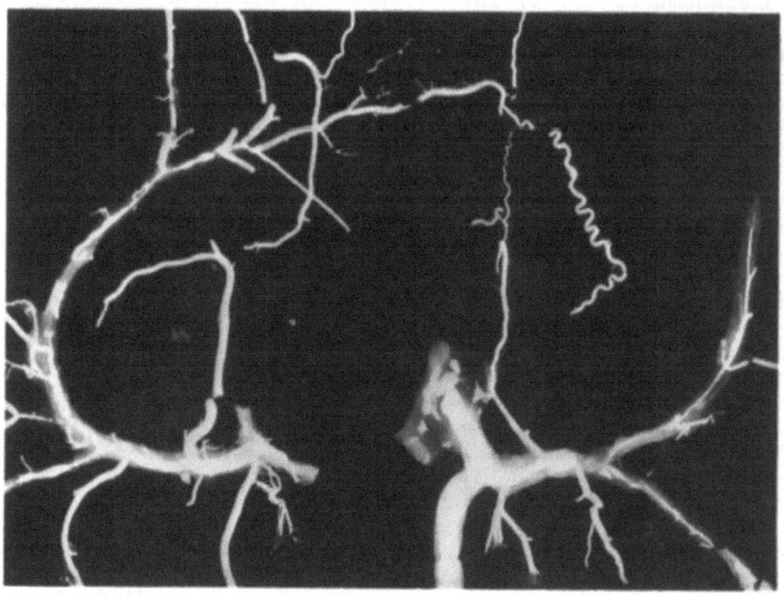

Fig. 2. X-ray of prepared coronary arteries, multiple occlusions and stenoses

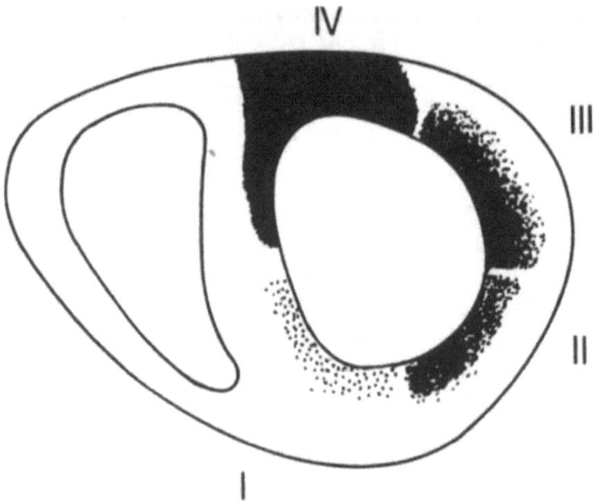

Fig. 3. Grading of myocardial infarctions

Results

I. State of the myocardium behind critical coronary stenoses
In the supply area behind critical coronary stenoses (n = 142), the myocardium is morphologically intact in 55.6% of cases; transmural (5.6%) and semitransmural (3.5%) infarctions are rare. In 26.1% of cases infarctions of grade I and in 9.2% infarctions of grade II were diagnosed. Thus, in 90.9% of cases of critical stenosis, more than half of the myocardium is morphologically intact (Fig. 4). No significant differences are evident in the three main supply areas, left anterior descending branch, circumflex branch and right coronary artery (Fig. 5).

II. State of the myocardium behind coronary occlusions
In supply regions behind coronary occlusions, the myocardium is not scarred in only 8.6% of the cases. In 21% and 23% of the cases, semitransmural and transmural infarctions were obtained respectively grade II infarctions were those most frequently found (30.5%). In 56.3% of the cases, more than one-half of the supply region behind coronary occlusions is not scarred (Fig. 6). With respect to the three main branches of the coronary arterial system, most myocardium is preserved in the region supplied by the circumflex branch (69.6%), while transmural infarctions are most frequent in the region supplied by the left anterior branch (34%); here the sum of the portions of intact myocardium and infarctions of grade I and II is only 48%, for the right coronary artery it is 58.2% (Fig. 7).

III. Relationship between size and degree of infarction
In the case of small infarction, a scarring of only the inner layer of the myocardium is found in the majority of cases; in medium-sized infarctions the degree of scarring also increases, and in large infarctions, the transmural scars clearly predominate (Fig. 8).

IV. Relationship between the number of diseased coronary vessels and the size and degree of infarction
The infarction is predominantly large (64.3%) when the infarction-triggering coronary obstruction is localized in the proximal third of the coronary branch involved.

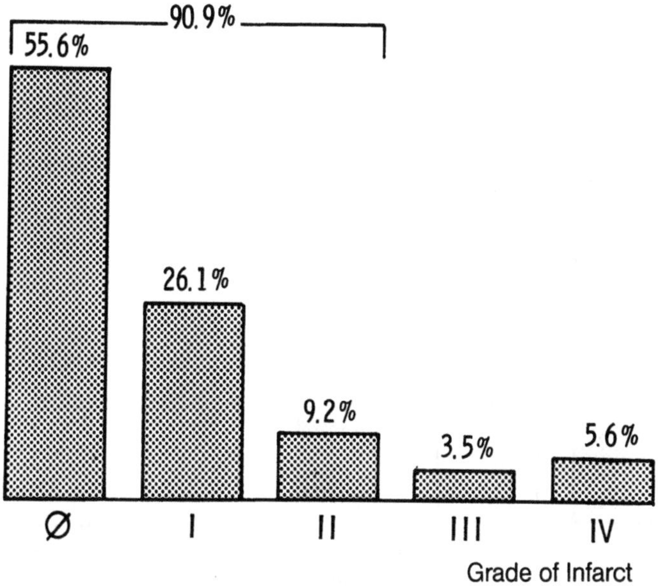

Fig. 4. State of the myocardium in the supply area behind critical stenoses. (n = 142)

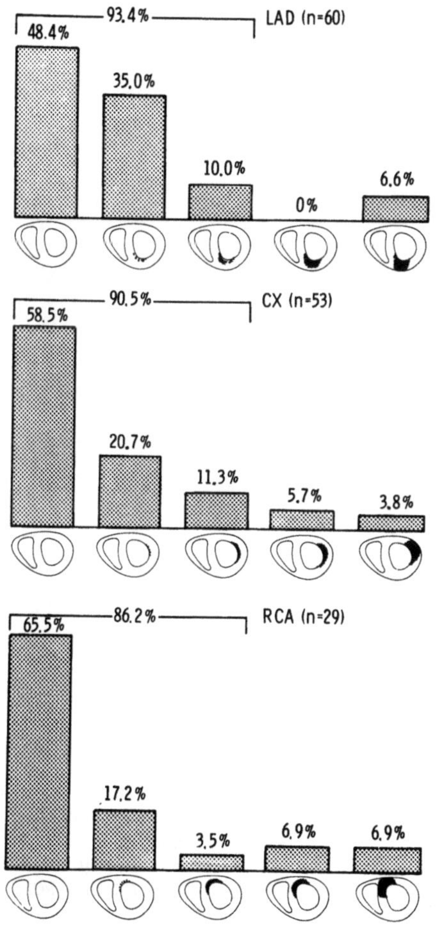

Fig. 5. State of the myocardium behind critical stenoses in the supply area of left anterior descending (LAD), left circumflex (CX) and right coronary artery (RCA)

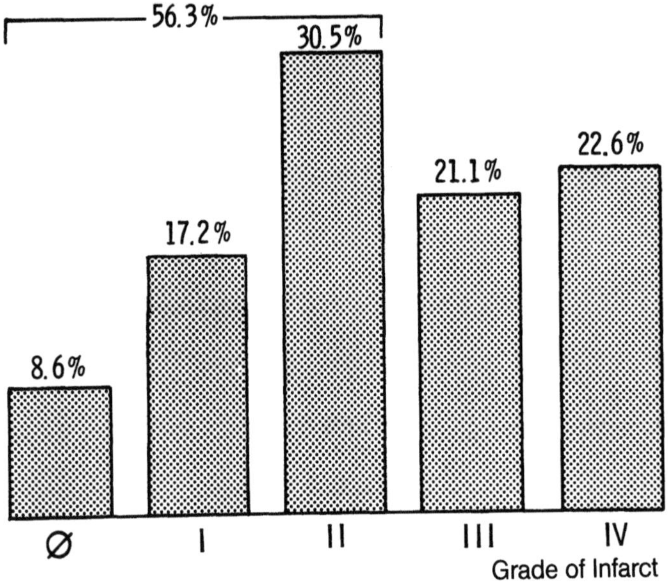

Fig. 6. State of the myocardium in the supply area behind coronary occlusions. (n = 128)

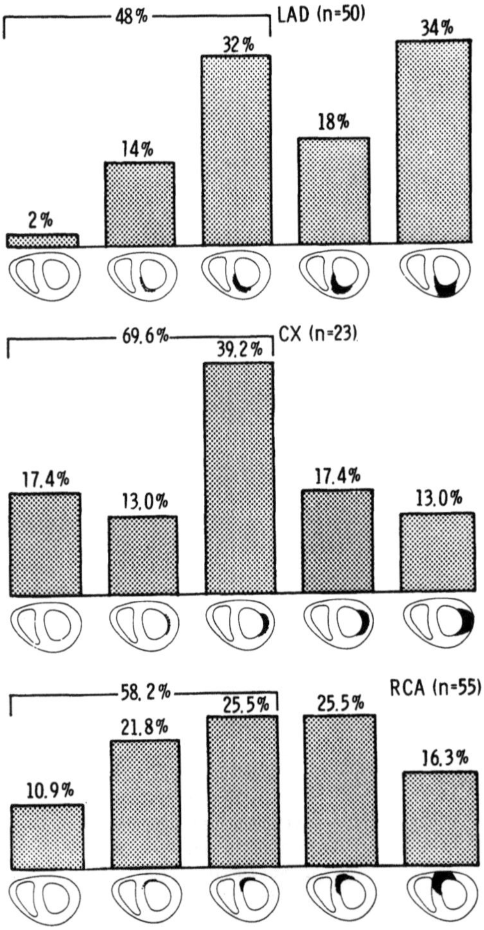

Fig. 7. State of the myocardium behind coronary occlusions in the supply area of LAD, CX and RCA

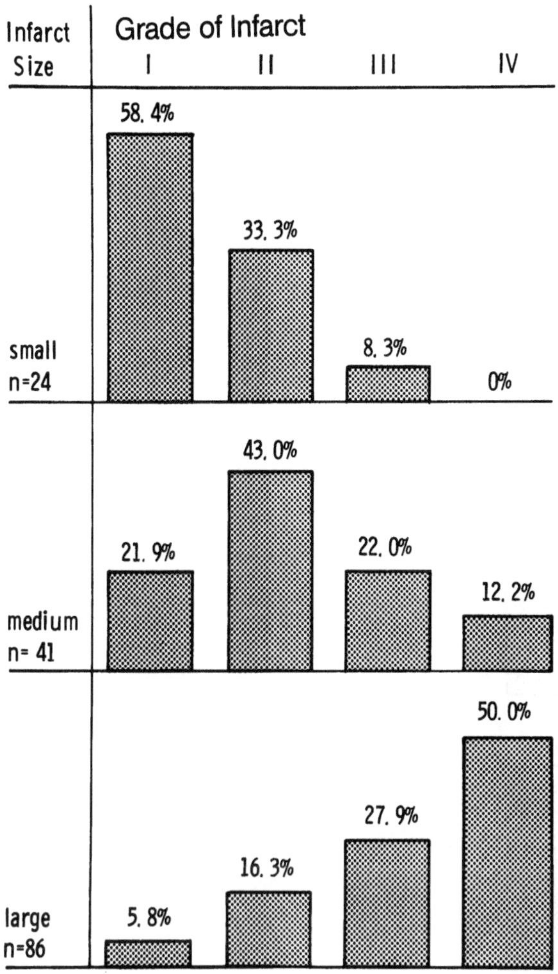

Fig. 8. Relationship between size of infarct and degree of wall involvement

When the obstruction is in the middle or distal third, the percentage of medium-sized and small infarctions increase to 50% and 66.7%, respectively.
However, no statistically significant correlation was found to exist between the number of critically stenosed vessels and the size of the infarction (Fig. 9). Nor did the number of diseased vessels have any influence on the grade of the infarction (Fig. 10).

V. Relationship between anastomoses and size and grade of infarction
It was not possible to establish an unequivocal relationship between the extent of intercoronary anastomoses and the size of the infarction (Fig. 11). There are certainly other, additional factors at work here, in particular the degree of the stenoses in the coronary arterial branch in which the region of supply is not yet scarred.
With respect to the relationship between the extent of anastomoses and the degree of wall involvement of the infarction, it is striking that in the case of transmural infarction the extent of anastomoses is less than in the other groups. Again, however, there are no differences between grade I-III infarctions (Fig. 12).

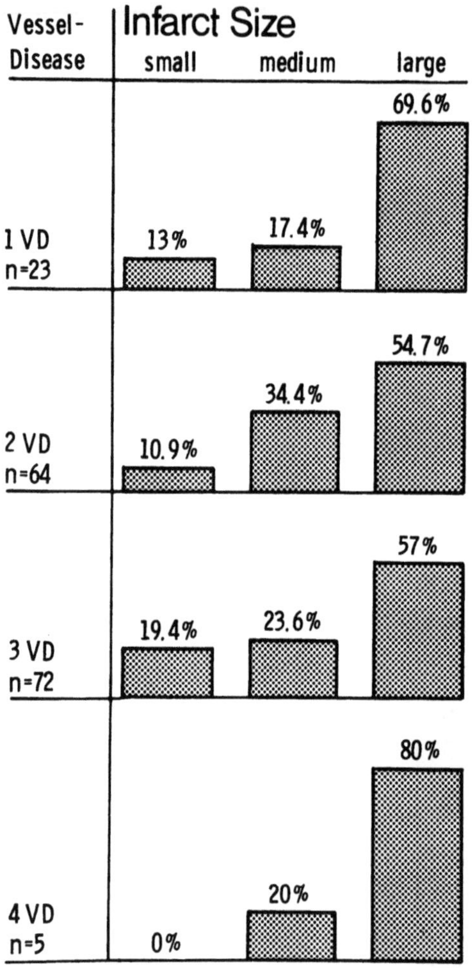

Fig. 9. Relationship between size of infarct and the number of diseased coronary artery branches

VI. Vascularization of the infarcted area

The degree of devascularization of the infarcted area depends upon the size of the infarction and on the degree of wall involvement. In small infarctions, the vascularization manifest in 61.1% of cases cannot be differentiated from the vascularization of intact areas of myocardium, and 11,1% present hypervascularization; devascularization in large infarctions is marked in 38.4% and complete devascularization in 20.5%. In the case of medium-sized infarctions, the percentage of hypervascularization in the marginal areas of the scars is at its highest at 32.5% (Fig. 13).

Even more clearly marked is the relationship between the vascularization of the area of the infarction and the degree of wall involvement. The degree of devascularization is only slight in infarctions of grade I and II and increases with increasing wall involvement (Fig. 14).

In the case of subendocardial infarctions, hypervascularization of the preserved myocardium is found in 16.6% and 26.0% of the cases, respectively (Fig. 14).

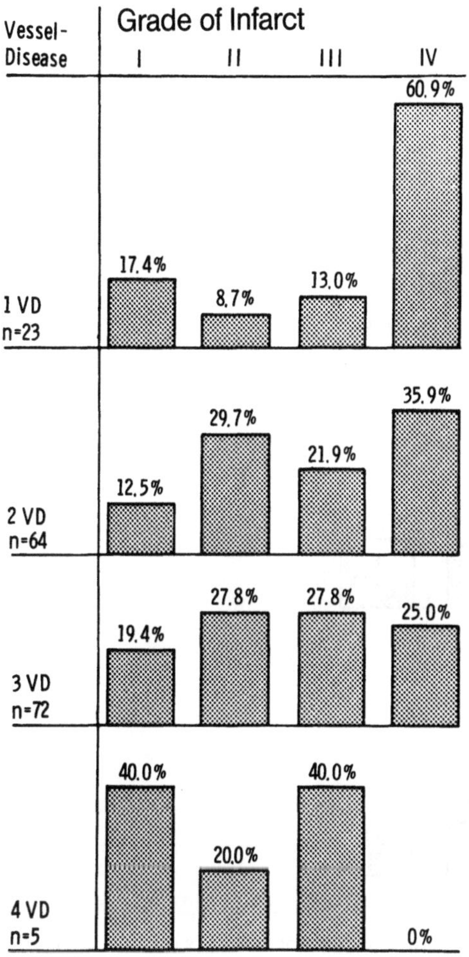

Fig. 10. Relationship between number of critically stenosed or occluded coronary vessels and grade of infarct

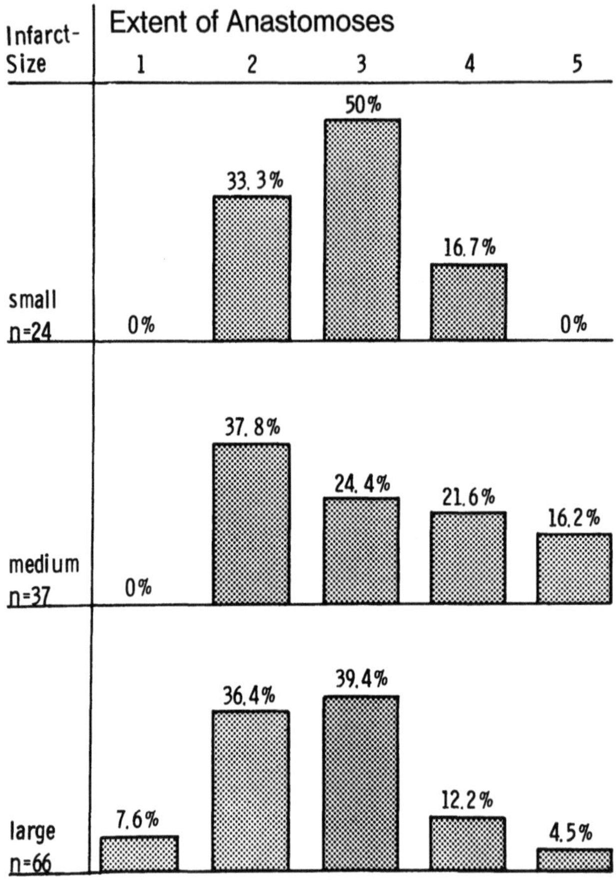

Fig. 11. Relationship between extent of coronary anastomoses and size of infarct

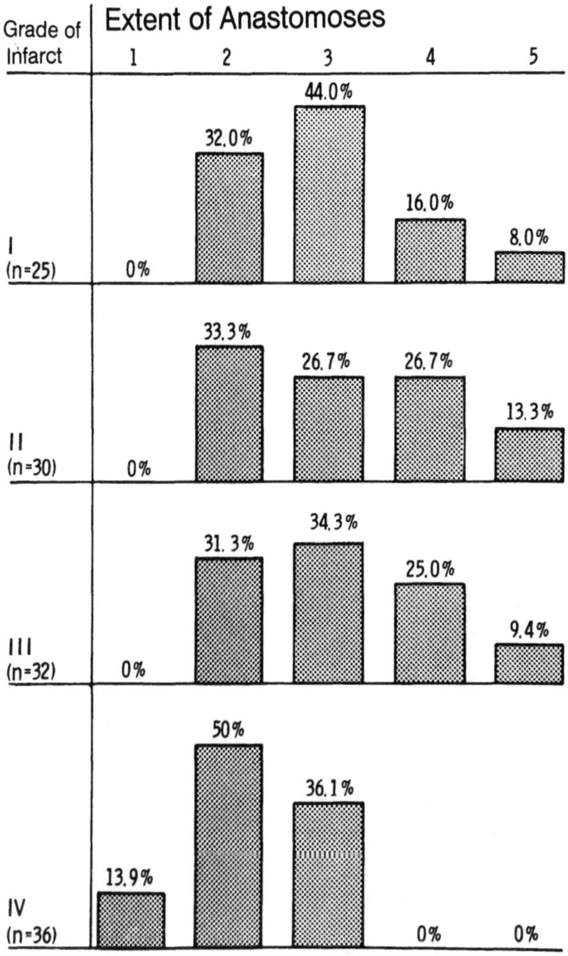

Fig. 12. Relationship between degree of coronary anastomoses and degree of wall involvement

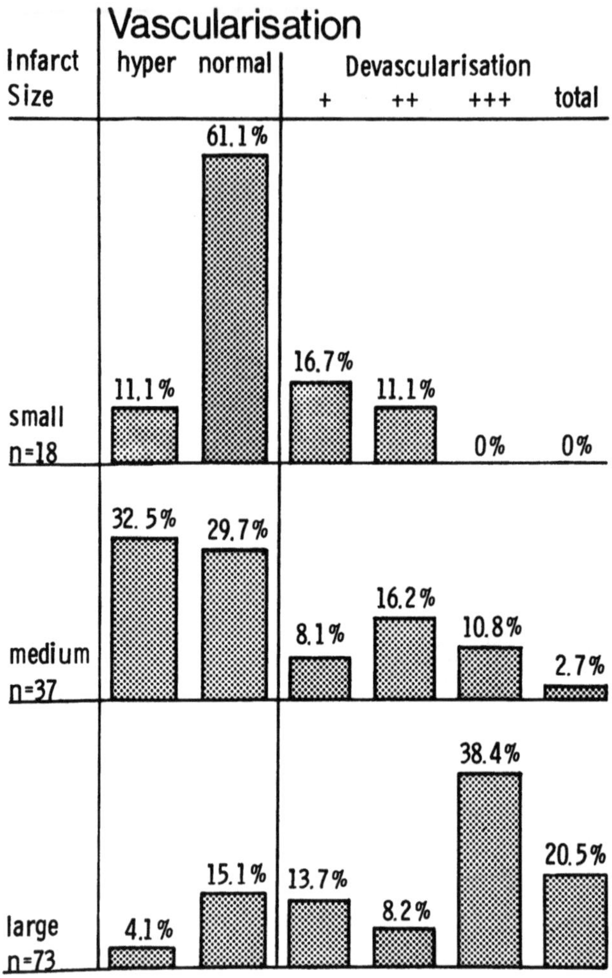

Fig. 13. Relationship between size of infarcts and vascularization in the infarcted supply area

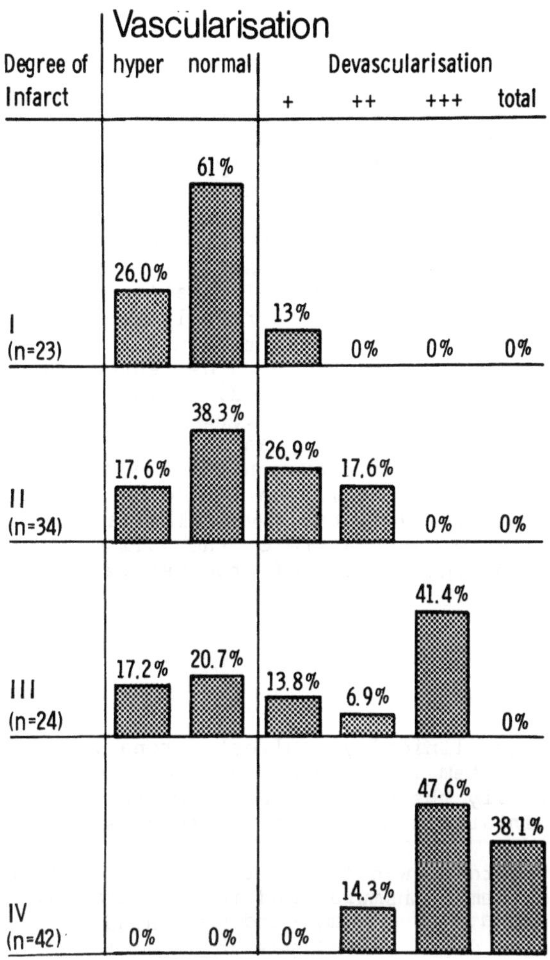

Fig. 14. Relationship between degree of infarcts (explantion see Fig. 3) and vascularization in the infarcted area

Discussion

Studies on the problem of operability of coronary heart disease from the point of view of pathologic anatomy are rare, and are usually concerned exclusively with the topography of the coronary arterial sclerosis [13-15]. We have already drawn attention to the myocardial aspects in the indication for revascularization [16,17]. The results of this study show that:

1) The state of the heart muscle in an area supplied by a coronary artery depends upon the degree and location of the stenosis in the particular branch of the artery.
2) There is a correlation between the size of the infarction and the degree of wall involvement.
3) The size of the infarction and the degree of wall involvement do not depend upon the number of additionally diseased vessels.

4) The extent of intercoronary anastomoses does not correlate with the size of the infarction and wall involvement. Only in transmural infarction is the extent of anastomoses less marked that in nontransmural infarctions.
5) The intramyocardial vascularization of the infarcted area depends upon the size of the area and on the degree of wall involvement. The larger the infarction and the more layers of myocardial wall involved, the more marked is also the degree of devascularization. In the case of subendocardial infarctions, the vascularization of the intact myocardium is however, normal or even more marked than in noninfarcted areas in a high percentage of cases.
Thus, from a morphologic standpoint, the revascularization of partially infarcted areas of myocardium would certainly seem to be a good approach. The hypervascularization of the intact myocardium in the infarcted area in a relatively high percentage of the cases of subendocardial infarctions is, indeed, an indication of the inadequate blood supply in these areas. Probably, the increase in the amount of blood brought about by an aortocoronary bypass in this region can result in an improvement of the contractility of the residual myocardium. But, even if the contractility of these areas can not be improved, the revascularization probably protects the noninfarcted musculature of the wall which are under increased tension from the results of progressive ischemic damage.

Summary

One hundred sixty-five hearts with clinically manifest coronary heart disease were subjected to a postmortem angiographic and pathologic examination in an attempt to clarify the question as to whether the revascularization of partially infarcted myocardial areas shows promise of success.
Behind critical stenoses the myocardium was intact in 55.6% of cases; in 35.3% subendocardial, in 3.5% semitransmural and in 5.6% transmural infarctions were found. The state of the myocardium behind coronary occlusions may be "broken down" as follows: 8.6% normal, 47.7% subendocardial, 21.2% semitransmural and 22.6% transmural infarctions. On the assumption that it is possible to effect revascularization in the presence of subendocardial scars, 90.9% of the supplied areas behind critical stenoses and 56.3% of the supplied areas behind occluded coronary arteries are capable of being revascularized. A further point in favor of revascularization is that in nontransmural infarctions, the degree of intercoronary anastomoses is marked. The vascularization in the region of the infarction is the most important argument for the indication for revascularization. In the case of subendocardial scars the preserved myocardium manifests a hypervascularization in 17%-26% of cases; in 40%-60% of cases vascularization is normal, devascularization is relatively seldom and only slight. In the case of semitransmural and transmural infarctions on the other hand, there is a considerable degree of devascularization. Thus, from the morphologic point of view, the revascularization of partially infarcted areas of the myocardium would certainly be justified. Even if increased blood supply were to effect no marked improvement on the contractility of these areas , it probably protects the remaining intact myocardium from progressive scarring.

References

1. Alderman, E.L., Sandler, H., Marquis, S., Harrison, D.C.: Segmental analysis of left ventricular wall motion following aortocoronary bypass surgery. Circulation *45* [Suppl. 2] 68 (1972)
2. Anderson, R.: Effects of coronary bypass graft occlusion on left ventricular performance. Circulation *44*, 507-513 (1972)
3. Bolooki, H., Rubinson, R.M., Michi, D.D., Jude, J.R.: Assessment of myocardial contractibility after coronary bypass grafts. J. Thorac. Cardiovasc. Surg. *62*, 543-552 (1971)
4. Isom, O.W., Spencer, F.C., Dembrow, J.M., Pasternack, B.S., Glassman, E.: Longterm survival following coronary bypass surgery in patients with significant impairment of left ventricular function. Circulation *50* [Suppl. 3], 131 (1974)
5. Johnson, W.D., Lepley, D.: An aggressive surgical approach to coronary disease. J. Thorac. Cardiovasc. Surg. *59*, 128-135 (1970)
6. Kay, J.H., Redington, J.V., Mendez, A.M., Zubiate, P., Dunne, E.F.: Coronary artery surgery for the patient with impaired left ventricular function. Circulation *46* [Suppl. 2], 49 (1972)
7. Kay, J.H., Zubiate, P., Mendez, A.: Five year follow-up-coronary artery surgery for patients with drastic impairment of left ventricular function. Circulation *50* [Suppl. 3], 182 (1974)
8. Kline, S., Apstein, C., Baltxe, H., Levin, D.: Left ventricular function after aorto-coronary bypass. Circulation *45* [Suppl. 2], 23 (1972)
9. Lefemine, A.A., Moon, H.S., Flessas, A., Ryan, T.J., Ramaswamy, K.: Myocardial resection and coronary artery bypass for left ventricular failure following myocardial infarction. Ann. Thorac. Surg. *17*, 1-15 (1974)
10. Shore, R.T., Johnson, W.D., Kayser, K.L.: Coronary surgery in patients with poor left ventricular performance. Circulation *50* [Suppl. 3], 205 (1974)
11. Spencer, F.C., Green, G.E., Tice, D.A., Wallsh, E., Mills, N.L., Glassman, E.: Coronary artery bypass grafts for congestive heart failure. J. Thorac. Cardiovasc. Surg. *62*, 529-540 (1971)
12. Hort, W., Kalbfleisch, H., Köhler, F., Milzner-Schwarz, U., Frenzel, H.: Kombinierte coronarangiographische, makroskopische und mikroskopische Untersuchungen an menschlichen Herzen. Verh. Dtsch. Ges. Pathol. *57*, 384-385 (1973)
13. Barmeyer, J., Baumeister, L., Blümchen, G.: Morphologie und postmortales Angiogramm bei Koronarsklerose, Eine vergleichende Studie. Z. Kreislaufforsch. *60*, 679-683 (1971)
14. Barmeyer, J., Reindell, H., Blümchen, G.: Konservative oder chirurgische Behandlung bei koronarer Herzerkrankung? Versuch einer krtischen Analyse der augenblicklichen Situation. Z. Kardiol. *63*, 697-712 (1974)
15. Berger, R.L., Stary, H.C.: Anatomic assessment of operability by the saphenous-vein bypass operation in coronary artery disease. N. Engl. J. Med. 285, 248-252 (1971)
16. Stolte, M.: Morphologische Analyse der Koronarchirurgie. Baden-Baden: Witzstrock 1975
17. Stolte, M.: Postmortale Untersuchungen nach Revaskularisations-Operationen. Thoraxchirurgie *25*, 181-186 (1977)

Revascularization of Partially Infarcted Myocardium

O. Pachinger, P. Probst, and F. Kaindl

From the cardiologist's point of view the question of surgery in patients with partially infarcted myocardium is extremely difficult. In this situation the indications have not been clarified and the role of bypass surgery with the goal of saving myocardium is highly controversial.

The main problem the clinician has to face is the assessment of the amount of ischemic myocardium at risk. Two examples can be considered (Fig. 1). One, where the infarct is large and only a small amount of myocardium is ischemic, and the other where the infarct is small and a large area of myocardium is at risk. Bypass surgery is likely to be of greater value in the latter group of patients. Thus, the problem becomes one of identification of the amount of jeopardized myocardium. This applies to the acute as well as chronic phase of coronary heart disease [1].

None of the current methods used is entirely satisfactory in identifying that subset of myocardial infarction patients in whom myocardial ischemia is both intense and potentially reversible.

Pain indicates ischemia but it is likely that it is not a good criterion of the amount of myocardium that is ischemic. Patients can have severe or recurrent pain even though only a small amount of myocardium may be ischemic and, thus, at risk of new infarction.

It would seem logical that the area of infarction on the ECG may be smaller with a nontransmural than with a transmural myocardial infarction. However, there are limitations to this simple concept because clinical electrocardiography is not precise and studies by Rahimtoola have shown that the amount of LV dysfunction can not be

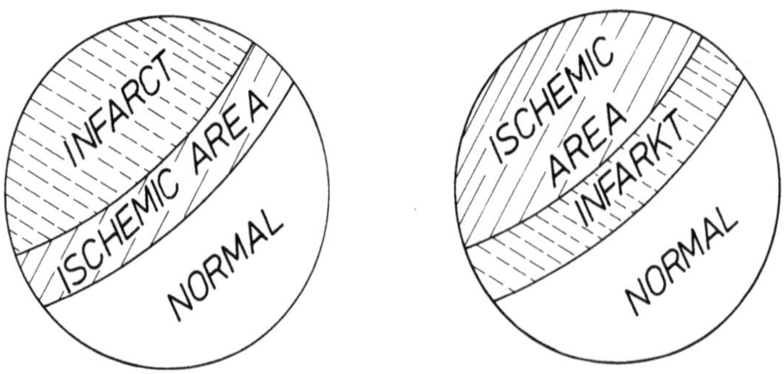

Fig. 1. Diagram representing partially infarcted myocardium. Bypass surgery is likely to be of greater value in the situation where the ischemic zone is large and the infarcted area is small

precisely predicted on the basis of electrocardiographic diagnosis of a nontransmural versus a transmural infarct [2,3]. The presence of pathologic Q waves on the surface ECG is generally recognized to be indicative of transmural infarction and correlates well with the presence of scar tissue in corresponding zones of the left ventricle at autopsy [4]. Banka and Bodenheimer showed that only 27% of akinetic segments with Q waves were responsive to nitroglycerin; however, if the pathologic Q waves were associated with collaterals, 70% improved [5]. The authors concluded that a significant amount of myocardium in or more likely surrounding these areas may be viable despite the presence of Q waves.

Clearly, the question of reversible ischemia can not be judged by clinical, electrocardiographic, or enzymatic evidence alone. Biochemical markers of myocardial ischemia such as transmyocardial lactate differences have been employed for establishing the presence of ischemia [6]. However, a number of theoretical objections have been advanced and in our experience it is a less sensitive indicator than mechanical changes.

There is also no specific coronary arteriographic pattern which characterizes ischemia or differentiates it from infarction: patients with previous transmural infarction have a higher incidence of total occlusion of a coronary artery and more collateral vessels than patients with angina alone [5]. Also, stenoses of greater than 90% are more often associated with irreversible asynergy than stenoses of less than 90%. Paradoxically, the presence of collateral vessels may increase the likelihood of surgical reversibility of function despite the fact that collateral vessels are more commonly associated with a history of transmural infarction.

Ischemia, partial infarction, and transmural necrosis cause a spectrum of abnormalities in regional wall motion for the assessment of which ventriculography is currently the best method. However, little is known about the underlying histopathologic characteristics of asynergic zones as defined ventriculographically. In this regard, methods have been devised to determine the potential improvement of abnormally contracting segments. Fundamental to all such methods is the assumption that noncontracting, but viable muscle can be induced to contract, whereas infarcted muscle can not. Where does partially infarcted muscle stand?

The reversibility of an asynergic zone is a function of the degree to which the contraction abnormality is due to chronically ischemic viable myocardium as opposed to the presence of irreversible fibrosis.

At the present time there are only two diagnostic procedures that facilitate an answer to that question preoperatively; on the one hand, intervention ventriculography using epinephrine, nitroglycerin, or postextrasystolic potentiation [7], and on the other hand, myocardial imaging techniques using radioisotopes. Two general classes of isotopes are used: Those which are assimilated by ischemic or infracted myocardium, such as 99 mTc-pyrophosphate, and those which are deposited in normally perfused myocardium, the most promising of which at present is Thallium-201.

In a previous study we analyzed the scintigraphic counterparts of responsive versus unresponsive asynergic segments as defined by nitroglycerin ventriculography [8]. There was an excellent qualitative correlation between the positive response of an asynergic segment to nitroglycerin and evidence of viable muscle on the perfusion scintigram (Table 1). Out of 29 segments which did not improve with

Table 1. Correlation of TNG-ventriculography and perfusion scanning

Asynergy	Number of segments	Pos. response to TNG	Scan	Neg. response to TNG	Scan
Hypokinesis	30	12	11/1	18	13/5
Akinesis	10	2	2/2	8	5/3
Dyskinesis	4	1	1/1	3	3/3

nitroglycerin, 21 had a negative scan indicating scar formation. Eight segments had scintigraphic evidence of ischemia although they did not respond to nitroglycerin.

In noninfarcted areas it was possible to unmask reversible asynergy by scintigraphic techniques. However, in partially infarcted areas it is not only more difficult to assess viability preoperatively, it is also much more difficult to assess the amount of myocardial salvage in these patients postoperatively (Fig. 2). Considering all the factors interacting postoperatively, it seems nearly impossible to prove that myocardium was saved by revascularization. The amount of preoperative scar formation, the number of grafts placed, the patency of the grafts, and possible intraoperative myocardial infarctions, are only a few of the major determinants of postoperative results (Fig. 3). And even if there is an increase in inward systolic motion of an asynergic area postoperatively, this improvement may occur as a passive accompaniment of enhanced contraction of its surrounding normal myocardium, especially in cases where multiple grafts are placed. In addition, we have to consider all the limitations of quantitative analysis of cineangiograms for wall motion assessment (superimposition of enddiastole and endsystole, reference system, shifts in the long axis within the ventricle, systolic rotation of the left ventricle with lifting up of the apex, etc.).

We analyzed the effect of revascularization on regional wall motion in 22 patients with partially infarcted areas evidenced by the following preoperative criteria: Abnormal ECG, abnormal wall motion preoperatively, abnormal myocardial perfusion scan (diminished, but not absent perfusion).

Table 2 summarizes the results: 63% of all segments showed no change in wall motion postoperatively, 27% improved slightly and 9% demonstrated a decreased function. These data indicate that enhancement of left ventricular performance by surgery is not a predictable or realistic goal in this subgroup of patients.

Table 2: Effect of revascularization on regional wall motion in partially infarcted areas

Asynergy	Number of segments	Improved	No change	Worsened
Hypokinesis	7	2 (28%)	3 (43%)	2 (28%)
Akinesis	15	4 (27%)	11 (73%)	-
Total	22	6 (27%)	14 (63%)	2 (9%)

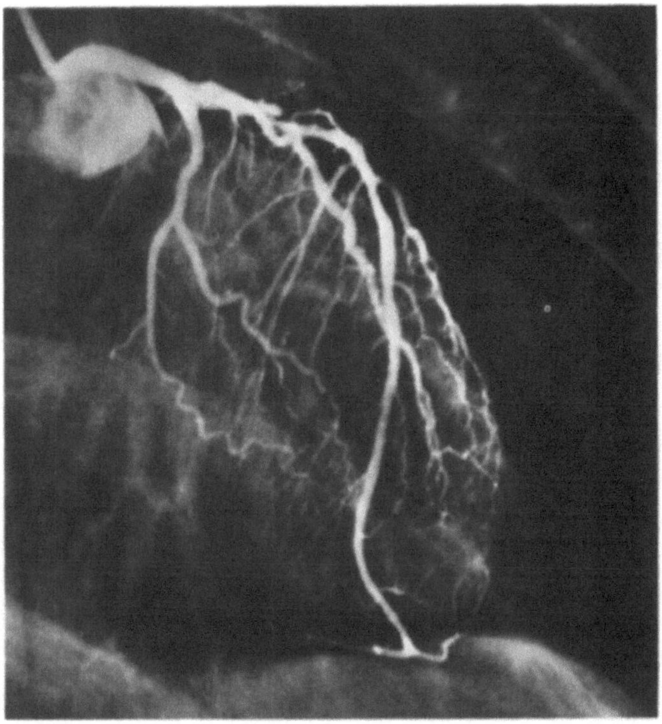

Fig. 2a

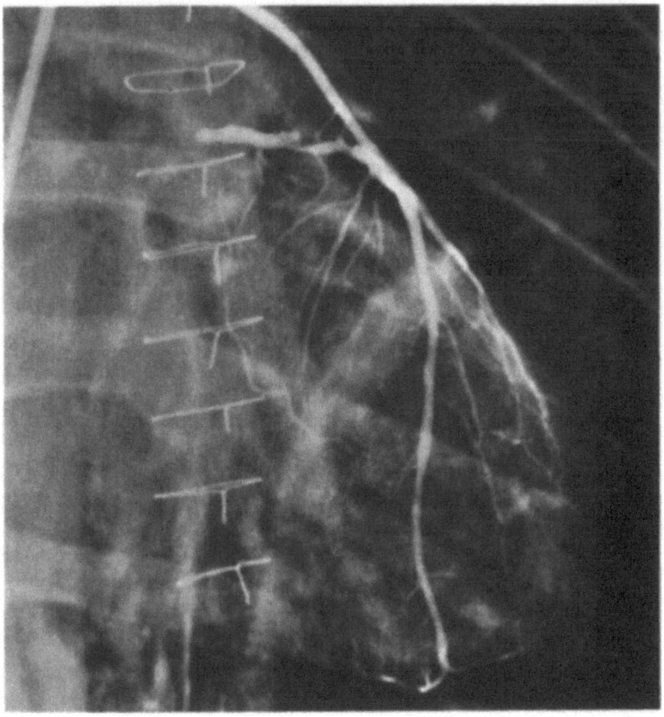

Fig. 2b

Fig. 2. a) A left coronary arteriogram viewed in the right anterior oblique projection showing critical obstruction of the proximal left anterior descending artery supplying a partially infarcted anterior wall (evidenced by ECG pattern and abnormal scan). b) Following coronary bypass surgery, the left anterior descending artery is now visualized via an internal mammary anastomosis. Despite successful myocardial revascularization wall motion of the anterior segment showed no change or improvement

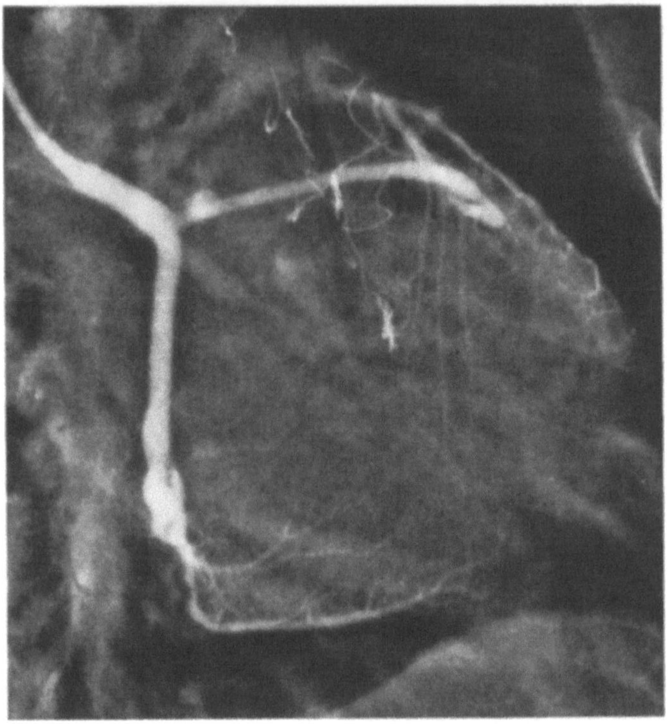

Fig. 3. An example of the multiple factors that interact postoperatively: as a result of an intraoperative myocardial infarction preoperatively good anterior wall motion diminished to a larger extent than inferior wall motion improved postoperatively. This example also reflects the difficulties of using global parameters (such as LVEF) as an indicator of postoperative results

Since there are so many factors that influence postoperative results, there is a great need for a method which allows the evaluation of the effects of revascularisation in patients with partially infarcted myocardium.

Postoperative perfusion scanning using microspheres injected into the vein grafts is of little or no value in evaluating possible salvage of myocardium.

We, therefore, have recently developed a quantitative approach to regional perfusion using Thallium-201 imaging [9]. This approach appeared very attractive to us because it might offer the possibility of correlating the function of the segment with its perfusion pre- and postoperatively [10].

A radial sweep emanating from the center of gravity is intersecting a Thallium image in 20° increments (Fig. 4). The Thallium uptake within this slice is averaged and expressed as ratio of activity of myocardium over reference area. Areas with intact myocardium can now be quantitatively compared with infarcted or partially infarcted zones (Fig. 5).

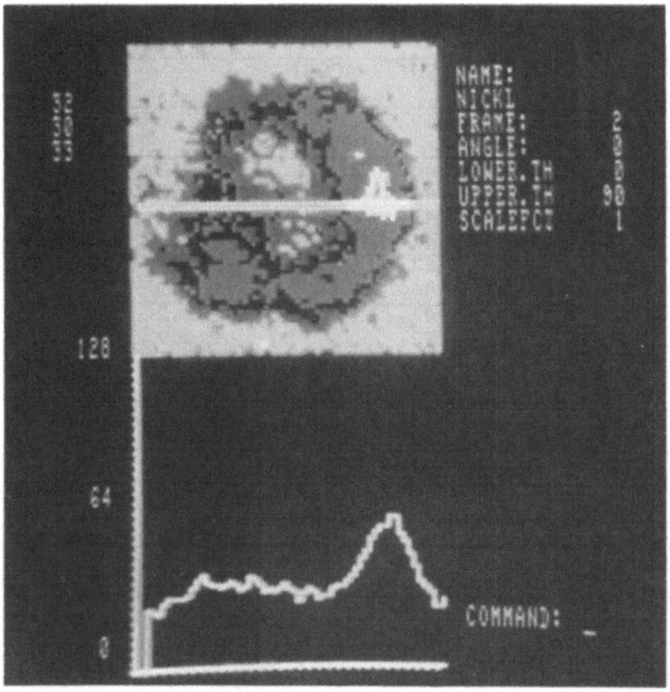
NAME:
NICK1
FRAME: 2
ANGLE: 0
LOWER.TH 0
UPPER.TH 90
SCALEFCT 1
128
64
0
COMMAND:

Fig. 4a

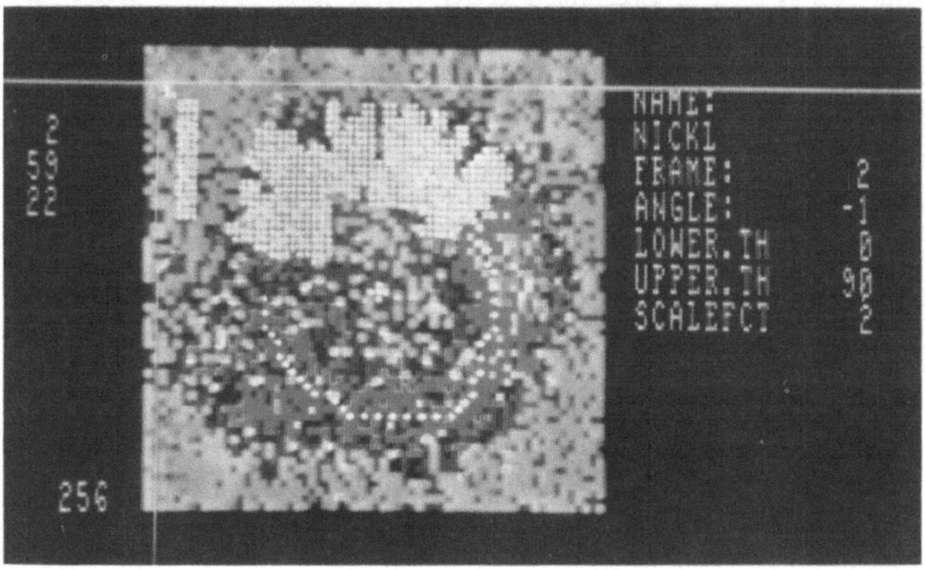
NAME:
NICK1
FRAME: 2
ANGLE: -1
LOWER.TH 0
UPPER.TH 90
SCALEFCT 2
256

Fig. 4b

Fig. 4c

THALLIUM 201 DISTRIBUTION... O=RIGHT X-ACHSIS
MARK REFERENCE AREA...
REFERENCE LEVEL: 23

ANGLE	CELLS	VALUE	PERC.
20	26	44.	192.3
40	22	44.	192.3
60	42	41.	176.1
80	25	41.	177.4
100	29	42.	180.7
120	43	46.	201.2
140	31	47.	202.2
160	28	48.	210.7
180	32	48.	208.7
200	26	51.	222.7
220	27	50.	216.7
240	26	50.	218.4
260	9	56.	242.5
280	24	56.	243.7
300	22	55.	239.9
320	23	51.	221.0
340	27	51.	223.5

Fig. 4a-c. Evaluation of regional perfusion using quantitative Thallium-201 imaging. a) The intersection of the horizontal axis through the center of gravity of the myocardial Thallium-image is used as starting point for a division of the silhouette in 360°. b) A radial sweep in increments of 20° is intersecting the Thallium-image like slices of a cake. The Thallium uptake within these slices is averaged and expressed as ratio of myocardial activity over reference area. The borders are automatically determined and the results are independent of operator interaction. c) A computer print out of regional Thallium-imaging. Areas with intact myocardium can be quantitatively compared with infarcted or partially infarcted areas; during stress testing reversible ischemia can be detected

With all limitations of quantifying Thallium images in mind, we established an uptake pattern in normal subjects, patients with transmural myocardial infarction and those with nontransmural myocardial infarction. Figure 6 summarizes the preliminary results in patients with anterior wall infarction in the segments of the RAO projection. Although the number of patients is small, there seems to be a difference in the reduction of Thallium uptake between transmural and nontransmural myocardial infarction.

Although our postoperative examinations are based on a small number of patients which do not yet allow any definite conclusions, we feel that our approach might be helpful in evaluating patients with partailly infarcted areas pre- and postoperatively.

Conclusions

At present, the application of coronary bypass surgery for patients with partially infarcted myocardium will continue to be controversial. The detection of ischemia versus fibrosis must be an important goal of clinical investigations. It appears that there are certain groups for whom a surgical approach is indicated: Those patients with continuing angina associated with a significant amount of viable myocardium, those with life-threatening arrythmias, and those where the

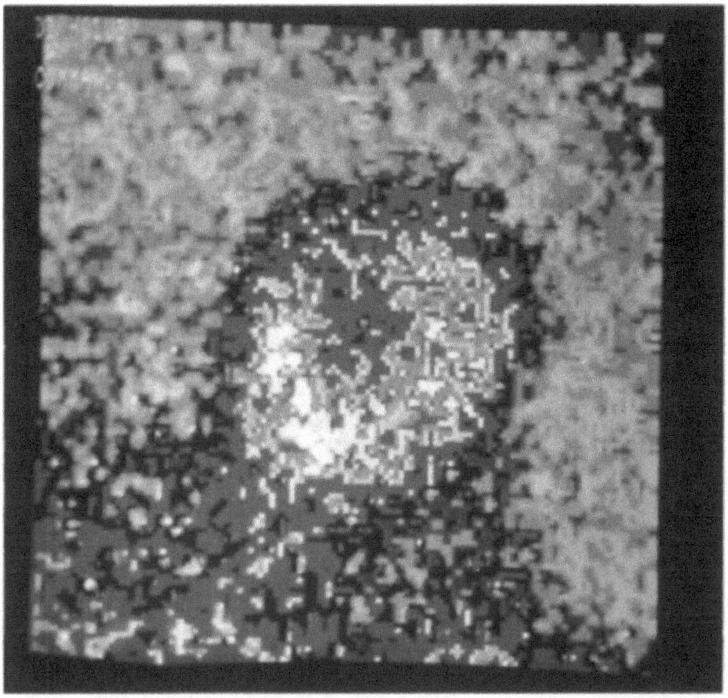

Fig. 5a

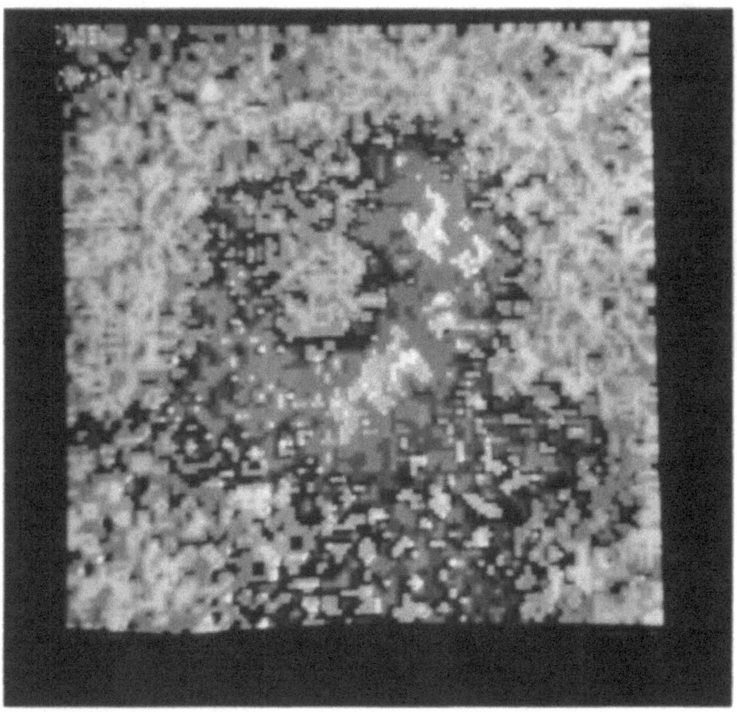

Fig. 5b

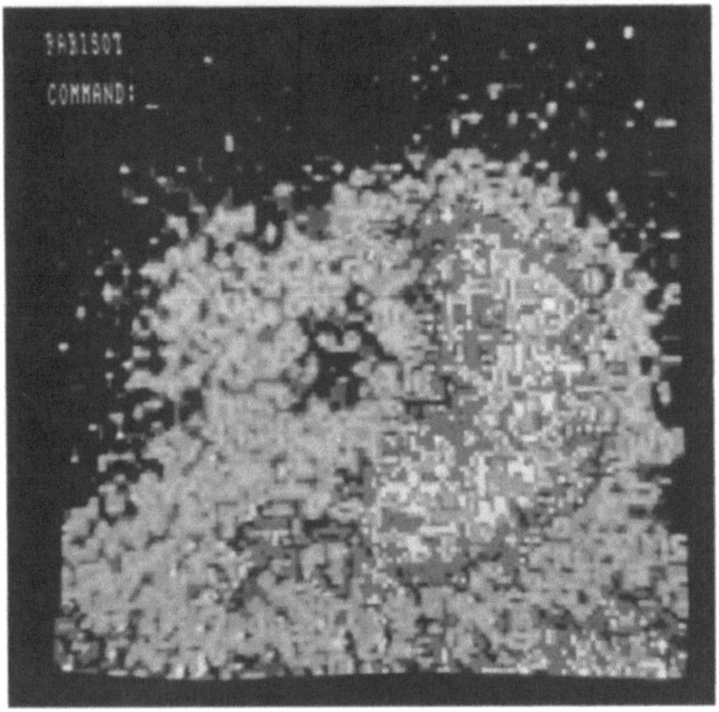

Fig. 5c

Fig. 5. a) LAO view of a normal Thallium-scan, b) LAO view of a patient with a nontransmural anterior wall infarction; c) LAO view of a patient with a transmural anteroseptal wall infarction

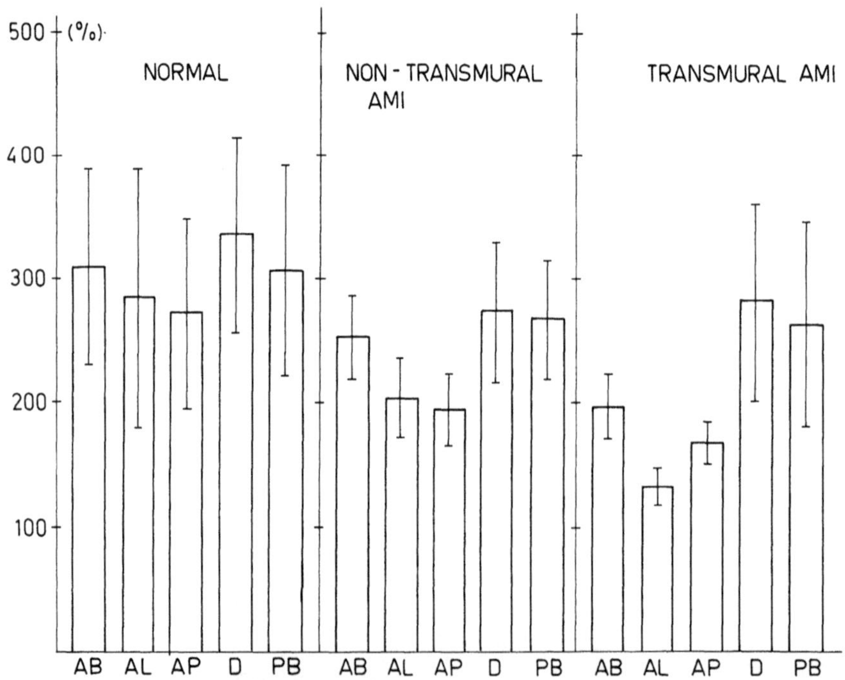

Fig. 6. Quantitative Thallium-uptake pattern in normal subjects, patients with transmural myocardial infarction and those with nontransmural anterior wall infarction. The columns represent the average Thallium-uptake in the five segments of the RAO projection. *AB* anterobasal; *AL* anterolateral; *AP* apical; *D* diaphragmatic; *PB* posterobasal

partially infarcted areas are part of a complete revascularization procedure. At present, we feel that each situation must be considered individually while awaiting more definitive analysis of the benefits of coronary revascularization in the treatment of this subgroup of patients.

References

1. Rahimtoola, S.H.: Coronary bypass: a perspective. In: Cardiovascular clinics Vol. 8/2: Coronary bypass surgery. Rahimtoola, S.H. (ed.). Philadelphia: Davis 1977
2. Abbott, J., Scheinman, M.M.: Non-diagnostic electrocardiogram in patients with acute myocardial infarction. Am. J. Med. *55*, 608 (1973)
3. Madia, J.E., Chahine, R.A., Gorlin, R., et al.: A comparison of transmural and non-transmural acute myocardial infarction. Circulation *49*, 498 (1974)
4. Bodenheimer, M.M., Banka, V.S., Herman, G.A., et al: Reversible asynergy. Histopathologic and electrographic correlations in patients with coronary artery disease. Circulation *53*, 792 (1976)
5. Banka, V.S., Bodenheimer, M.M., Helfant, R.H., et al: Determinants of reversible asynergy. Circulation *52*, 810 (1975)
6. Waters, D.D., Forrester, J.S., Swan, H.J.C.: Detection of myocardial ischemia. In: Cardiovascular clinics. Vol. 8/2: Coronary bypass surgery. Rahimtoola, S.H. (ed.). Philadelphia: Davis 1977
7. Banka, V.S., Bodenheimer, M.M., Shah, R., et al: Intervention ventriculography: Comparative value of nitroglyzerin, post-extrasystolic potentiation and nitroglyzerin plus post-extrasystolic potentiation. Circulation *53*, 632 (1976)
8. Pachinger, O., Probst, P., Powischer, G., et al: Wertigkeit des Nitroglyzerin-Ventrikulogramms im Vergleich mit der Perfusionsszintigraphie bei der Identifikation reversibelasynerger Myokardbezirke. Verh. Dtsch. Ges. Kreislaufforsch. *42*, 389 (1976)
9. Pachinger, O.: Quantitative Erfassung regionaler Störungen der Myokardfunktion bei koronarer Herzerkrankung. Wiener Klin. Wochenschr. *90*, [Suppl. 85] (1978)
10. Ogris, E., Pachinger, O., Probst, P., Sochor, H., et al: Evaluation of global and regional left vetricular function by radioisotope techniques. In: Radioaktive Isotope in Klinik und Forschung. (Höfer, R.) (ed.), Vol. 13, p. 227. H. Egermann: 1978

Indications for Distal Coronary Artery Endarterectomy and Proximal Coronary Artery Bypass Grafts

H. C. Urschel and M. A. Razzuk

For patients with coronary artery insufficiency and myocardial ischemia, coronary artery bypass grafts using saphenous vein or internal mammary artery have been successful in managing short, localized, or proximal obstructions in the coronary artery with patent distal vessels [26-27]. For patients with diffuse or long obstructions without adequate distal vessels, endarterectomy either with carbon dioxide or mechanical techniques combined with proximal saphenous vein bypass graft has been an adjunctive substitute procedure where simple bypass alone could not be performed [1-27].

Previously, endarterectomy alone had a high incidence of failure and occlusion and was limited primarily to the right coronary artery [10, 16]. The development of distal endarterectomy with closure of proximal arteriotomy by insertion of saphenous vein bypass graft eliminated the disadvantages of simple arteriotomy closure with its higher failure rate, and also expanded the application of this technique to the left anterior descending system without jeopardizing the circumflex system. The early patency of endarterectomy distally with saphenous vein bypass grafts has been as good as bypass grafts alone [8, 24,25]. However, over the long term, they have shown a higher incidence of occlusion. With low mortality and morbidity rates even though the patency of the long term endarterectomy is not as good as bypass grafts alone. This procedure is only employed when bypass grafts can not be utilized. Therefore, the alternative would be to leave such a diffusely diseased vessel alone, and not revascularize it. As long as no damage is done with the technique, many collaterals may be opened that may subsequently persist even if the main vessel occludes. This procedure is always applied in conjunction with bypass grafts in other vessels. It is never used alone or as a primary procedure. Vessels should be at least 1.5 mm or larger in diameter.

Table 1. Objectives of surgical revascularization of the heart

1) Technical
Re-establish adequate blood flow to viable myocardium that is jeopardized by significant artherosclerotic obstructive coronary artery disease.
2) Clinical
Improve quality of life
Postpone or prevent:
Death
Myocardial infarction
Complications of coronary atherosclerotic occlusive disease

Table 2. Indications for direct coronary artery surgery

Significant stenosis (75% of one or more major coronary arteries in a "rehabilitable" patient)

1) Angina pectoris
   a. Disabling
   b. New or progressive
   c. Pre-infarctional
   d. Stable with positive exercise stress test
2) "Intractable" cardiac arrhythmias
3) Myocardial Infarctions
   a. "Impending"
   b. Previous infarctions with "high risk" stenosis (not occlusion) and positive exercise stress test
   c. Complications (significant)
      (1) Mitral regurgitation
      (2) IVSD
      (3) Ventricular aneurysm
4) Impaired left ventricular function (CHF) with angina pectoris and lactate production with atrial pacing

Table 3. Critical variables in decision for surgical revascularization

1) Clinical or symptomatic status
2) Coronary pathology
3) Ventricular function
4) Status of other physiological systems

Table 4. Selection of surgical procedures for patients with severe coronary disease

Localized	Diffuse disease
Vein bypass graft (Proximal stenosis with patent distal vessel)	Gas (CO_2) coronary endarterectomy of distal vessel + Proximal vein bypass graft (Diffusely occluded or stenotic vessel)

Myocardial Infarction

Complications

Ventricular aneurysm or localized areas of ventricular asynergy Resection plus revascularization procedure	Mitral insufficiency secondary to rupture of papillary muscle of chordae tendineae Mitral valve replacement	Interventricular septal defect (IVSD) Closure of IVSD

Table 5. Distal CO_2 endarterectomy proximal vein bypass graft technique

1)	Cardiopulmonary bypass - left atrial or ventricular vent
2)	Elective ventricular fibrillation
3)	Vein graft sutured to nonendarterectomized coronary arteries - vent
4)	Tournequet isolation of artery for CO_2 endarterectomy
5)	Aortic cross clamp and proximal vent
6)	Multiple artery punctures - 26 gauge needle - CO_2 15 L/M flow
7)	Single arteriotomy - distal spatula dissection - CO_2
8)	Mechanical wire loop dissection
9)	Plaque removal - smooth blind end and branches
10)	Removal of aortic cross clamp - vent
11)	Vein graft anastomosis to arteriotomy site
12)	Defibrillation
13)	Vein graft anastomosis to aorta

Review of recent literature revealed 605 distal endarterectomies with proximal coronary artery vein bypass grafts which were recatheterized with a patency rate of approximately 80%. In our own series there were approximately 200 distal endarterectomies and approximately 100 recatheterized with an early patency rate of about 90%.

The incidence of perioperative myocardial infarction in the literature varies from 5% - 35%. Using the technique described in meticulous fashion, our perioperative myocardial infarction rate is 3%.

In conclusion, distal endarterectomy is indicated in vessels larger than 1.5 mm in diameter that are diffusely occluded. If performed properly, morbidity and mortality will be minimal and even though it itn't as good as bypass alone, any improvements will be of some advantage to the revascularization of the myocardium.

References

1. Bailey, C.P., May, A., Lewman, W.M.: Survival after coronary endarterectomy in man. JAMA *164*, 641 (1957)
2. Bartley, T.D., Bigelow, J.D., Page, U.S.: Aortocoronary bypass grafting with multiple sequential anastomoses to a single vein. Arch. Surg. *105*, 915 (1972)
3. Cheanvechai, C., Groves, L.K., Reyes, E.A., Shirey, E.K., Sones, F.M. (Jr.): Manual coronary endarterectomy. J. Thorac. Cardiovasc. Surg. *70*, 524 (1975)
4. Dumanian, A.V.: Endarterectomy of the branches of the left coronary artery in combination with an aorta-to-coronary artery reversed saphenous vein graft. J. Cardiovasc. Surg. *15*, 154 (1974)
5. Effler, D.B., Groves, L.K., Sones, F.M. (Jr.), Shirey, E.K.: Endarterectomy in the treatment of coronary artery disease. J. Thorac. Cardiovasc. Surg. *47*, 98 (1964)
6. Groves, L.K., Loop, F.D., Silver, G.M.: Endarterectomy as a supplement to coronary artery-saphenous vein bypass surgery. J. Thorac. Cardiovasc. Surg. *64*, 514 (1972)
7. Harjola, P.T., Valla, M.: Fate of gas endarterectomized coronary artery segments. J. Cardiovasc. Surg. [Spec. issue] *95* (1975)
8. Hochberg, M.S., Michaelis, L.L.: Results of combined coronary endarterectomy and coronary bypass for diffuse coronary artery disease. J. Thorac. Cardiovasc. Surg. *75*, 38 (1978)

9. Kaplitt, M.J.: Discussion of Urschel et al [25]
10. Kaplitt, M.J., Robinson, G.: Coronary gas endarterectomy. Am. Heart J. *81*, 136 (1971)
11. Keon, W.J.: Distal Endarterectomy. Its role in coronary artery bypass surgery. Ann. Thorac. Surg. (in press) (1978)
12. Klie, J.H., Johnson, L., Smulyan, H., Potts, J.L., Obeid, A.I., Fruehan, C.T., Eich, R.H., Parker, F.B., Webb, W.R.: Gas endarterectomy of right coronary artery. The importance of proximal bypass surgery. Circulation *49*, 63 (1974)
13. Kuijpers, P.J., Lacquet, L.K., Skotnicki, S.H., Linssen, G.H., Vonk, J.T.C.: Distal gas endarterectomy and venous bypass in coronary artery surgery. J. Cardiovasc. Surg. *15*, 158 (1974)
14. Leatherman, L.L., Rochelle, D.G., Dawson, J.T., Terneny, O., Hallman, G.L., Cooley, D.A.: Coronary angiography after coronary artery bypass (CAB) surgery. Circulation *45/46* [Suppl. 2], 181 (1972)
15. Longmire, W.P. (Jr.), Cannon, J.A., Kattus, A.A.: Direct vision coronary endarterectomy for angina pectoris. N. Engl. J. Med. *259*, 993 (1958)
16. Robinson, G., Kaplitt, J., Philips, P., Patel, B.: Complete surgical correction of the totally occluded and diffusely diseased right coronary artery. J. Thorac. Cardiovasc. Surg. *60*, 504 (1970)
17. Robinson, G., Kaplitt, M.J.: Combined gas endarterectomy and saphenous vein graft. Adv. Cardiol. *9*, 119 (1973)
18. Sabiston, D.C. (Jr.), Ebert, P.A., Friesinger, G.C., Ross, R.S., Sinclair-Smith, B.: Proximal endarterectomy, arterial reconstruction for coronary occlusion at aortic origin. Arch. Surg. *91*, 758 (1965)
19. Sawyer, P.N., Kaplitt, M.J., Sobel, S., Karlson, K.E., Stuckey, J., Wechsler, B.M., Summers, D.N., Dennis, C.: Experimental and clinical experience with coronary gas endarterectomy. Arch. Surg. *95*, 736 (1967)
20. Sawyer, P.N., Kaplitt, M.J., Sobel, S., Dimaio, D.: Application of gas endarterectomy to atherosclerotic peripheral vessels and coronary arteries. Circulation *35/36* [Suppl. 1], 163 (1967)
21. Sawyer, P.N.: Direct revascularization with coronary gas endarterectomy. NY State J. Med. *70*, 1195 (1970)
22. Sawyer, P.N., Zufi, D., Wslowski, S.A., Burrowes, C.B.: Electrical surface change as a factor in maintenance of patency of endarterectomized aorta. Surgery *59*, 1019 (1966)
23. Sewell, W.H.: Improved coronary vein graft patency rates with side to side anastomoses. Ann. Thorac. Surg. *17*, 538 (1974)
24. Urschel, H.C., Razzuk, M.A.: Reconstruction of the left anterior descending coronary artery. JAMA *216*, 141 (1971)
25. Urschel, H.C. (Jr.), Razzuk, M.A., Wood, R.E., Paulson, D.L.: Distal CO_2 coronary artery endarterectomy and proximal vein bypass graft. Ann. Thorac. Surg. *14*, 10 (1972)
26. Urschel, H.C. (Jr.), Razzuk, M.A., Nathan, M.J., Miller, E.R., Nicholson, D.M., Paulson, D.L.: Combined gas (CO_2) endarterectomy and vein bypass graft for patients with coronary artery disease. Ann. Thorac. Surg. *10*, 119 (1970)
27. Yacoub, M.H., Fawzy, E., Anyanwu, H., Towers, M.: Combined gas endarterectomy and coronary artery bypass graft. Circulation *51/52* [Suppl. 1], 182 (1975)

Patency Rate and Functional Results of Left Anterior Descending Bypass Surgery by Internal Mammary Artery

P. Mathieu, C. Giorgi, J. Helmer, and Ch. Goepfert

Abbreviations

IMA: Internal mammary artery
SVG: Saphenous vein graft
LAD: Left anterior descending artery

From 1970 to 1977 we operated on 599 patients with coronary artery disease. Of these patients 410 had an IMA bypass, 400 on the LAD and 10 on its diagonal branch. A single IMA bypass was performed on 189 patients and 221 had an IMA bypass associated with one or several SVG on the circumflex or the right coronary artery.

We could not compare the results of IMA bypass to SVG on the LAD: we performed 97 SVG on the LAD, but whereas IMA bypass was performed since December 1972, half of the SVG were performed before that time; since 1973 we have used SVG on the LAD only when an IMA bypass was not possible or contraindicated.

Patency of the IMA bypass in our experience was much higher than that of the SVG performed on the three main coronary trunks; for this reason we prefer this technique.

During the first 3 years of our practice, postoperative angiographies were carried out as systematically as possible: 97 postoperative angiographies out of 121 patients operated on. Patency rate in this group was 92.78%, and in the same period, SVG patency rate was only 74.19%.

We must say that our recent experience did not show the same difference of results between SVG and IMA bypass: 86.75% and 76.53%, but these series could not be considered because angiographic controls were no longer systematic. We performed them especially on patients who were not completely relieved after operation (Table 1).

Table 1. Patency rate

	1972	1973	1974	1975	1976	1977
IMA	2	42	77	95	104	90
Angiographic control	2	36	59	63	49	25
Patent	2	32	56	54	38	21

Patency rate: 92.78% Global: 86.75%

	1972	1973	1974	1975	1976	1977
SVG (all vessels)	45	55	86	117	102	83
Angiographic control	42	44	69	69	50	20
Patent	28	34	53	58	37	15

Patency rate: 74,19% Global: 76,53%

Table 2. Comparative results

		IMA		SVG	
		Number angiographic control	Patency	Number angiographic control	Patency
Green	1968-1971	70	97%	67	70%
Kay	1968-1971	137	98.5%	32	84.3%
Loop	1972-1975	644	95.8%	1208 (LAD)	86%
Edwards	1972		98%		80%-85%
Geha	1973-1974		99%		81%
Barner	1972-1975	215	90%	88	88%

The superior results of the IMA bypass as compared to SVG, are similar to those of different surgical teams (Table 2).

For the angiographic controls performed within 6 months or 1 year, the patency of the IMA bypass was 10% - 15% higher than that of the SVG.

We must now try to answer two questions:

1) Is the IMA bypass superior to SVG in the long run?
2) As a consequence of the lower IMA bypass flow, are the functional results less satisfactory?

As far as the long-term patency is concerned the slow but progressive deterioration of SVG with mural fibrosis or possibility of late thrombosis is well known. On the contrary, the long-term development of the IMA remains unknown. In our experience, among 203 angiographically patent IMA bypasses, we made no further investigations; we had no evidence at all of late thrombosis.

The second question concerns the functional results of the IMA bypass. To evaluate these results, we selected 91 patients who had a single graft patent, and who had been rehabilitated and tested in the same center (Hôpital Jeanne d'Arc); therefore this study concerns only a small group of 25 patients, more or less in the same condition.

Their ages ranged from 30 to 60 years, (among them only one woman). Regarding the development of the coronary disease, ten patients suffered from unstable angina. They had only postoperative tests; the 15 patients who had a chronic coronary artery disease had pre- and postoperative tests. In this group, eight patients had complete revascularization. All but one had a good left ventricle. Seven patients had only partial revascularization; all but one had an impaired left ventricle.

On all our patients, the test was performed using a constant workload calibrated bicycle ergometer. The first stage consisted of: 40 W, 3 min; then regular increments, 30 W, 3 min.

Each stage must have a 3 min duration. Endpoints of the exercise test were leg fatigue, predicted maximal effort reached, or positive test (chest pain, failure of blood pressure, dyspnea, ventricular arrhythmia, 1 mm at least segmental ST depression).

Table 3. Chronic disease complete revascularization in 8 patients 3-8 months postoperatively

	Max. workload (watts)		Max. heart rate		Max. rate pressure product x 10^2		Max. O^2 consumption		Chest pain		ST de-pression	
	preop	postop	preop	postop	preop	postop	preop	postop	preop	postop	preop	postop
1	80	125	85	155	144.5	294.5	960	1980	++	-	1 mm	O
2	80	145	142	180	255.6	378	1300	1890	++	-	1 mm	O
3	95	135	142	175	298.2	402.5	1680	1800	++60w	-	2 mm	1 mm
4	70	115	115	160	184	256	-	-	++	-	3 mm	O
5	80	100	118	112	177	212.8	1270	1300	++	-	2.5 mm	O
6	150	160	175	185	402.5	370	2280	2240	-	-	O	O
7	110	130	120	152	204	281.2	-	-	++90w	-	O	O
8	135	130	160	142	272	255.6	2220	1920	-	-	1 mm	O
Mean	100	130	132	158	242.2	306.3	1618	1855	6/8	O/8	6/8	1/8

Table 4. Complete revascularization (IMA bypass). Exercise test data before and after IMA bypass (mean values)

	Max. workload (W/min)	Max. heart rate	Rate pressure product (x 10^{-2})	Max. oxygen consumption (ml/min)	Chest pain	ST de-pression
Preop test	100	132	242.2	1618	6/8	6/8
Early postop (3-8 months)	130	158	306.3	1855	O	1 (1 min)
Late postop >1 year	159	174	379.8	2080	O	2
Change +	+59	+42	+137.6	+462	++	+

Table 5. Chronic disease: Partial revascularization in 7 patients 3-8 months postoperatively

	Max. workload (W/min.)		Max. heart rate		Max. rate pressure product x 10^{-2}		Chest pain		ST depression	
	preop	postop	preop	postop	preop	postop	preop	postop	preop	postop
2-vessels	140	180	140	160	195	304	-	-	1.5 mm	O
Stenosis	80	110	135	134	189	227.8	++	-	3 mm	O
Ventricular	90	110	165	178	264	427.2	++	dyspnea	2 mm+Pvc	O
Function ↘	120	115	160	175	264	367.5	-	-	1 mm	1 mm
3-Vessel stenosis--ventricular function ↘	110	130	115	165	184	297	++	-	O	O
	145	170	130	165	234	264	-	-	O	O
3-Vessel stenosis--normal ventricular function	120	150	142	116	291.1	235.2	-	-	4 mm[a]	O
Mean	115	138	141	156	231.7	303.2	3/7	0/7	5/7	1/7

[a] 1 mm with 120 heart rate.

Table 6. Unstable angina in 10 patients 3-8 months postoperatively

	Revascularization	Max. workload (W/min)	Max. heart rate	Max. rate pressure product x 10^{-2}	Chest pain	ST depression
Prinzmetal angina	Complete + normal ventricular function	110	138	241.5	-	0
		165	142	312.4	-	0
		160	125	212.5	-	0
Other unstable angina	Complete + normal ventricular function	120	162	372.6	-	1 min
		165	178	338.2	+	1.5 min
		150	175	367.5	-	1 min
		130	180	370.8	-	0
		140	160	272.8	-	0
	Partial + poor ventricular function	145	163	326	-	0
		160	170	391	-	0
Mean		145	159	320.5	1/10	3/10

The results of the eight patients with complete revascularization show that the maximal work load increases significantly, just as maximal heart rate and maximal rate and pressure product, which is paralleled to maximal oxygen consumption (Table 3).

There was no angina during the postoperative test, although most of the patients reached the predicted maximal heart rate. With regard to ECG, six of the patients had an exercise-induced segmental ST depression preoperatively only one patient had postoperatively an ST abnormality, but at a lesser degree for a maximal test.

After a longer time period postoperatively, the results became still better (Table 4).

In the group of partially revascularized patients, the results were similar: no postoperative angina and a marked improvement of ST abnormality (Table 5).

In the group of unstable angina, the postoperative functional results were also good, considering that all these patients presented severe chest pain and marked ST depression before operation (Table 6).

Finally, in all these groups, the exercise tests showed:

- Relief of spontaneous or exercise-induced angina in all patients except one.
- Suppression of spontaneous or exercise-induced segmental ST depression in 80% of the patients.
- Significant improvements or good level reached in physical work capacity, maximal heart rate, and maximal rate-pressure product.

The results suggest the presence of excellent coronary blood flow and very satisfactory ventricular function (unless it was impaired before the operation) at rest and during testing.

In spite of these satisfactory results, we are aware that the IMA bypass is criticized by some surgeons:

- The dissection is more tedious, but in many different surgical series, operative and postoperative morbidity and mortality are similar with IMA bypass and SVG.
- The anastomosis is more difficult, but with IMA bypass, patency rate is better.
- The main opposition to this procedure concerns the blood flow which is lower with IMA bypass than with SVG.

For many reasons (spasm, postoperative dilation) the validity of preoperative measurements is doubtful. With regard to the postoperative measurements, there is also a certain controversy because these measurements are difficult to perform and to evaluate.

The functional results are considered to be unsatisfactory by some surgeons (Flemma, Wakabayashi...). This is not the opinion of other physicians, who consider the functional results excellent (Geha, Loop, Vogel...).

In conclusion, our views on the contraindications and indications of IMA bypass on the LAD artery are as follows:

- Contraindication would be for example, emergency situations, very large LAD, too small IMA, subclavian stenosis, patients over 65 years.
- In any other situation, the IMA bypass seems to be the best LAD artery bypass, better than SVG: functional results are similar and patency rate is better. Internal mammary artery bypass is especially interesting in situations in which low graft blood flow is anticipated.

References

1. Amrein, D.: L'anastomose mammaro-coronarienne avec l'artère inter-ventriculaire antérieure. Mise au point à propos de 316 cas opérés à la Clinique chirurgicale cardio-vasculaire de Nancy de 1972 à 1976. Nancy, Thesis 1978
2. Angell, W.W., Sywak, A.: The saphenous vein versus internal mammary artery as a coronary by pass graft. Circulation *56* [Suppl. 2], 22-25 (1977)
3. Barner, H.B., Kaiser, G.C., Jellinek, M., Hahn, J.W., Amako, H., Ohtsubo, M., Willman, V.L.: Aorto-coronary vein graft and internal mammary-coronary anastomosis. Arch. Surg. *105*, 908-911 (1972)
4. Barner, H.B., Mudd, J.G., Mark, A.L., Ahmad, N., Dickens, J.F.: Patency of internal mammary coronary grafts. Circulation *54* [Suppl. 3], 70-73 (1976)
5. Bartel, A.G., Behar, V.S., Peter, R.H., Orgain, E.S., Kong, Y.: Exercise stress testing in evaluation of aorto-coronary by pass surgery. Report of 123 patients. Circulation *48*, 143-148 (1973)
6. Bode, R.F., Zajtchuk, R.: Evaluation of saphenous vein by pass surgery with multistage treadmill test and ventricular function studies. J. Thorac. Cardiovasc. Surg. *74*, 44-46 (1977)
7. McCormick, J.R., Kaneko, M., Baue, A.E., Geha, A.S.: Blood flow and vasoactive drug effects in internal mammary and venous by pass grafts. Circulation *51/52* [Suppl. 1], 72-80 (1975)
8. Crochet, P.D.: Résultats de la chirurgie de revascularisation myocardique directe. Analyse de 1000 cas opérés à l'Institut de Cardiologie de Montréal. Nantes, Thesis 1976
9. Dobrin, P., Canfield, T., Moran, J., Sullivan, H., Pifarre, R.: Coronary artery bypass. The physiological basis for differences in flow with internal mammary artery and saphenous vein grafts. J. Thorac. Cardiovasc. Surg. *74*, 445-454 (1977)

10. Dodek, A., Kassebaum, D.G., Griswold, H.E.: Stress electrocardiography in the evaluation of aorto-coronary by pass surgery. Am. Heart J. *86*, 292-307 (1973)
11. Edwards, W.S., Blakeley, W.R., Lewis, C.E.: Technique of coronary by pass with autogenous arteries. J. Thorac. Cardiovasc. Surg. *65*, 272-275 (1973)
12. Flemma, R.J., Singh, H.M., Tector, A.J., Lepley, D., Frazier, B.L.: Comparative hemodynamic properties of vein and mammary artery in coronary by pass operations. Ann. Thorac. Surg. *20*, 619-626 (1975)
13. Geha, A.S., Krone, R.J., McCormick, J.R., Baue, A.E.: Selection of coronary bypass. Anatomic, physiological and angiographic considerations of vein and mammary artery grafts. J. Thorac. Cardiovasc. Surg. *70*, 414-431 (1975)
14. Geha, A.S., Baue, A.E., Krone, R.J., Kleiger, R.E., Oliver, G.C., McCormick, J.R., Salimi, A.: Surgical treatment of unstable angina by saphenous vein and internal mammary artery by pass grafting. J. Thorac. Cardiovasc. Surg. *71*, 348-354 (1976)
15. Giorgi, C.: Contribution à l'évaluation des pontages aorto-coronarients. A propos de 667 observations relevées à l'Institut de Cardiologie de Montréal. Nancy, Thesis 1974
16. Green, G.E.: Role of blood flow from the internal mammary artery. Surgery *70*, 809-813 (1971)
17. Green, G.E., Spencer, F.C., Tice, D.A., Stertzer, S.H.: Arterial and venous microsurgical by pass grafts for coronary artery disease. J. Thorac. Cardiovasc. Surg. *60*, 491-503 (1970)
18. Green, G.E.: Internal mammary artery to coronary artery anastomosis. Three year experience with 165 patients. Ann. Thorac. Surg. *14*, 260-271 (1972)
19. Grondin, C.M., Lesperance, J., Bourassa, M.G., Campeau, L.: Coronary artery grafting with the saphenous vein or internal mammary artery. Ann. Thorac. Surg. *20*, 605-617 (1975)
20. Guiney, T.E., Rubenstein, J.J., Sanders, C.A., Mundth, E.D.: Functional evaluation of coronary by pass surgery by exercise testing and oxygen consumption. Circulation *47/48* [Suppl. 3], 141-145 (1973)
21. Hamby, R.I., Aintablian, A., Wisoff, G. Hartstein, M.L.: Comparative study of postoperative flow in the saphenous vein and internal mammary artery by pass grafts. Am. Heart J. *93*, 306-315 (1977)
22. Hirose, J., Marshall, D.: A comparative Study of the direct internal mammary-to-coronary artery anastomosis and the aortocoronary vein by pass graft. Ann. Thorac. Surg. *16*, 471-479 (1973)
23. Irarrazaval, M.J.: Use of the internal mammary artery for myocardial revascularisation. Clev. Clin. Q. *43*, 109-112 (1976)
24. Jahnke, E.J., Love, J.W.: By pass of the right and circumflex coronary arteries with the internal mammary artery. J. Thorac. Cardiovasc. Surg. *71*, 58-63 (1976)
25. Kay, E.B., Naraghipour, H., Beg, R.A., De Maney, M., Tambe, A., Zimmerman, H.A.: Internal mammary artery by pass graft. Long-term patency rate and follow-up. Ann. Thorac. Surg. *18*, 269-279 (1974)
26. Knoebel, S.B., Mc Henry, P.L., Phillips, J.F., Lowe, D.K.: The effect of aortocoronary by pass grafts on myocardial blood flow reserve and treadmill exercise tolerance. Circulation *50*, 685-693 (1974)
27. Kolessov,.: Mammary artery-coronary artery anastomosis as method of treatment for angina pectoris. J. Thorac. Cardiovasc. Surg. *54*, 535-544 (1967)
28. Lapin, E.S., Murray, J.A., Bruce, R.A., Winterscheid, L.: Changes in maximal exercise performance in the evaluation of saphenous vein bypass surgery. Circulation *47*, 1164-1173 .(1973)
29. Loop, F.D., Effler, D.B., Spampinato, N., Groves, L.K., Cheanvechai, C.: Myocardial revascularization by internal mammary artery grafts. A technique without optical assistance. J. Thorac. Cardiovasc. Surg. *63*, 674-680 (1972)
30. Loop, F.D., Spampinato, N., Cheanvechai, C., Effler, D.B.: The free internal mammary artery by pass graft use of the IMA in the aorta-to-coronary artery position. Ann. Thorac. Surg. *15*, 50-55 (1973)
31. Loop, F.D., Irarrazaval, M.J., Bredee, J.J., Siegel, W., Taylor, P.C., Sheldon, W.C.: Internal mammary artery graft for ischemic heart disease. Effect of revascularization on clinical status and survival. Am. J. Cardiol. *39*, 516-522 (1977)

32. Marcantoni, J.P., Blondeau, M.: L'électrocardiogramme d'effort après pontage aorto-coronarien. Coeur *6*, 1087-1093 (1975)
33. Merril, A.J., Thomas, C., Schechter, E., Cline, R., Armstrong, R., Stanford, W.: Coronary bypass surgery. Value of maximal exercise testing in assessments of results. Circulation *51/52* [Suppl. 1], 173-177 (1975)
34. Rossiter, S., Brody, W.R., Kosek, J.C., Lipton, M.J., Angell, W.W.: Internal mammary artery versus autogenous vein for coronary artery by pass graft. Circulation *50*, 1236-1243 (1974)
35. Sheldon, W.C., Loop, F.D.: Direct myocardial revascularization - 1976. Progress report on the Cleveland Clinic experience. Clev. Clin. Q. *43*, 97-108 (1976)
36. Sheldon, W.C., Rincon, G., Pichard, A.D., Razavi, M., Cheanvechai, C., Loop, F.D.: Traitement chirurgical de la maladie artérielle coronarienne par pontage isolé: étude de 741 malades suivis de 3 à 7 ans. Acquisitions Nouvelles en Pathologie Cardio-Vasculaire *18*, 429-462 (1976)
37. Siegel, W., Loop, F.D.: Comparison of internal mammary artery and saphenous vein by pass grafts for myocardial revascularization. Exercise test and angiographic correlations. Circulation *54* [Suppl. 3], 1-3 (1976)
38. Siegel, W., Lim, J.S., Proudfit, W.L., Sheldon, W.C., Loop, F.D.: The spectrum of exercise test and angiographic correlations in myocardial revascularization surgery. Circulation *51/52* [Suppl. 1], 156-162 (1975)
39. Singh, H., Flemma, R.J., Tector, A.J., Lepley, D., Walker, J.A.: Direct myocardial revascularization. Determinants in the choice of vein graft or internal mammary artery. Arch. Surg. *107*, 699-703 (1973)
40. Westphal, J.C.: Notre expérience du pontage coronarien (A propos d'une série consécutive de 225 cas avec étude d'une courbe de survie actuarielle). Nancy, Thesis 1976

The Internal Mammary Artery as a Coronary Artery Bypass Graft

J. L. Ochsner, J. W. Jones, and N. L. Mills

Men in medicine, and particularly surgeons, are known to heavily support a particular idea or operative procedure. Frequently, this nonrelenting attitude leads to a dogmatic opinion, which in turn results in biased thinking. This may act to the detriment of the patient's health. With the amount of data available today, in regard to the various conduits used for bypass grafts in myocardial revascularization, one would think that controversy or question would not exist; yet this is not fact.

After 10 years of experience with direct myocardial revascularization, we believe that today one can make an intellectually honest selection of which graft should be used in reference to a particular situation. It is only natural that in selection of the proper conduits each particular artery to be bypassed needs to be studied in reference to various factors. It is important to take into consideration the size of the coronary artery, the structure and pathology of this particular vessel, the amount of myocardium supplied by the vessel, the degree of proximal stenosis or occlusion, the status of the other coronary arteries, and the collateral circulation associated with the particular artery. Of equal importance is the status of the various conduits that are available, that is whether they are autogenous, homologous, or heterologous, their physical characteristics in relation to the internal and external diameter, the morphological state of a vessel wall, the length of bypass that need be performed, the number of such conduits that are needed or available, whether the conduit is to arise from its natural habitat; whether the conduit is to take origin from the aorta or elsewhere; and the physical condition of the ascending aorta or wherever the conduit is to originate. Also, one must take into account the condition and function of the myocardium supplied by the coronary arteries in question. With these variables taken into account, a surgeon should be able to make the proper selection of a graft.

Clinical Data

The two most common types of grafts used today are the autogenous saphenous vein graft (SVG) and the left internal mammary artery (IMA). The IMA has shown a better patency rate, but the SVG has demonstrated higher flow rates and better hemodynamics. In order to determine which of these grafts is superior when there is a choice for a similar situation, we studied the first 1,000 consecutive patients who underwent direct coronary artery bypass at the Ochsner Clinic. An analysis of these patients was performed by computerizing the available data. The operative procedures were performed between 1968 and 1974, and thereby followed from 3 to 9 years. Follow-up averaged over 5 years and was complete to the present in 99% of cases.

Table 1. Cross-tabulation between IMA and SV grafts and variables* in unbiased patient population

Variable	Graft type	No. with variable (%)	No. without variable (%)			Chi square	*P* value
Age	IMA	Below 50	50-59 yrs.	60-69 yrs.	70-79 yrs.		
		117 (35%)	159 (47%)	57 (17%)	2 (1%)	5.128	0.27443
	SV	89 (35%)	114 (45%)	44 (18%)	5 (2%)		
Valve repair	IMA	3 (1%)	332 (99%)			0.017	0.8951
	SV	2 (1%)	250 (99%)				
Elevated cholesterol	IMA	30 (9%)	305 (91%			1.352	0.2444
	SV	16 (6%)	236 (94%)				
Elevated triglycerides	IMA	151 (45%)	184 (55%)			0.266	0.6057
	SV	119 (47%)	133 (53%)				
Hypertension	IMA	124 (37%)	211 (63%)			1.264	0.26089
	SV	82 (33%)	170 (67%)				
Diabetes	IMA	47 (14%)	288 (86%)			1.435	0.2309
	SV	27 (11%)	225 (89%)				

*Partial listing of variables analyzed.

Success of the operation was judged by relief of angina, overall survival, prevention of congestive heart failure, and nonfatal myocardial infarction rates. All deaths were included in the analysis regardless of cardiac relationship. Those patients requiring treatment for chronic failure were included as such, and the patients classified as having myocardial infarctions had to have electrocardiographic evidence supporting the diagnosis.

In order to compare the clinical success of all patients who had the two types of grafts, a study was made of any variable indicating clinical result. A cross-tabulation was made of the two types of grafts among 195 independent clinical variables. There was found to exist an uneven distribution in a number of independent variables, and those maldistributed variables were then cross-tabulated with increased mortality. The following variables were found to be associated with increased mortality: (1) female sex; (2) concomitant ventricular aneurysmectomy; (3) preoperative congestive heart failure; (4) generalized ventricular dysfunction by ventriculogram; (5) acute myocardial infarction. In order to eliminate bias, these subgroups were removed and the distribution analysis was repeated. Table 1 shows that the distribution of the two groups among the independent variables is now uniform. Also, the anatomic severity of disease in the coronary artery is quite similar in the redefined subsets. Internal mammary artery patients average 2.06 major arteries with 70% or greater obstruction and saphenous vein graft patients average 2.01 arteries similarly involved. The internal diameter of the coronary arteries bypassed was 1.98 mm for the internal mammary artery group and 2.0 mm for the saphenous vein group. Also, the ventricular function as estimated by ventriculogram was almost identical after exclusion of those in the generalized dysfunction category. Therefore, after removing the maldistributed subsets, groups for comparison had similar severity of clinical disease, anatomical location of disease, and other variables.

Table 2. Comparison of clinical results between IMA and SV grafts in total patient population

Variable	Graft type	No. not having variable (%)	No. having variable (%)	Chi square	*P* value
Angina	IMA	398 (94.1%)	25 (5.9%)	7.601	0.00583
	SV	345 (91.0%)	44 (9.0%)		
Myocardial infarction	IMA	417 (98.5%)	6 (1.5%)	13.842	0.0020
	SV	364 (93.6%)	25 (6.7%)		
Death	IMA	404 (95.5%)	19 (4.5%)	22.242	0.00001
	SV	338 (86.9%)	51 (13.1%)		
Postoperative CHF	IMA	408 (96.4%)	15 (3.6%)	6.718	0.00954
	SV	359 (92.3%)	30 (7.7%)		

CHF = Congestive heart failure.

Results

The comparison of the clinical results of the entire group is shown in Table 2. In each clinical variable examined, the patients who had internal mammary artery bypasses had significantly better clinical results than those with saphenous vein grafts. When study of the clinical success of patients in whom all bias subsets were removed showed again that patients with internal mammary grafts had a better course, anginal relief and postoperative congestive heart failure were not improved to a statistically significant extent (Table 3). In the unbiased groups, survival rates again were improved in the internal mammary group - 97.3% survival in the internal mammary group compared to 91.7% in the saphenous vein group. These results were highly significant ($P = 0.000862$) in favor of increased survival in those patients who had an internal mammary graft.

Cumulative survival curves comparing the two groups emphasize the continued attrition rate in the group who had saphenous vein bypass grafts and a remarkably stable survival of patients with internal mammary grafts (Fig. 1). When the two curves are compared with the expected survival curve of white males of 53 years of age (the average age of the patients in this study) in Louisiana, the results in-

Table 3. Comparison of clinical results between IMA and SV grafts in unbiased patient population

Variable	Type	No. not having variable (%)	No. having variable (%)	Chi square	*P* value
Angina	IMA	316 (94.3%)	19 (5.7%)		
	SV	227 (90.1%)	25 (9.9%)	3.744	0.0530
MI	IMA	331 (98.8%)	4 (1.2%)		
	SV	242 (96.0%)	10 (4.0%)	4.754	0.02923
Death	IMA	326 (97.3%)	9 (2.7%)		
	SV	231 (91.7%)	21 (8.3%)	9.508	0.00862
Postop CHF	IMA	331 (98.8%)	4 (1.2%)		
	SV	248 (98.4%)	4 (1.6%)	0.165	0.68447

CHF = Congestive heart failure.

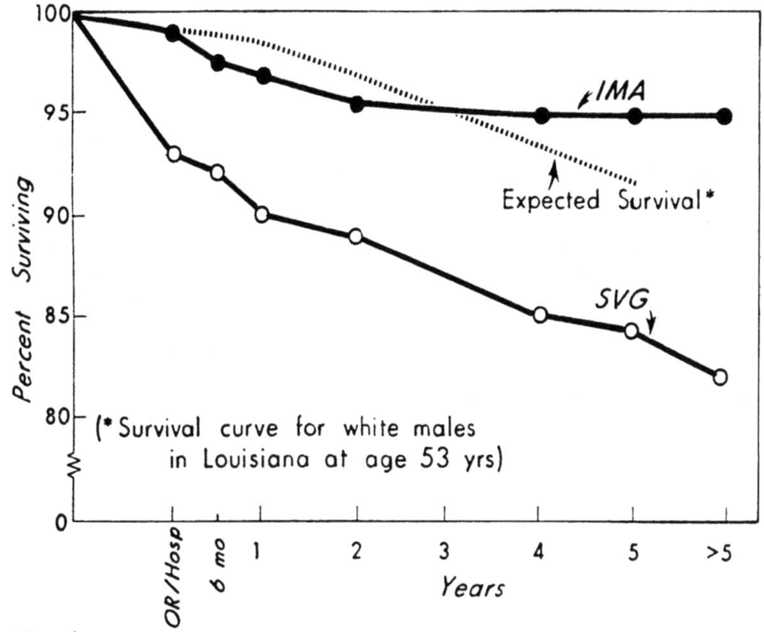

Fig. 1

dicate that the longevity of patients with internal mammary grafts equals or exceeds that of a normal man at 3 years after operation and survival in the patients with saphenous vein graft does not.

Discussion

Despite the differences of the physical and hemodynamic characteristics of the two grafts, it is logical that if a graft remains patent longer and is able to supply enough blood to the affected area, a longer life span will result. In this regard, one must consider the graft that yields the longest life to be superior.

It becomes evident that the internal mammary artery is a suitable graft as long as it is able to supply an adequate volume of blood to the myocardium in question. Unsuitable grafts will produce a high percentage of technical failures. One must be sure that the diameter of the vessel is adequate, that is greater than 2 mm in diameter, that there is free flow of more than 100 ml/min, that there is no damage to the artery during operative preparation, that there is operative dilatation of smaller arteries by diluted papaverine solution, that there is no proximal obstruction of flow from subclavian stenosis or stenosis of the origin of the internal mammary, and that there is avoidance of postoperative stretching of the graft by hyperinflated lungs.

Both preoperative and operative precautions are necessary to prevent these pitfalls and to thereby assure the highest possible long-term patency. Selective internal mammary angiography is routine in all patients considered for myocardial revascularization at the Ochsner Clinic. There are other criteria that are necessary for the assured successful internal mammary coronary artery bypass. There must be a critical proximal stenosis and the internal mammary artery should not compete with a larger conduit such as a saphenous vein of 4 mm or greater in diameter. In essence, where an internal mammary is used, it should be into a vessel that has greater than a 75% stenosis. The internal mammary does have an advantage over other conduits for bypassing small coronary arteries less than 1.5 mm in diameter and to an area of myocardium in which there is only a small amount of flow. The chances for continued patency under these conditions are greater than with a larger conduit of another type.

In summary, no one conduit is acceptable for all situations. Therefore, the surgeon must be knowledgeable of the advantages, disadvantages, and limitations of each type. Utilizing this knowledge, one is able to select the best conduit for a particular vessel and thereby allow a higher patency rate with the best hemodynamics possible. Where a situation exists for an equal choice, the internal mammary artery appears to be the best.

Does the Choice of Grafts (Veins or IMA) Influence Patency Rate and Functional Results?

R. J. Flemma

Experience and time have shown that the left internal mammary artery (IMA) and saphenous veins are the two best coronary bypass conduits. It remains to determine the proper usage of each by utilizing their unique characteristics. It is the purpose of this paper to discuss the results of their usage in over 1500 patients in hopes that this may elucidate the appropriate circumstances for their use.

The factors that we consider in selecting a coronary bypass conduit are physiologic adequacy, patency, durability, availability, ease of handling, and the myocardial bed to be perfused by that conduit. Durability for both conduits has been observed over 9 years.

There is usually greater availability of saphenous vein except in those patients who have undergone greater saphenous vein stripping. The IMA then becomes of paramount importance along with lesser saphenous and arm veins in cases requiring multiple bypass grafts.

The IMA is originally more difficult to work with but with experience and meticulous technique soon make vein or IMA anastomatic methodology equally simple.

The study of Kay [1], et al. demonstrated that the IMA in situ is "protected" from atherosclerotic involvement. In a study of 100 autopsy patients they showed that atherosclerosis was rare even in the presence of atherosclerotic disease elsewhere in the body.

While reassuring in consideration of the availability of the IMA, it remains to be seen whether atherosclerosis may affect the IMA in a different manner when it is removed from the chest wall and placed in the coronary bypass position.

Studies on patency have generally reported superior results for the IMA. However, these studies have compared patency of all veins to patency in good IMA anterior descending bypasses. They thus have not been fair comparisons. A closer look at the patency reported by Grondin [2], et al. showed a 1 year cumulative patency of 88% for the IMA and 85% for the vein bypasses. This is not a significant difference. One must also recall that from the IMA implant era that IMA may remain patent with little or no forward flow. There is also a higher incidence of anastomotic stricture with small IMA's. Barner [3] also reported that veins with higher flows had a 90% patency. We had long measured flows in all bypass conduits and early reported an average mean flow of 64 ml/min in saphenous vein bypasses and 45 ml/min in IMA's. We also noted that with increased LVEDP the average IMA mean flow dropped further to 35 ml/min. We also observed that the flow in the right internal mammary artery was approximately 10 ml less than the mean flow in the left internal mammary artery. In order to better study the comparison of flow and physiologic adequacy between the IMA and saphenous vein, we utilized a model that eliminated all variables and compared the flow in both of these conduits to the same coronary artery.

Fourteen patients who were undergoing myocardial revascularization for atherosclerotic coronary heart disease were selected for the study. All anterior descending coronary vessels were involved with severe proximal atherosclerotic lesions. The vessel was normal distally and supplied a normally contracting myocardium. We described this as a Class I vessel in which we would anticipate a high bypass flow. The left internal mammary artery was taken down from the chest wall in the usual manner. In order to qualify for the study the internal mammary had to be 2 mm or greater in internal diameter at the site of anastomosis, and the free flow measured at least 100 ml/min into a beaker. Diluted papaverine was externally applied to ensure maximum dilatation of the internal mammary artery.

The lower leg saphenous vein was utilized and the proximal end sutured into the aorta. The site of vein-coronary anastomosis with the proper measurement of the vein graft was carried out prior to instituting cardiopulmonary bypass. Following heparinization, the isolated IMA was sutured to the vein bypass graft 1-1.5 cm from the proposed venous anastomotic site. We called this the vein-mammary additive graft (V-MAG). The adequacy of the anastomosis was then checked, and we also passed a probe in a retrograde manner up the mammary artery. After the institution of cardiopulmonary bypass, the vein at the preselected site was anastomosed to the anterior descending coronary artery utilizing 6-0 Prolene. At the conclusion of the procedure, with the patient still heparinized and in a stable hemodynamic state, the physiological studies were carried out.

Flow Studies

With the patient in a stable hemodynamic state, flow probes were placed on the vein bypass and flows determined in sequence. Vein flow was measured with both the IMA and the vein open and flowing. The mammary was then occluded so that we could record vein graft flow alone. Next the vein was occluded reflecting mammary flow alone (Fig. 1). These studies were all repeated and the range and mean flow recorded.

Flow Results

Flow in the vein grafts of the 14 patients averaged 117 ml/min and flow in the internal mammary artery was 43 ml/min. Therefore, the vein graft flow averaged 2.7 times greater than the IMA flow in the same coronary bed.

Physiologic Study

In order to determine how each bypass conduit best meets the supply-demand ratio, we placed a flexible No. 18 needle into the left ventricle to record intraventricular pressure. A No. 20 flexible needle was inserted into the vein and threaded down to lie just above the V-MAG coronary anastomosis (Fig. 2). Care was taken to ensure that no venous valve existed between the end of the needle and the IMA-vein-coronary anastomosis. These needles were attached to pressure

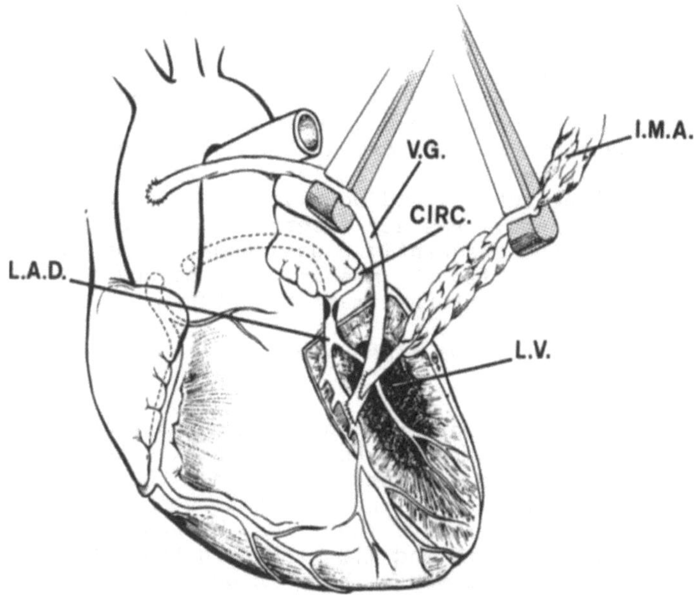

Fig. 1. V-MAG preparation and flow probes on vessel. When mammary flow is recorded, vein graft is occluded in proximal portion, when vein graft flow is recorded, IMA is occluded. [5]

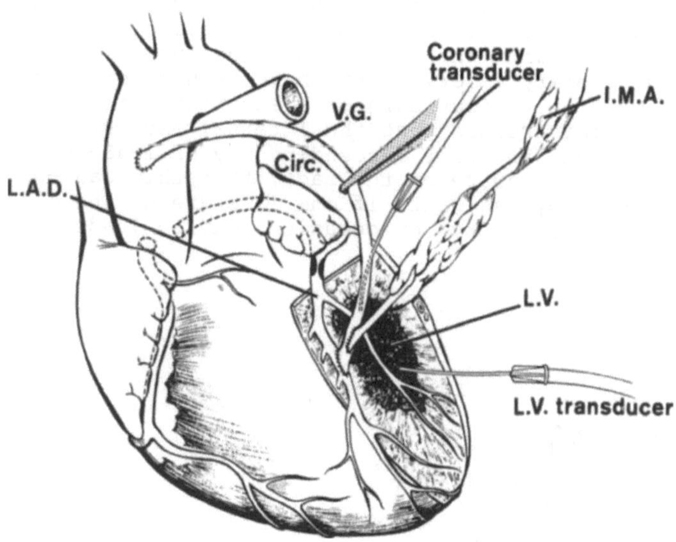

Fig. 2. V-MAG preparation with transducer in LV and in vein adjacent to the tripartite anastomosis. This enables the recording of pressures in vein or mammary and simultaneously in the LV. [5]

transducers. The needle in the vein reflected coronary pressure hemodynamics, and that in the left ventricular cavity showed intraventricular pressure and essentially approximated subendothelial pressures. Pressures were simultaneously recorded in the left ventricle and vein while the electrocardiogram was monitored with both bypasses functioning. The mammary was occluded to obtain pressure tracings reflecting the simultaneous vein bypass left ventricular pressure characteristics. The vein was then occluded proximal to the site of pressure recording and we determined the simultaneous IMA-left ventricular pressure. These measurements were done in duplicate and with comparable cardiovascular hemodynamics. At the conclusion of the study the needle holes in the left ventricle and vein graft were easily closed with 6-0 Prolene suture, and both vein and IMA were left intact and flowing. The needle was not inserted into the internal mammary artery as this quite frequently causes hematous and disruption of the arterial surface. Also the needle would occupy a large portion of the lumen of the internal mammary artery.

The mean DPTI/TTI ratio was nearly two times greater with the vein grafts than with the IMA.

A further study was taken in which both the internal mammary artery and saphenous vein were sutured separately to the same anterior descending coronary artery and in two patients showed that the flows were app ximately three times higher in the saphenous vein than they were in the internal mammary artery. The flows in these two vessels were 35 ml/min in the mammary and 110 ml/min in the vein. Further evidence that this has occurred has been in personal experiences where the internal mammary artery was sutured into the anterior descending. At the conclusion of bypass after flows have been measured, the patient began to have arrhythmias and fibrillation. The patient was placed back on cardiopulmonary bypass and a saphenous vein was placed into the anterior descending when it was shown that there was absolutely no obstruction to the mammary artery flow. It was assumed that there was inadequate flow to meet physiologic needs and these patients were saved when the vein bypass was inserted into the anterior descending coronary artery. There have been other anecdotal reports given to me from various surgeon's experience in the same situation. It is for this reason that the internal mammary artery as the sole bypass to the anterior descending may be inadequate, that we wish all surgeons to be aware of the fact, that this can be remedied by inserting a vein bypass graft if one is aware of the fact that the internal mammary artery, on occasion, may be inadequate to meet physiologic needs.

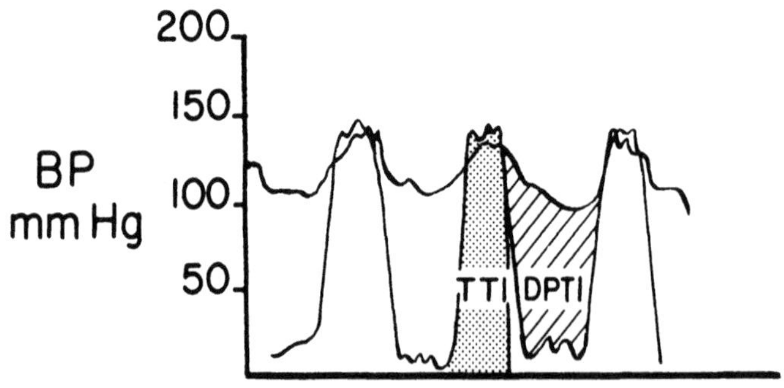

$$\frac{\text{DPTI}}{\text{TTI}} = \frac{\text{SUPPLY}}{\text{DEMAND}}$$

Fig. 3. Schematic shows the theoretical basis for estimating supply/demand ratio. The TTI (*demand*) is the area under the LV pressure trace (*dotted area*) that approximates the O_2 demands of the LV. The DPTI is the area under arterial curve over the LV pressure and the *striped area* represents the driving force to diastolic coronary blood flow. This is the period of supply of O_2 to the LV in diastole. [5]

Discussion

The data that we have accumulated on flow show that the differences between the mammary artery and vein bypass grafts have been substantiated in numerous series in our own institution and are generally accepted by others. The physiologic data showing the supply-demand ratios has been carried out in this unique model, which to our knowledge is the only study that shows the relative efficacy of the mammary and the vein when supplying the same coronary artery. This drop-off has been partially explained by Dobrin [4], et al. who showed that at 2-3 mm there is a pressure drop across the conduit. It is well known that resistance is inversely proportional to the fourth power of the radius. These two physical facts when combined with the demonstration that the diastolic pressure drops precipitously in the mammary, but much more physiologically in the vein to afford an adequate explanation of the decrease of flow. The rapid drop in diastolic pressure in the IMA leads to a smaller driving force to coronary flow. The vein maintains a much more physiologic diastolic pressure and gives it much greater driving force which is depicted as DPTI in the schematics. To further accentuate this, four patients had this same procedure carried out at basal heart rates and with atrial pacing. Atrial pacing led to a shorter diastolic interval and there was actually a decrease in the DPTI/TTI ratio in the mammary which was in a greater excess than the decrease in the vein DPTI/TTI ratio.

It would seem that the only advantage that the mammary has is a very slight increase in patency, which when in comparable vessels may not truly be substantiated. The physiologic adequacy of the vein is far greater than that of the mammary, and in extreme instances the IMA may be totally inadequate and lead to ischemia and catastrophe immediately. It has therefore, been our policy to use the internal mammary artery in those patients in whom we expect a low flow situation where an average of 45 ml/min which the mammary can deliver will suffice. An example of this would be a diagonal vessel or a small circumflex branch that will not accept more than this flow, nor does it need more than the flow that the mammary can provide. We call this a low flow situation. In the high flow situation, with a proximal lesion in a large vessel going to a large area of myocardium, such as an anterior descending or a major circumflex, we have continued to use the saphenous vein. It not only has approximately the same patency, but in a far better manner will match the physiologic needs of the myocardium to be supplied.

We have found it helpful to classify each vessel that we bypass to a potential high flow - low flow situation, and with experience, this has been borne out in the vast majority of bypassed vessels. By utilizing this knowledge, we feel that we have made optimal usage of the best characteristics of both of these bypasses and provide the patient with optimal long-term myocardial revascularization.

References

1. Kay, H., Korns, M., Flemma, R.J., Tector, A., Lepley, D. (Jr.): Atherosclerosis of the internal mammary artery. Ann. Thor. Surg. *21*, 504 (1976)
2. Grondin, C.M., Lesperance, Jr., Bournassa, M.G.: Coronary artery grafting with the saphenous vein or internal mammary artery: Comparison of late results in two consecutive series of patients. Ann. Thor. Surg. *20*, 605 (1975)
3. Barner, H.B., Mudd, J.G., Mark, A.L., Ahmad, N., Dickens, J.: Patency of internal mammary-grafts cardiovascular surgery. Circulation *54* [Suppl.], III-71 (1976)
4. Dobrin, P. et al.: Coronary artery bypass. J. Thoracic Cardiovasc. Surg. *74*, 445 (1977)
5. Flemma, R.J., Singh, H.M., Tector, A.J., Lepley, D., Jr., Frazier, B.L.: Comparative hemodynamic properties of vein and mammary artery in coronary bypass operations. Ann. Thorac. Surg. 20, 619-627 (1975)

Intra-operative Estimation of Technical and Functional Causes of Limited Aortocoronary Bypass Flow*

P. Walter, W. Flameng, F. Schwarz, and F. W. Hehrlein

Intra-operative basal graft flow measurements are of predictive value in determining the fate of aorto-coronary artery vein bypass grafts. In patients with a graft flow less than 20 ml/min at the time of operation an early closure rate of 50%-100% was established [1-3]. Because different factors may be involved in graft closure occurring in the perioperative period, it was the purpose of this study to investigate the functional causes of a limited graft flow in order to distinguish them intra-operatively from technical factors related to the construction of the bypass.

Material and Methods

In 68 patients with a significant LAD stenosis the degree of coronary artery stenosis (CAS) was measured according to the method of Brown and Dodge [4]. From the biplane cinecoronarogram the diameters of the left anterior descending coronary artery proximal to the obstructive lesion and the narrowed diameter of the stenosis were measured during diastole and calibrated by the size of the coronary catheter of known dimension. The lumen of the vessel was assumed to have an elliptical shape. The two hemiaxes determined from the cineangiogram represent the hemiaxes of the ellipse. The coronary obstruction therefore is defined as percentage luminal narrowing.

The motion of the anterior part of the left ventricle (AWM) was investigated by the percentage shortening of the left ventricular anterior hemiaxes as described by Herman and Gorlin [5].

For this purpose the long axis L was drawn from the mid-aortic root to the apex and 3 hemiaxes (R_1, R_2, R_3) perpendicular to L were constructed dividing L into four segments of equal lengths. The percentage shortening was calculated as diastolic axis minus systolic axis, divided by diastolic axis times 100%. Anterior wall motion was then determined as $AWM = R_1 + R_2 + R_3 + L/4$ in percentage shortening. The basal graft flow (BF) was registered with a Hellige pulse square wave electromagnetic flowmeter. The hyperemic response was determined as hyperemic flow after 30 s graft occlusion divided by basal flow times 100 = RH%. The poststenotic pressure (PSP) and the peripheral coronary pressure (PCP) were measured via a small PVC tube inserted into a side branch of the vein graft during open and closed coronary artery (Fig. 1).

With the knowledge of the AWM and the characteristics of the coronary artery stenosis, functional causes of a limited graft flow can be distinguished intra-operatively from technical factors related to the construction of the bypass.

* Published in "The Thoracic and Cardiovascular Surgeon", Vol. 27, No. 1, Georg Thieme Verlag, Stuttgart, 1979.

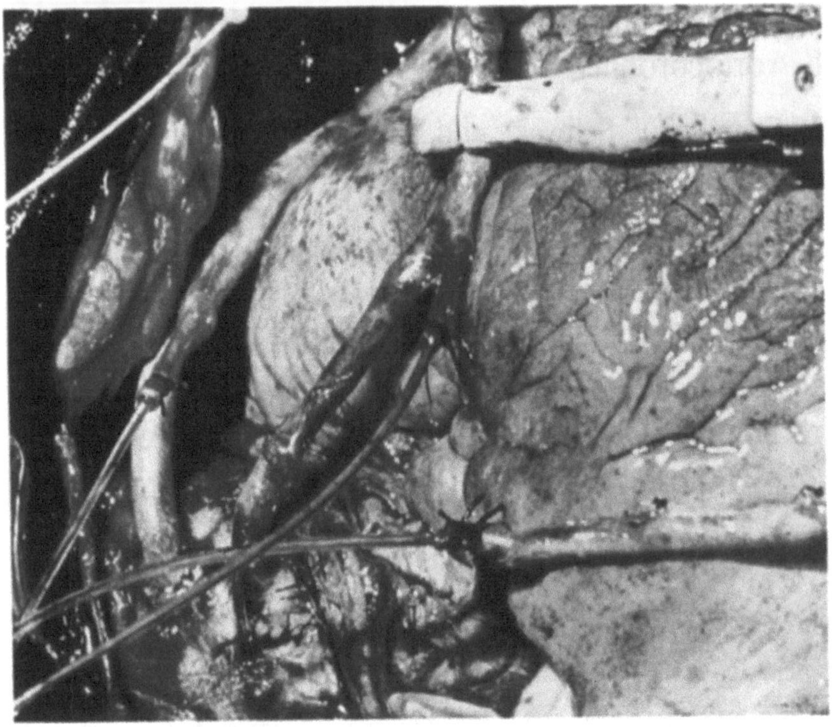

Fig. 1. Demonstration of intra-operative flow- and pressure measurements. The PSP and PCP are recorded via a small PVC tube inserted into a side branch of the vein graft

Results

The following technical factors leading to a low graft flow have been found (Fig. 2).

An impaired reactive hypermia in a graft with a stenosis of the proximal and distal anastomosis due to tension of the graft is demonstrated in the lower left panel of Fig. 2. Interposition of a vein segment of adequate length results in an unrestrained reactive hyperemia of more than 100%.

A limited graft flow may result from a distortion of the aortocoronary bypass graft. Under these circumstances the anastomosis at the recipient artery or the lumen of the vein may become stenotic. Transection of the vein and anastomosis of the distal and proximal segment in the correct axis restores the graft flow completely which is shown in the right upper panel of Fig. 3.

Fig. 4 demonstrates the blood flow tracings in case of an incorrect proximal anastomosis in combination with a relative unimportant coronary artery stenosis of less than 60%. A short occlusion of the artery and graft results in an impaired reactive hyperemia after graft release. Opening of the coronary artery led to a further decrease of graft flow because of an unsignificant coronary artery stenosis.

Technical factors related to the construction of the bypass can be distinguished from functional causes of a limited graft flow.

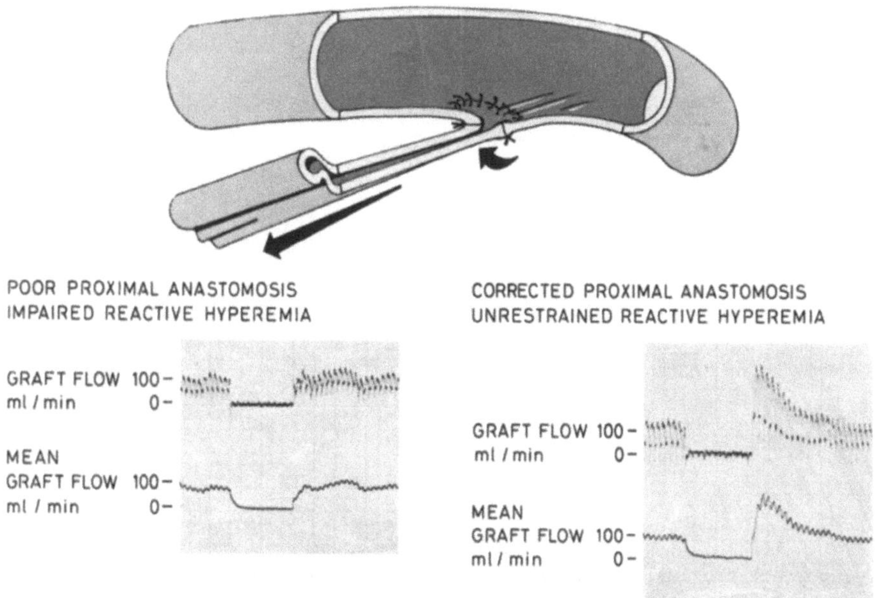

Fig. 2. Impaired reactive hyperemia in a graft with a stenosis of the proximal and distal anastomosis due to tension of the graft

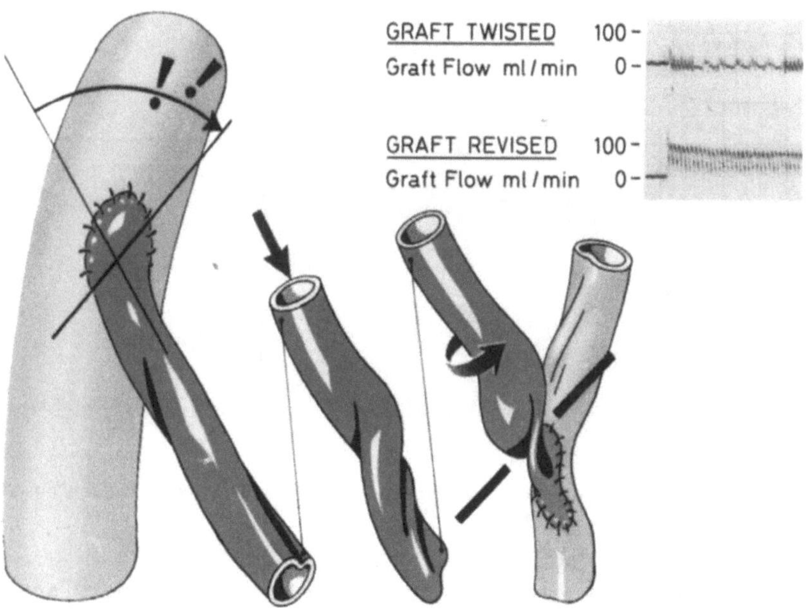

Fig. 3. Distortion of the aortocoronary bypass graft resulting in a limited flow

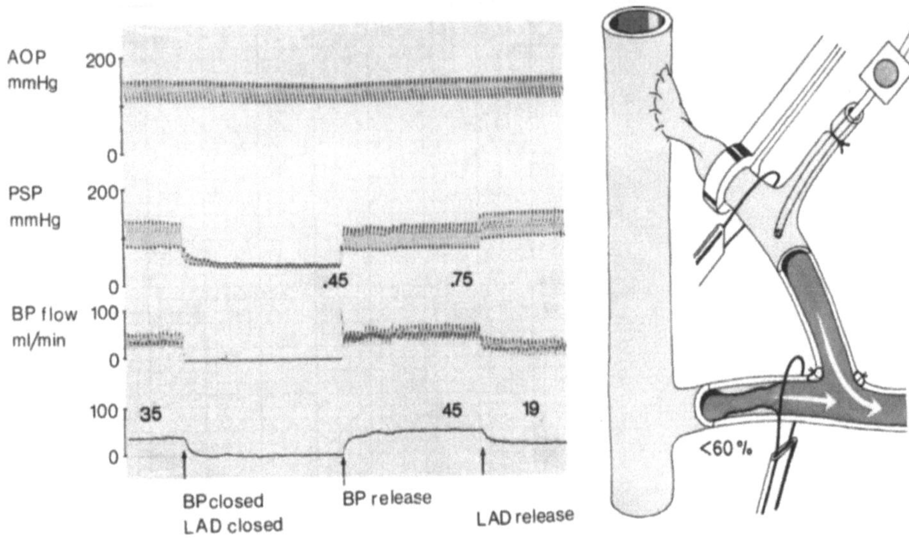

Fig. 4. Incorrect proximal anastomosis in combination with a coronary artery stenosis less than 60% as cause of reduced graft flow

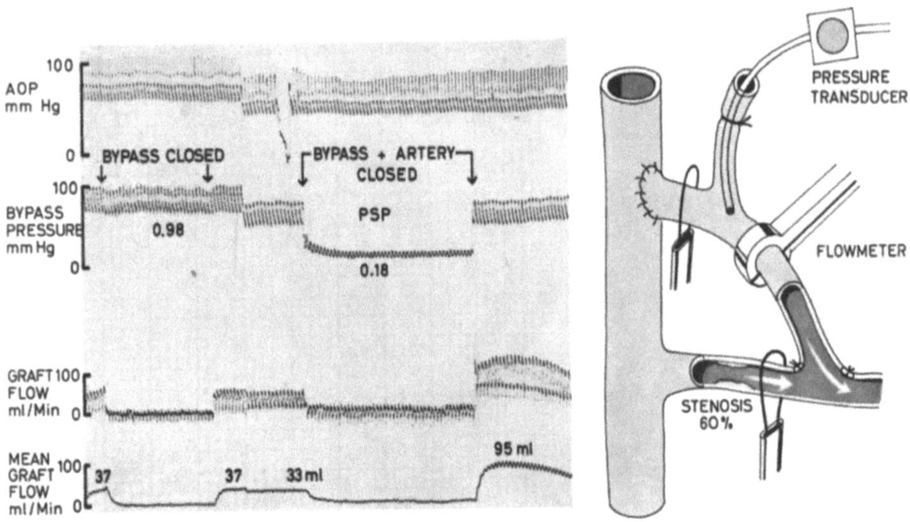

Fig. 5. Competition of flow in a case of stenosis of 60% leading to a reduction of flow both in the artery and the graft

Figure 5 demonstrates the competition of flow between coronary artery and graft in a case of 60% coronary artery stenosis. Occlusion of the graft does not result in a reactive hyperemia and a fall of the poststenotic pressure. If bypass and artery were shortly closed (right side of the tracings) a fall of the PSP and the subsequent reactive hyperemia can be recognized.

When two or more stenotic branches of a main coronary tree were bypassed, a competition of flow may result leading to a relative low flow in each of these grafts. This condition is demonstrated in the lower right panel of Fig. 6.

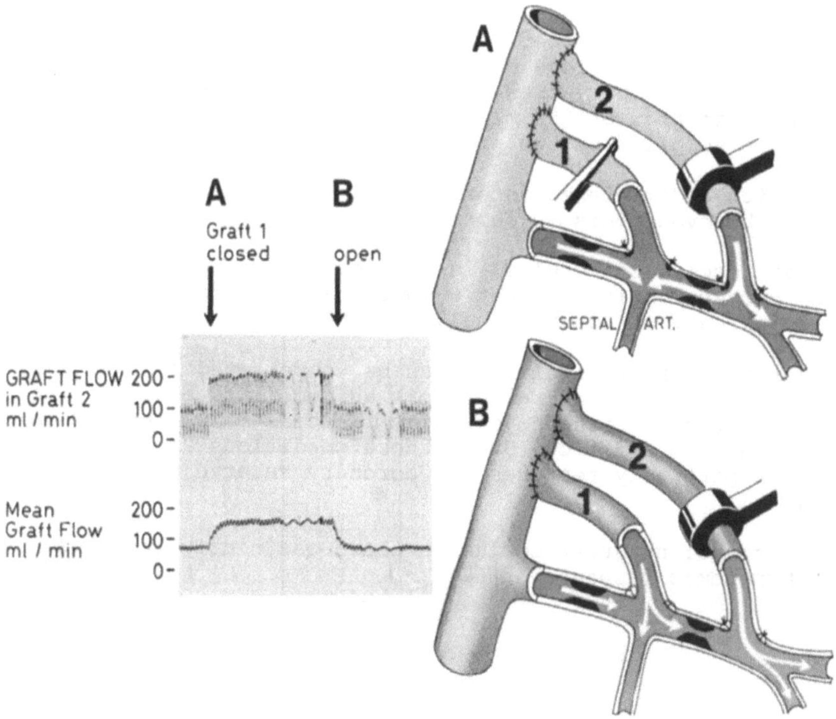

Fig. 6. Competition of flow between multiple grafts to different branches of a main coronary tree

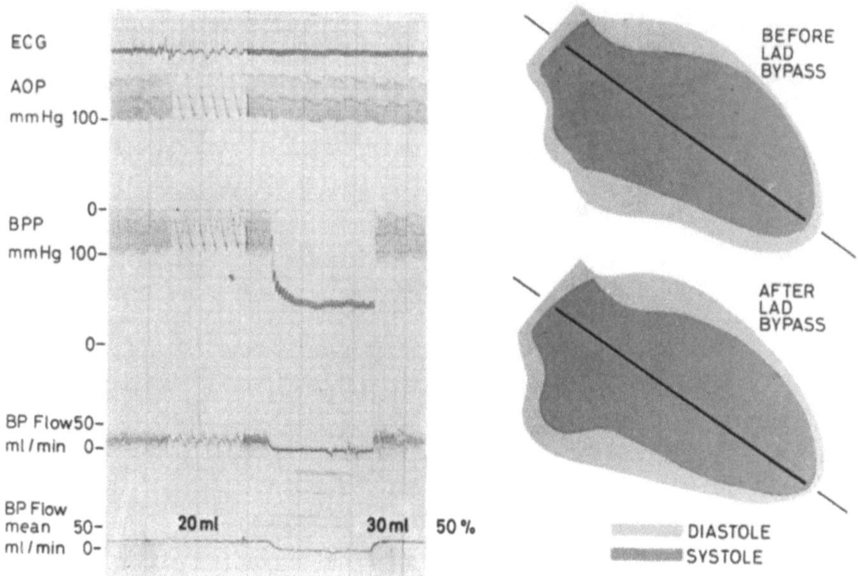

Fig. 7. Reactive hyperemia of 50% in a patient with a low basal graft flow of 20 ml/min and a reduced anterior wall motion

The competition of flow can be demonstrated by clamping one of these grafts, shown in the right upper panel under A. Changes of graft flow under these two conditions can be seen in the left part of the panel. If the whole coronary tree is supplied by one graft (condition A) there is a graft flow of 150 ml/min which will be reduced to 50% when the area is supplied by two grafts (condition B).

In a patient with a diminished anterior wall motion a low mean graft flow could be observed. This is demonstrated in Fig. 7.

Temporary graft occlusion resulted in a reactive hyperemia of 50%. Although the bypass remained patent 6 months after surgery there was only a small increase of anterior wall motion.

A complete coronary artery occlusion can be compensated by the development of an extensive collateral network as demonstrated in Fig. 8. The viability of the concerned myocardium is still maintained by an adequate collateral blood flow. Under these conditions an aortocoronary bypass partially restores the coronary reserve which is shown in Fig. 9.

After a short transient graft occlusion there was nearly the same increase of hyperemic response of 62%.

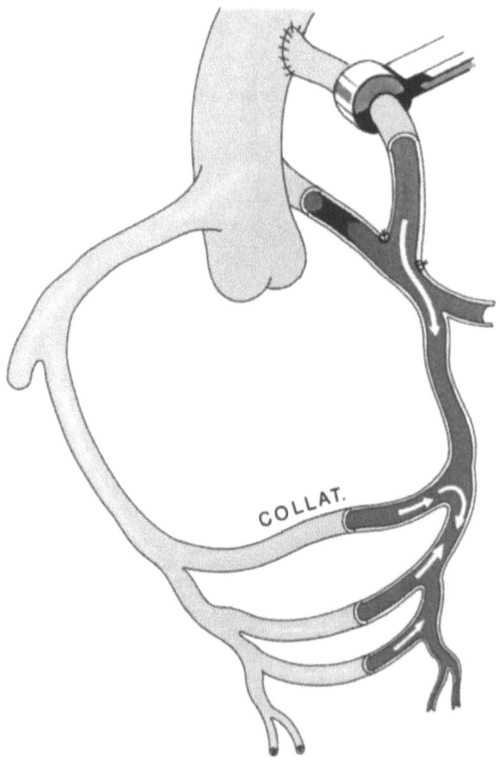

Fig. 8. Demonstration of an extensive collateral network as an important factor for the maintenance of myocardial viability

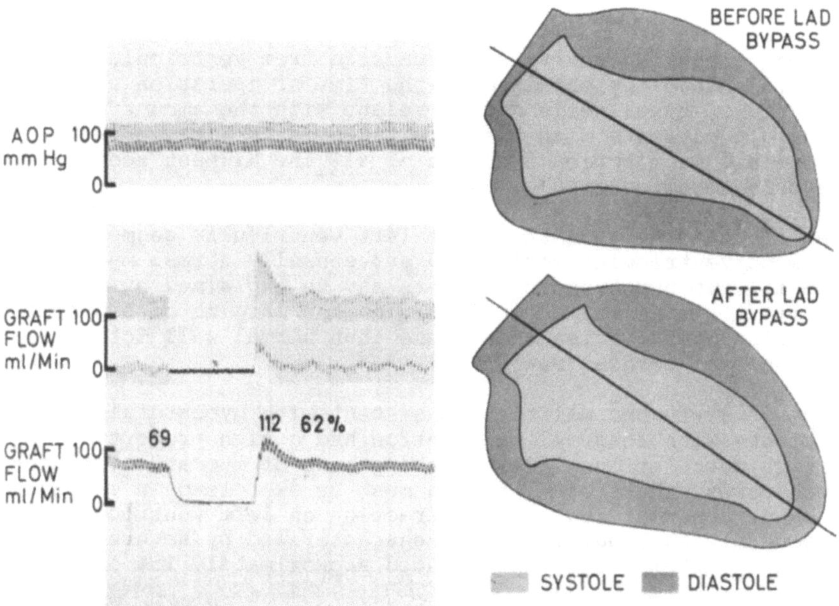

Fig. 9. Improvement of anterior wall motion due to a high graft flow in a case of a complete occlusion of the LAD and the development of collateral vessels

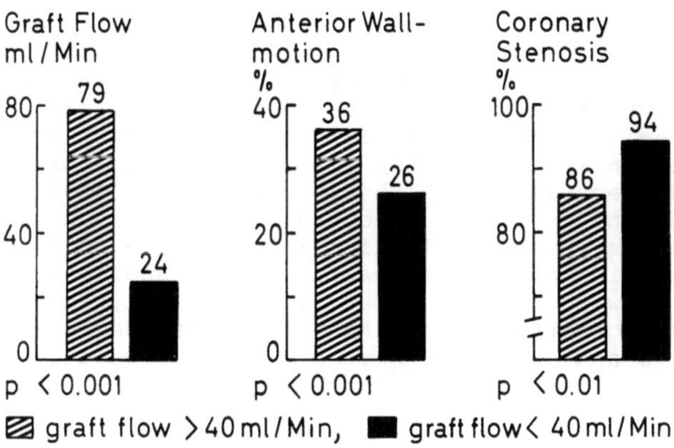

Fig. 10. Correlation between the graft flow, the anterior wall motion and the degree of coronary artery stenosis

The importance of the anterior wall motion for the extent of the graft flow was investigated in these 68 patients. Patients with a BF >40 ml/min were compared with those with a BF of <40 ml/min. The results are demonstrated in Fig. 10.

Fig. 10 demonstrates the relation between graft flow, anterior wall motion, and coronary artery stenosis. Results of patients with a graft flow below 40 ml/min (group II) are represented by black columns and those with a blood flow above 40 ml (group I) by striped columns. The mean graft flow of patients in group I was 79 ml/min and was significantly higher than that of group II which was 24 ml/min.

Discussion

A recent study comparing ventricular function from ventriculography with myocardial histology obtained at the time of operation suggests that the degree of hypokinesis did correlate with the amount of myocardial scar. In patients with a severely depressed anterior wall motion of 16% and an ejection fraction of 41% the highest scores of tissue fibrosis were found [6].

Hutchins et al. have shown that 41% of left ventricular segments with poor and absent ventricular motion had structurally normal myocardium. Such normal but hypodynamic segments may be explained by transient ischemia. Or they may occur either on the margins of scars or throughout dilated ventricles where less than normal wall motion is adequate for normal cardiac output [7].

The presence of ST-T abnormalities consistent with myocardial ischemia in patients with abnormal wall motion had a high proportion of false positive correlations (50%) to the amount of myocardial fibrosis. In such cases, therefore, caution must be exercised in the interpretation of abnormal regional contraction on left ventriculography. In general, such patients were characterized by severe unstable anginal symptoms. They constituted approximately 15% of that study [8].

The demonstration of an increase in inward systolic motion of asynergic segments of the left ventricle following nitroglycerin has given impetus to the concept that these "responsive" asynergic zones consist of viable, chronically ischemic myocardium possessing residual contractile ability [9].

The present study has shown a correlation between a reduced anterior wall motion (AWM) with a mean of 26% and a low mean graft flow of 24 ml/min. It can be assumed that the graft flow to hypokinetic areas which respond to nitroglycerin is higher than to areas with a fibrosis induced diminished AWM. Because of a high closure rate of grafts with a low flow it is important to select preoperatively left ventricular hypokinetic zones for revascularization which show a good responsiveness to nitroglycerin. After eliminating other functional causes of a limited graft flow such as a competition of flow, technical factors related to the construction of the bypass can be recognized by flow measurements and should be corrected intra-operatively.

Summary

Intra-operative measurements of aortocoronary bypass flow are of great predictive value because of a high closure rate of grafts with a small flow rate. In 68 patients with a significant LAD stenosis, the degree of coronary artery stenosis, the anterior wall motion, the basal graft flow, the hyperemic response, and the poststenotic pressure were measured. The anterior wall motion in patients with a low graft flow of 24 ml/min was significantly more reduced than in patients with a graft flow of 79 ml/min. The competition of flow was found to be another functional cause of a limited graft flow. They can be distinguished from technical factors related to the construction of the bypass which should be recognized and corrected intra-operatively.

References

1. Grondin, C.M., Lapage, G., Castongnay, Y.R., Meere, C., Grondin, P.: Aortocoronary bypass graft. Initial blood flow through the graft and early post-operative patency. Circulation *44*, 815-819 (1971)
2. Marco, J.D., Barner, H., Kaiser, G., Codd, J., Mudd, G., Willman, V.: Operative flow measurements and coronary bypass graft patency. J. Thorac. Cardiovasc. Surg. 545-547 (1976)
3. Walker, J., Friedberg, H., Flemma, R., Johnson, D.: Determinants of angiographic patency of aortocoronary vein bypass grafts. Circulation *45/46* [Suppl. 1], 86-90 (1972)
4. Brown, B.G., Bolson, E., Frimer, M., Dodge, H.T.: Quantitative coronary arteriography: Estimation of dimensions, hemodynamic resistance and atheroma mass of coronary artery lesions using the arteriogram and digital computation. Circulation *55*, 329-337 (1977)
5. Herman, M.V., Heinke, R.A., Klein, M.D., Gorlin, R.: Localized disorders in myocardial contraction. N. Engl. J. Med. *277*, 222-232 (1967)
6. Walter, P., Flameng, W., Thiedemann, K., Schwarz, F., Hehrlein, F.: Correlation between regional left ventricular function and myocardial ultrastructure in patients with coronary artery disease. Proceedings of the 13th World Congress of the International Cardiovascular Society. Tokyo 1977
7. Hutchins, G.M., Buckley, B.H. Ridolfi, R.C., Griffith, L.S., Lohr, F.T. and Piaso, M.A.: Correlation of coronary arteriograms and left venticulograms with postmortem studies. Circulation *56*, 32-37 (1977)
8. Stinson, E.B., Billingham, M.E.: Correlation study of regional left ventricular histology and contractile function. Am J. Cardiol. *39*, 378-383 (1977)
9. Helfant, R.H., Pine, R., Meister, S.G., Feldman, M.S., Tront, R.G. Banka, V.S.: Nitroglycerin to unmask reversible asynergy: Correlation with postcoronary bypass ventriculography. Circulation *50*, 108-113 (1974)

3. Indications for and Results of Aneurysmectomy

Tachyarrhythmia as an Indication for Cardiac Surgery

J. W. Lister, A. J. Gosselin, Th. O. Gentsch, P. B. Larsen,
E. A. Traad, and P. S. Swaye

Abstract

From January, 1975 to August, 1977 twelve patients ranging in age from 37-73 years presented with the presumptive diagnosis of life-threatening ventricular tachycardia (VT). All had cardiac catheterizations and electrophysiologic studies. Cardiac catheterization revealed ten to have coronary artery disease and nine of these had associated ventricular aneurysms. Two had congestive cardiomyopathies. Electrophysiologic evaluation showed three to be suffering from supraventricular tachycardias (SVTs) rather than VTs, and seven to have atrioventricular accessory pathways (AVAP). In three cases, electrophysiologic observations suggested bundle of His (BH) - bundle branch reentry played a role in the initiation of their VTs.

Six cases were treated surgically and six medically. At surgery, five had aneurysmectomies; four of these had associated coronary revascularization and one had coronary reconstruction only. Also, one had a complete AVAP successfully cut and one had an unsuccessful attempt at creating complete atrioventricular block. The six medical cases were treated with standard medications.

All patients were alive and contacted in the last week of February 1978. During an average follow-up period of 27.6 months (20-37 months), none of the surgical group had experienced a recurrence of their tachyarrhythmias (TA) and, during an average follow-up period of 14.3 months (6-25 months) only one of the medical group has had a symptomatic bout of TA requiring specific therapy. Overall, the surgical patients had significantly poorer ventricular function and more severe symptoms than did the medical patients. The criteria used for selecting patients for surgery was [1] an anatomically correctable lesion, [2] a high probability that the TAs would be eliminated by correction of the surgically remedial lesions, and [3] life-threatening symptoms and/or uncontrollable TAs.

An integrated clinical, hemodynamic, angiographic, and electrophysiologic approach in evaluating this high risk group of patients has been stressed. Although thus far, our surgical results have been satisfactory up to the present, the overall results of surgery for VT do not warrant an aggressive surgical approach. Should, however, newer electrophysiologic mapping techniques prove reliable in localizing the site of origin of VTs, the surgical results should improve and surgery may be more aggressively pursued in this high risk group of patients.

Introduction

In spite of advances in therapy, including pacemaking and surgery, the results of the treatment of ventricular tachycardia (VT) associated with severe symptoms has not been consistently salutary [1-8]. Since the early reports of Steinberg [9], Parade [10], and Parkinson [11] associating ventricular aneurysms, coronary artery disease, and a poor prognosis, clinicians have tended to assume the presence of VT, when a tachyarrhythmia (TA) exhibiting a wide QRS complex on the electrocardiogram (ECG), is associated with profound hemodynamic deterioration. Newer techniques, such as, endocardial and epicardial mapping and programmed pacing have helped to define more precisely rhythm disturbances and their electrophysiologic mechanisms. The present communication describes the evaluation, treatment, and follow-up of 12 patients who had the presumptive diagnosis of episodic life-threatening VTs, and stresses the importance of an integrated clinical, hemodynamic, and angiographic, as well as, electrophysiologic approach in their investigation.

Clinical Investigations

From January, 1975 to August, 1977 (a period of 32 months) 12 patients, 11 males and one female, ranging in age from 37-73 years presented with the presumptive diagnosis of life-threatening paroxysms of VT. Using standard techniques, cardiac catheterization, and angiography were carried out in each patient. In 11 of the 12 cases, endocardial electrophysiologic studies, including programmed stimulation of the heart were performed. In one patient, M.S., in whom an endocardial electrophysiologic study was not done, epicardial mapping was performed at surgery to localize a complete atrioventricular accessory pathway (AVAP), Kent bundle (KB), and in another patient, R.K., endocardial mapping was done to localize the bundle of His (BH).

Electrophysiologic Studies

Ten of the 11 patients who underwent endocardial electrophysiologic studies were taken to the cardiac catheterization laboratory in a nonsedated postabsorptive state. Patient J.K. was studied during his tachycardia while receiving an intravenous infusion of lidocaine. One, patient R.R.J., had both a pre- and postoperative electrophysiologic study. Under local anesthesia three bipolar electrode catheters with electrode rings 1 cm apart were positioned via the femoral veins in the right heart. Two of the catheters were used for recording bipolar electrograms and one for electrical stimulation. The latter catheter was attached to a triple pulse generator[1]. The recording electrodes were positioned in the high right atrium in proximity to the sinus node and adjacent to the septal leaflet of the tricuspid valve to record, respectively, the high right atrial (HRA) and BH electrograms. In some of the cases, the BH electrode was used to pace the BH, as well as, for recording. The recording catheters were attached to a distribution box, which in turn was connected to a multichannel photographic oscilloscopic recorder. During the studies, the electrograms simultaneous with standard electrographic leads 1, 3, and V1 were continuously monitored. All recordings were obtained at a paper speed of 50 or 100 mm/sec. The electrograms were obtained at filter settings of 40-200 Hz and the electrocardiographic leads at 1-20 Hz.

In each case atrioventricular conduction was evaluated by atrial and ventricular pacing at progressively shortened cycle lengths (CLs) and, either during normal sinus rhythm and/or programmed pacing, by pro-

---

[1] Medtronic Model # 1349A Triple Pulse Generator, Medtronic, Inc., Minneapolis, Minnesota.

gressive increase in the prematurity of premature atrial and ventricular beats. Also, in an effort to initiate a TA, the ventricles were paced at increasingly shortened CLs up to 300 ms (rate 200/min). If this proved unsuccessful, programmed atrial and ventricular pacing using up to three different basic rates and single, pairs, or three consecutive premature beats at multiple intervals were tried. In those cases, in which there was a sustained VT, the following efforts were made to terminate the rapid rhythm: (1) atrial pacing at a rate slightly greater than the VT; (2) single, pairs, or three consecutive premature ventricular beats at multiple intervals; (3) ventricular pacing at a rate slightly greater than the rate of the VT from three different right ventricular sites (apex, outlfow, and inflow tract) and from the BH [12]; and (4) if none of the above pacing techniques terminated the TA, then the patient was DC cardioverted. The pacing techniques used in these studies were similar to those reported by others [13-16].

In two patients, M.S. (who did not have an endocardial electrophysiologic study) and R.K., the heart was mapped at surgery by recording bipolar electrograms. In M.S., in order to localize a complete AVAP, close bipolar electrograms were obtained from 20 predetermined right ventricular and ten right atrial epicardial sites during atrial and ventricular pacing, respectively. In R.K., endocardial mapping was carried out in order to localize the BH. Standard techniques, previously reported from this [17] and other laboratories [18-22], were used in both cases.

Results

Electrocardiograms showing the paroxysms of TA were available for ten of the 12 patients (Tables 1 and 2). In the remaining two instances, they were unobtainable (Table 1). Review of tracings showed, that in case M.S., recurrent supraventricular tachycardia (SVT), rather than VT, to have been present (Fig. 1). In the other nine cases, the tracings were consistent with VT and in two of these, there had been both VT and ventricular fibrillation (VF) (Tables 1 and 2).

Table 1. Tachyarrhythmias - surgical therapy - clinical presentation

Date	Pt.	Age	Sex	Remote MI	T.A.	Hemodynamic effect	DC shock	Comments
1/75	M.S.	73	F	Yes	SVT[a]	Hypotension	x 20+	Pacemaker implanted
7/75	J.K.	64	M	Yes	VT	Tolerated well	x 10+	
11/75	A.B.	60	M	Yes	VT[b]	Syncope, hypotension	x 2	
12/75	R.K.	47	M	Yes	VT-VF	Syncope, hypotension	x 8	
1/76	R.R.J.	58	M	No	VT[b]	Syncope, hypotension	x 3	
5/77	O.R.	59	M	Yes	VT	Chest pain	x 3	

[a]Reported as VT

[b]ECGs showing TAs not available

Table 2. Tachyarrhythmias - medical therapy - clinical presentation

Date	Pt.	Age	Sex	Remote MI	T.A.	Hemodynamic effect	DC shock	Comments
1/76	G.M.	37	M	Yes	VT	Tolerated well	x 2	
5/76	A.C.	52	M	No	VT-VF	Cardiac arrest	x 1	Chronic AF
11/76	G.F.	61	M	Yes	VT	Tolerated well	0	Drug Therapy
3/77	H.P.	57	M	Yes x 2	VT	Tolerated well	x 1	
4/77	C.G.	69	M	No	VT	Tolerated well	x 3	
8/77	D.F.	57	M	Yes	VT	Tolerated well	x 4	

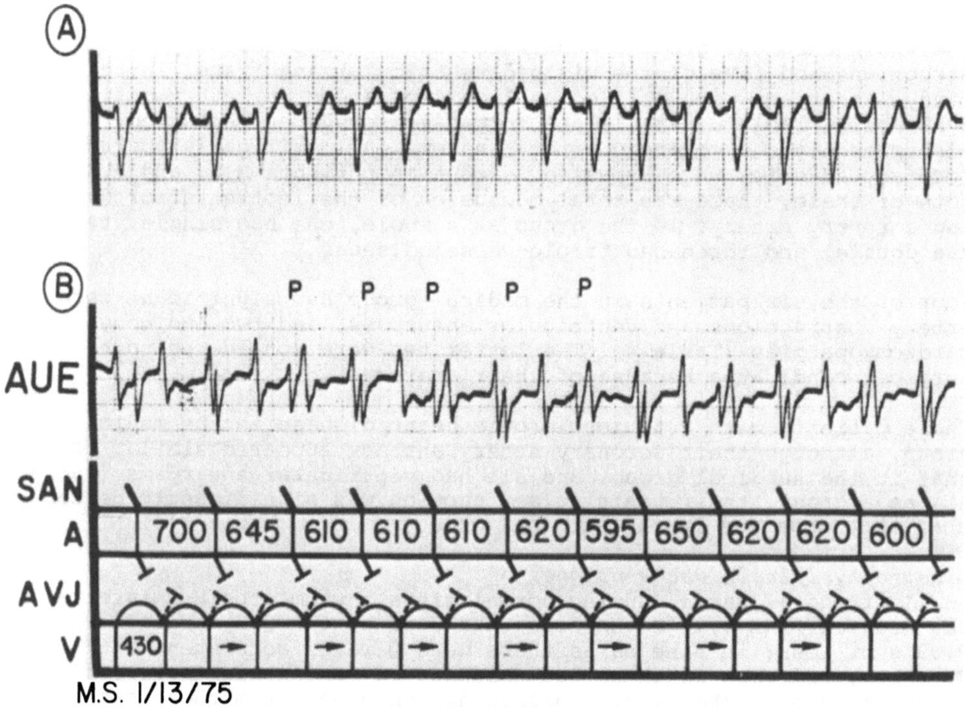

Fig. 1. A and B. Pt. M.S.: SVT and WPW syndrome. (A) Lead-2 ECG showing a TA at a rate of 140/min (CL 430 ms) with a regular rhythm. (B) A right atrial unipolar electrogram (AUE) recorded during the same TA as in (A), shows complete A-V dissociation. The complete A-V dissociation was taken to document the presence of VT (see text). However, upon comparison of the QRS complexes recorded in (A) to the second QRS complex of lead-2 in Fig. 2 and the QRS of lead-2 in the postoperative ECG (Fig. 5), it is seen that they are identical. This indicates that this TA is an A-V junctional tachycardia rather than a VT. The form of initiation of the TA depicted in Fig. 1, the configuration of the QRS complexes, and the presence of complete A-V dissociation are consistent with an A-V nodal reentrant tachycardia. In this case with WPW, the KB is not a part of the reentrant pathway. Key to ladder digram: *AUE* atrial unipolar electrogram; *SAN* sinoatrial node; *A* atrium; *AVJ* atrioventricular junction; *V* ventricles

Clinical Presentation
None of the patients had experienced a myocardial infarction during the six months prior to being seen. However, nine had histories of remote infarctions – five in the surgical group and four in the medical group (Tables 1 and 2, respectively).

The group selected for surgery had far more ominous clinical symptoms in association with their TAs than the group which was continued on medical management. In the surgical group (Table 1), four of the six, associated with their TAs, had signs of profound hemodynamic deterioration. In contradistinction, five of the six in the medical group (Table 2) tolerated their TAs with little difficulty. Only one had VF – a truly life-threatening event. Also, as a group, their TAs were easier to control and the episodes fewer than in the patients who were selected for surgery.

Cardiac Catheterization and Angiography
The whole surgical group demonstrated significant coronary artery obstructions and five of the six had ventricular aneurysms. In this study, aneurysms were defined as localized areas of left ventricular dyskinesis. Table 3 details the surgical procedures performed, and also presents the coronary artery anatomy. All critically obstructed coronary arteries were bypassed, except in patients M.S. and J.K. In both of these, there was total occlusion of the left anterior descending coronary artery. In the group as a whole, one had single, two had double, and three had triple-vessel disease.

Four of the six patients in the medical group had significant coronary artery obstructions and ventricular aneurysms, and two had congestive cardiomyopathies (Table 4). The latter two were considered to be nonsurgical candidates because of their anatomy.

Those patients with arteriosclerotic heart disease in the medical group, although their coronary artery anatomy appeared similar to that in the surgical group, and all had ventricular aneurysms (Table 4), as a group, their ventricular function was significantly better than that observed in the surgical group.

Electrophysiologic Observations
In 11 of the 12 cases, during normal sinus rhythm, the P-R interval was greater than 0.12 s and less than 0.20 s; the QRS duration was 0.09 s or less; in nine cases there were Q waves consistent with infarction, and none of these had evidence of ventricular preexcitation. Although none of the electrocardiograms obtained from these cases during sinus rhythm exhibited patterns consistent with bilateral bundle branch block, in eight of the 11, H-V conduction was abnormally depressed. In seven instances, resting H-V times were prolonged (Tables 5 and 6). In patient G.M., who had a normal resting H-V time, atrial pacing and atrial premature depolarizations exposed the abnormality in H-V conduction (Fig. 8). In patient M.S., old tracings showed a delta wave-ventricular preexcitation (see below) (Fig. 2).

Surgical Group
Patients M.S. and J.K. presented with unrelenting TAs. Both were emergency transfers to our institution and will be discussed separately.

Case Summaries:
M.S.: Fourteen days prior to transfer, this patient had had a VVI pacemaker implanted as therapy for her TAs. At the time of implantation of the pacemaker, it had not been appreciated that she had the Wolff-Parkinson-White syndrome (WPW)

Table 3. Tachyarrhythmias - surgical therapy - surgical procedure

Date	Pt.	Aneurysm-ectomy	Bypasses			Mortality	Recurrence of symptoms
			LAD	RCA	Circ.		
1/75	M.S.[a]	Yes	0	0	0	-	-
7/75	J.K.	Yes	0	+	0	None	None
11/75	A.B.	Yes	+	+	0	-	-
12/75	R.K.[b]	Yes	+	+	+	-	-
1/76	R.R.J.	No	+	+	+		
5/77	O.R.	Yes	+	+	0		

[a]Cut complete AVAP and removed pacemaker.

[b]Cut BH implanted Atricor pacemaker.

All patients were contacted in February, 1978. Follow-up period 20-37 months. Average 27.6 months.

Table 4. Tachyarrhythmias - medical therapy - cardiac catheterization

Date	Pt.	LV aneurysm	Coronary artery obstruction		
			LAD %	RCA %	Circ.%
1/76	G.M.	Yes	100	0	0
5/76	A.C.[a]	No	0	0	0
11/76	G.F.	Yes	100	50	60
3/77	H.P.	Yes	100	90	0
4/77	C.G.[a]	No	0	0	0
8/77	D.F.	Yes	<50	100	90

[a]Congestive cardiomyopathy

Table 5. Tachyarrhythmias - surgical therapy - electrophysiologic study

Date	Pt.	H-V[b]	AVAP	Accelerated VA conduction, VAAP	Observed arrhythmias
1/75	M.S.	-	Complete AVAP	Yes	SVT - AVN reentry
7/75	J.K.	60	None	No	VT - sustained - PF
11/75	A.B.	-	Complete ANAP	Yes	Ventricular & supraventricular echoes
12/75	R.K.	20-60	AVN-BHAP	No	VT - self-terminating, VT initiated by supraventricular echoes
1/76	R.R.J.	60	Complete ANAP	Yes	SVT terminated by APDs followed by 10 s cardiac standstill, hypotension and pain[a]
5/77	O.R.	40	Complete ANAP	Yes	VT - sustained - PF

[a]Study terminated. Postoperative study - normal sinus node function.

[b]H-V upper limit of normal 50 ms. *AVAP* = atrioventricular accessory pathway. *ANAP* = atrionodal accessory pathway. *AVN-BHAP* = A-V nodal - BH-accessory pathway. *VAAP* = ventriculoatrial accessory pathway.

Table 6. Tachyarrhythmias - medical therapy - electrophysiologic study

Date	Pt.	H-V	AVAP	Accelerated VA conduction VAAP	Observed arrhythmias	Recurrence of symptoms
1/76	G.M.	40	Complete ANAP	Yes	VT self-terminanting Critical V-H delay required to initiate (Fig. 10) two types of SVTs (Fig. 11)	None
5/76	A.C.[a]	65	Complete ANAP	Yes	Ventricular echoes, atrial fibrillation	None
11/76	G.F.	70	None	No	VT - three beats, V-H Wenckebach block	None
3/77	H.P.	50	None	No	SVT - LBB	None
4/77	C.G.	90	None	No	VT, PF	None
8/77	D.F.	40	None	No	None	One episode

[a]Cardioverted to NSR prior to study. All patients were contacted in February 1978. Follow-up period 6-25 months, average 14.3 months.

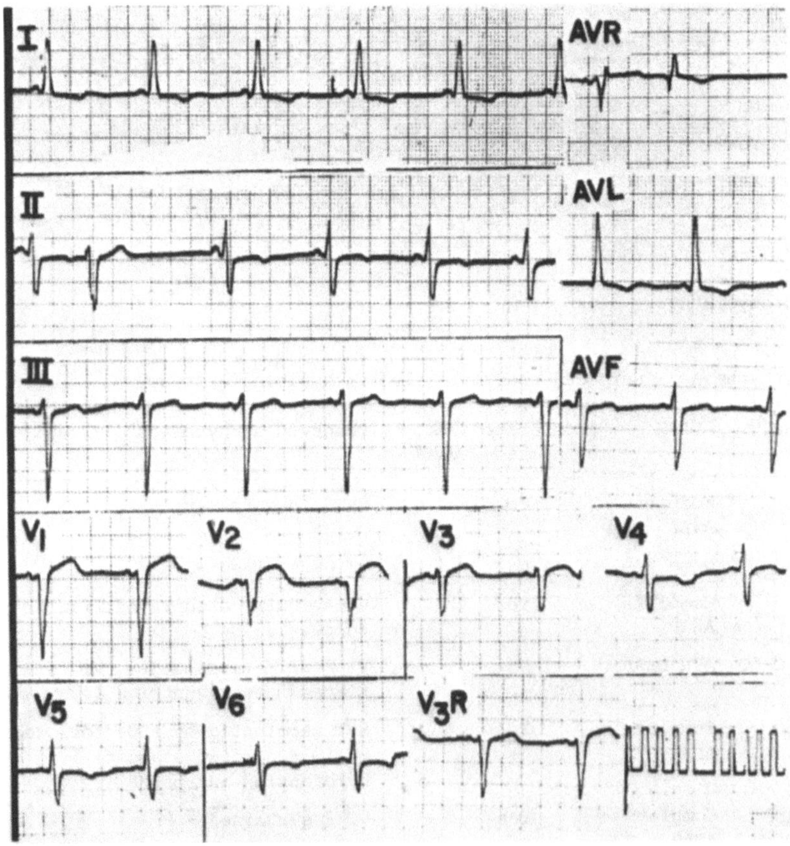

M.S. 8/21/71

Fig. 2. PT. M.S.: Wolff-Parkinson-White syndrome type B. The 12-lead ECG recorded 3.5 years previously showing ventricular preexcitation, WPW type B. In lead-2 the second beat is an atrial premature depolarization which is blocked in the complete AVAP and conducted to the ventricles solely via the normal atrioventricular conduction system (Fig. 1)

(Fig. 2), and just before implantation, a unipolar right atrial electrogram had been recorded, showing a tachycardia with complete A-V dissociation (Fig. 1). This had been interpreted as documenting the presence of VT. However, review of tracings (Fig. 1-3) revealed this patient to be suffering from A-V nodal reentrant tachycardias [23] rather than VT.

After the pacemaker was implanted, the TAs (Fig. 3) became more frequent and each episode was associated with profound hypotension. It was under these circumstances, several hours after admission, that her cardiac anatomy was defined by cardiac catheterization. Because of the precarious clinical situation, an endocardiac electrophysiologic study was not done. Instead, she was taken to surgery where the right atrium and ventricle were mapped and a complete AVAP, connecting the anterolateral right atrium to the right ventricle, was localized and cut, a calcified aneurysm resected, and the pacemaker removed. The postoperative course was uneventful and electrocardiograms (Fig. 4) up to the present have shown no evidence of a return of ventricular preexcitation.

J.K.: Shortly before entering our institution this patient had been DC cardioverted several times. On arrival at our hospital, he was in stable condition. His electrocardiogram was consistent with an old anteroseptal myocardial infarction with a ventricular aneurysm (Fig. 5). He remained stable until approximately 48 h after his cardiac anatomy had been defined by cardiac catheterization. Then, he again exhibited VT, which was unresponsive to pharmacologic and DC countershock therapy. Because of the unresponsiveness of the TA, he was taken to the cardiac catheterization laboratory for endocardial electrophysiologic study.

The VT could not be terminated, but the ventricles could be completely captured by pacing from the BH [12,24,25] (Fig. 6a and b) and three right ventricular sites at CLs shorter than the intrinsic CL of the VT. The tachycardia immediately reappeared as soon as the pacemaker CL was increased to a CL greater than that of the tachycardia (Fig. 7). This indicated the presence of entrance block to the site of origin of the VT (protected focus [PF]) for the paced beats. After pacing was found to be ineffective in terminating the VT, DC cardioversion was tried and was successful, and the study was completed. The ability to completely capture the ventricles by BH pacing and not terminate the VT suggests that the BH and bundle branches are not the site of origin of the rhythm disturbance (not a critical part of the reentry pathway). Upon completion of the study, the patient was taken to surgery and successfully operated upon (Table 3).

Enhanced A-V conduction and a partial or complete atrionodal accessory pathway (ANAP), was assessed to be present when either or both of the following criteria were met [26-28]: (1) 1:1 A-V conduction was maintained up to atrial-paced CLs as short as 300 ms (rate 200/min) and (2) maximum A-H interval prolongation during atrial pacing above that of normal sinus rhythm was equal to or less than 100 ms. A complete ANAP was assumed to be present when there was no significant increase in the A-H interval at atrial-paced rates up to 200/min (Fig. 8). A functional ventriculoatrial accessory pathway (VAAP) was assessed to be present when the criteria, established by Narula [29], were fulfilled. Ventriculoatrial conduction times remained relatively unchanged up to ventricular-paced rates which resulted in second degree ventriculoatrial block (Fig. 8).

Five of the surgical patients had enhanced A-V conduction, and four of these also had enhanced V-A conduction (Table 5). One had a complete AVAP, three had a complete ANAP, and one had an accessory A-V nodal to BH or bundle branch accessory pathway (AVN-BHAP). In this latter case, H-V conduction time exhibited rate-dependent variation (R.K. – Table 5). However, the BH deflection always preceded the onset of ventricular activation and there was no evidence of ventricular preexcitation (delta wave). This is consistent with an AVAN-BHAP (Mahaim fiber bypass tract) [30]. In the three with complete ANAPs,

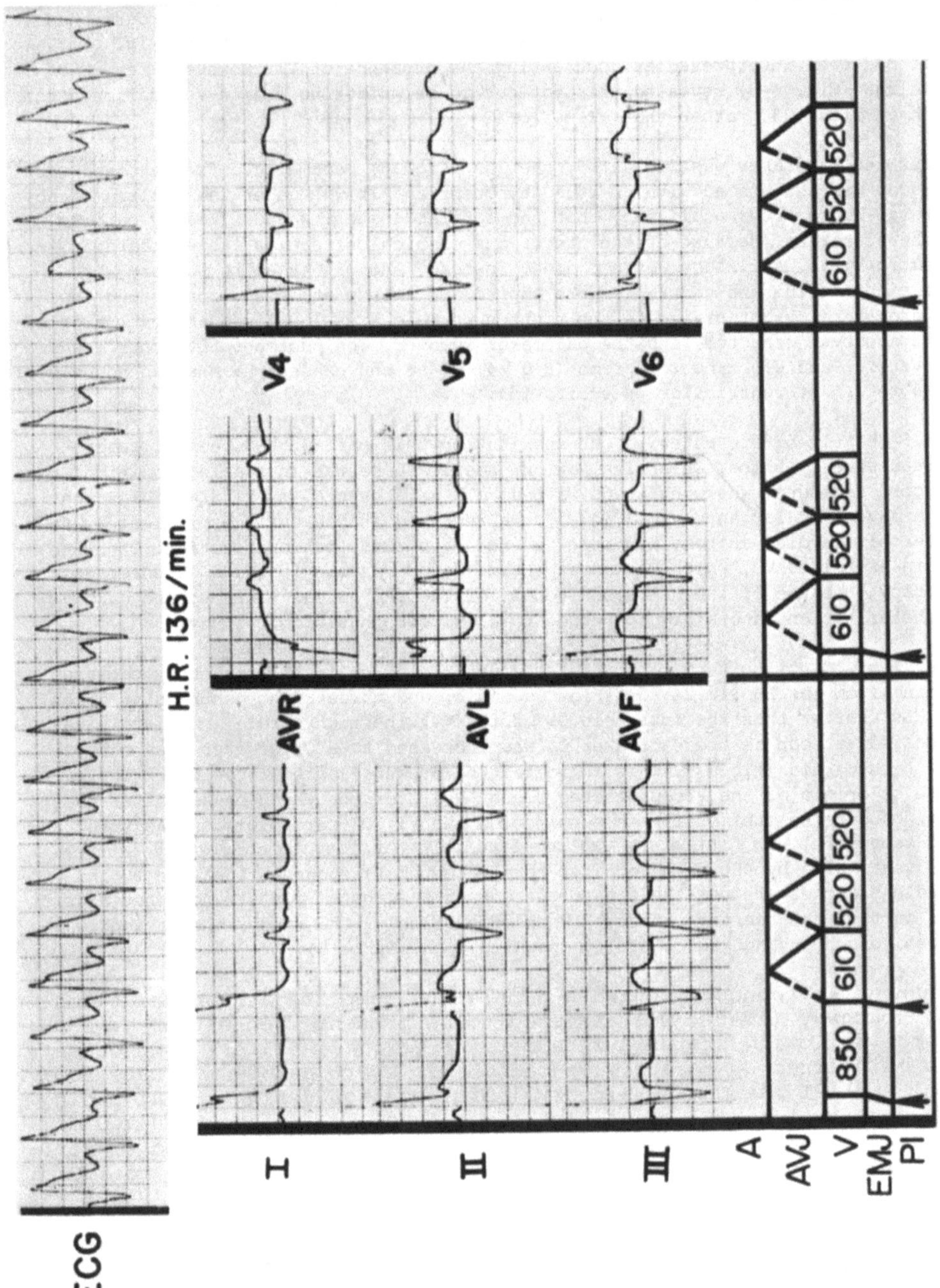

Fig. 3. Pt. M.S.: Recurrent SVT. The rhythm strip showing the SVT is a bipolar monitor lead. The 12-lead ECG shows repeat initiation of short paroxyxms of SVT by ventricular-paced beats. The interval between the first beat of the SVTs and the last paced beat is constant at 610 ms. The constancy of this interval suggest a reentrant mechanism (legend, Fig. 1). Key to ladder diagram: *PI* pacemaker impulse; *EMJ* electrode-myocardial junction

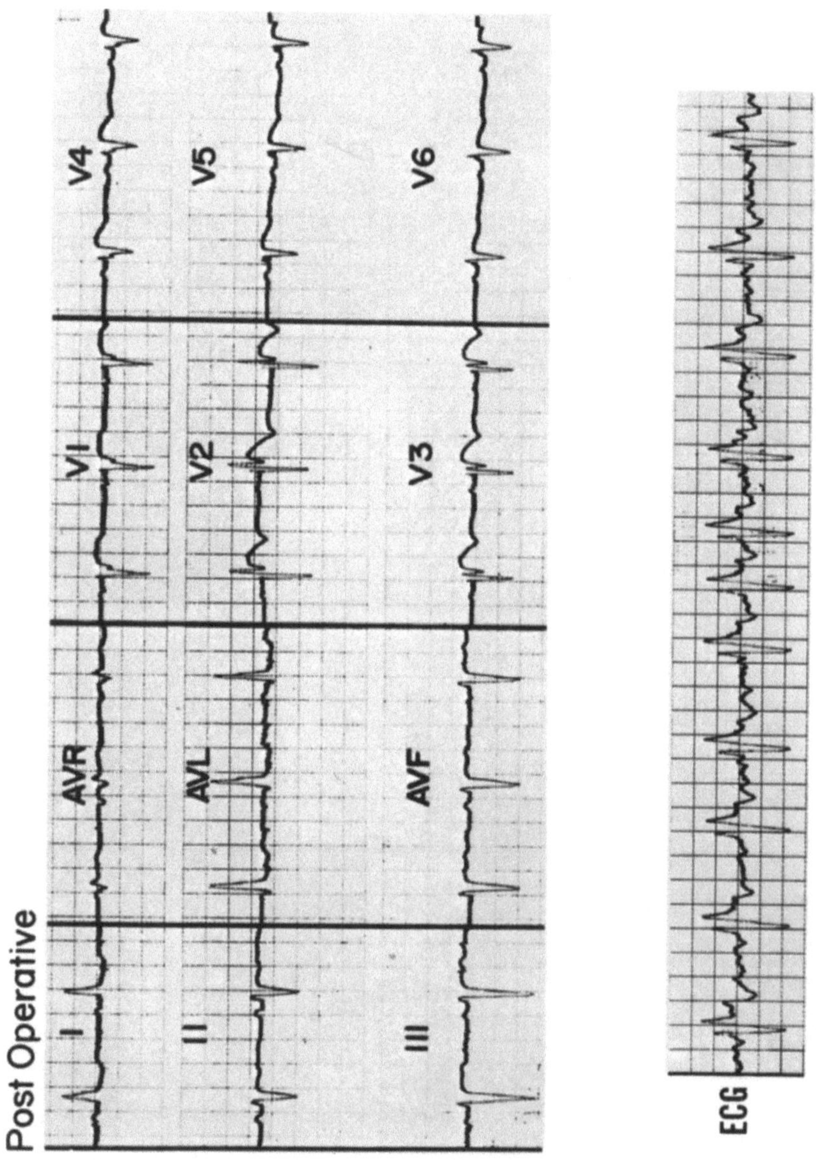

Fig. 4. Pt. M.S.: ECGs obtained after cutting of complete AVAP and left ventricular aneurysmectomy. The 12-lead tracing shows the P-R interval to have normalized, 0.16 s, and there is no longer evidence of ventricular preexcitation. The bipolar electrocardiographic monitor rhythm strip obtained during a paroxysm of atrial fibrillation also confirms the absence of ventricular preexcitation. The ventricular rate is controlled. It is approximately 82/min

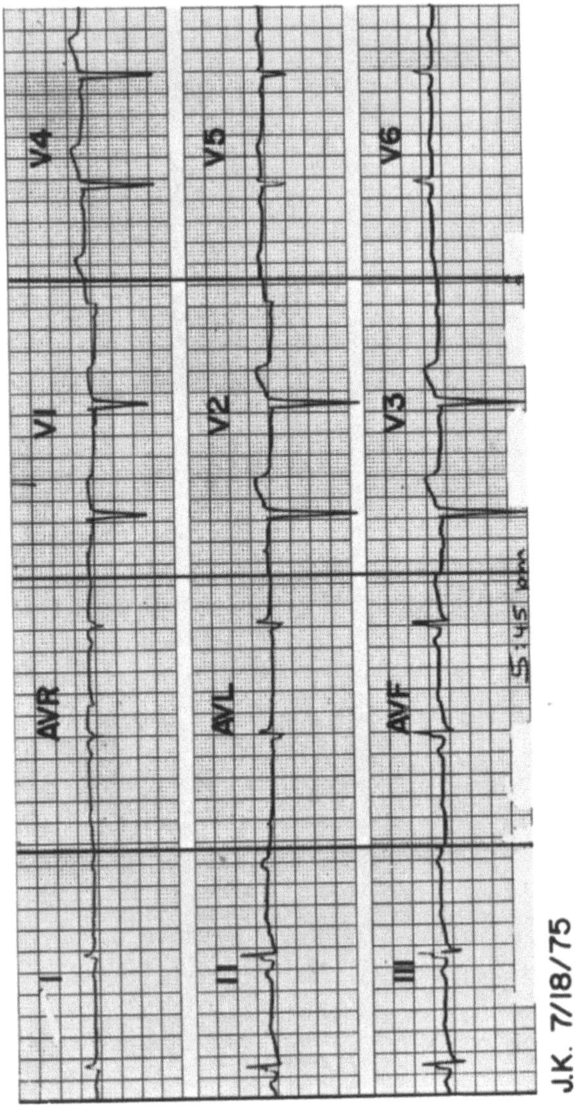

Fig. 5. Pt. J.K.: Preoperative 12-lead ECG. The tracing shows normal sinus rhythm with an anteroseptal myocardial infarction and elevated ST segment consistent with a ventricular aneurysm

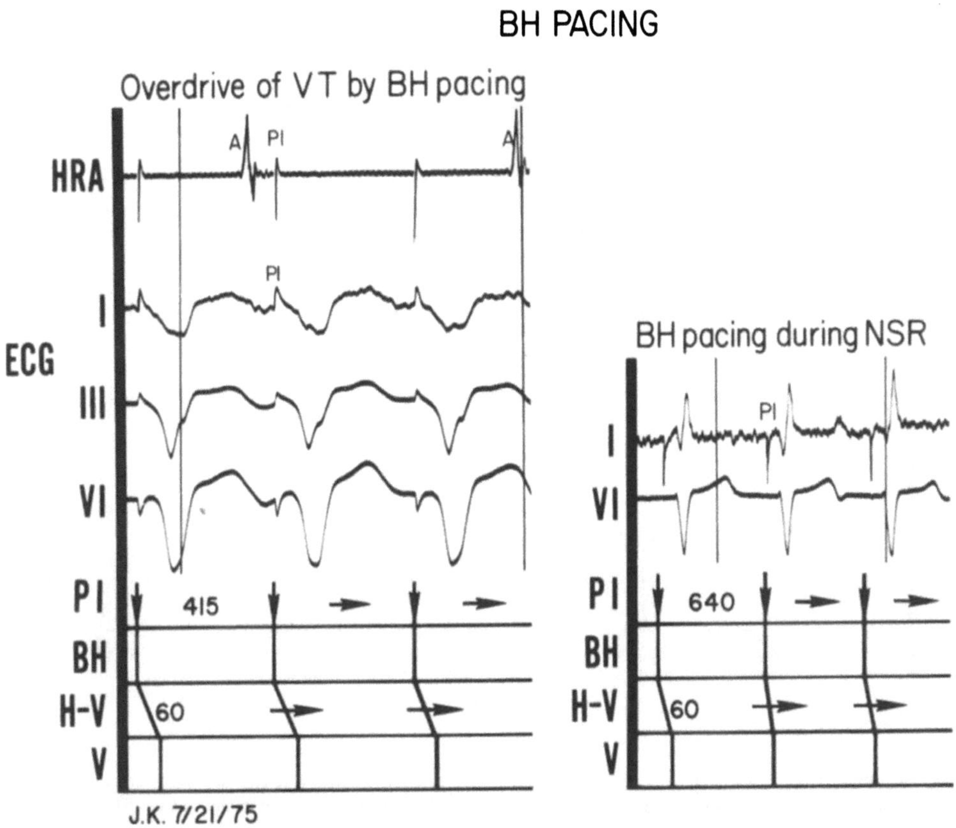

Fig. 6. Pt. J.K.: BH pacing. (A) Complete capture of the ventricles by BH pacing at a shorter CL than the VT. The VT was not terminated by the rapid pacing (Fig. 7). (B) BH pacing after the VT had been converted to NSR by DC countershock. The PI to onset of QRS interval is identical to this patient's H-V interval (Table 5), and the QRS configuration of leads 1 and V1 identical to the QRS complexes of these leads during normal sinus rhythm as shown in Fig. 5. Although the PI to onset of QRS interval is the same in (A), as in (B), the QRS complexes in (A) are widened and aberrant. The aberrancy may be due to simultaneous BH and septal pacing and/or a rate-dependent intraventricular conduction block

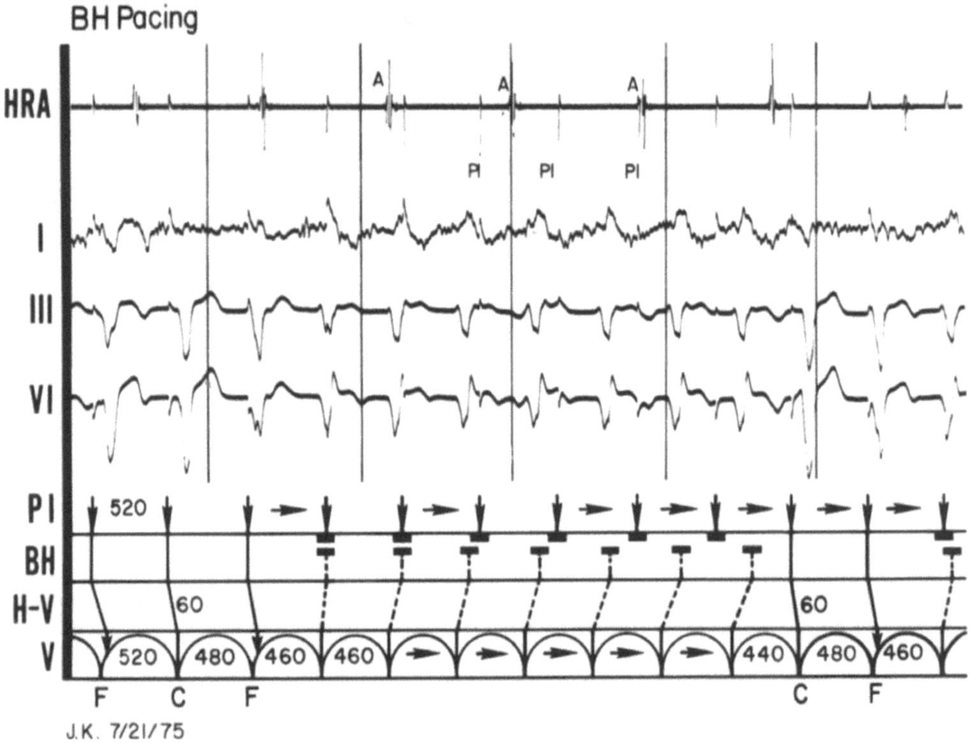

Fig. 7. Pt. J.K.: VT with PF — slowing of BH pacing. The pacing CL was increased (rate decreased) stepwise to 520 ms. At this CL, 60 ms longer than that of the VT, there is competition between the depolarizations of the VT and the paced beats. The first, third, and next to last depolarizations are fusion beats (*F*). The second, and third from last beat are completely pacemaker captured (*C*). There is entrance block for the paced beats PF to the site of origin of the VT. The lead-1 ECG is distorted by artifact paper speed 50 mm/s

the changes in A-H and ventriculoatrial conduction times during pacing were similar to the changes in these conduction times as shown for patient G.M. in Fig. 8. In the four cases with accelerated ventriculoatrial conduction, only in one, M.S., who had a complete AVAP, was the rapidly conducting retrograde tract localized electrophysiologically. This was done at surgery. In the other three cases with accelerated ventriculoatrial conduction, the rapidly conducting pathways were not localized electrophysiologically. The atria were not mapped during ventricular pacing or during the tachycardias. Therefore, in these cases, the pathway for accelerated retrograde conduction may have been the same as, or different from, the pathway used for accelerated antegrade conduction.

Only in three of the six surgical patients could recurrent paroxysms of VT be definitely documented (Table 5). In one case, R.K., the VTs initiated by programmed pacing terminated spontaneously. The VTs in this case were initiated by a supraventricular echo (Table 5), suggesting the possibility of BH - bundle branch reentry. In the other two cases, J.K. and O.R., the VTs were sustained; in both, the ventricles could be completely captured by pacing from various sites, but the VTs could not be terminated. J.K. was described above (Figs. 6 and 7). In O.R., because of the presence of a complete ANAP, the

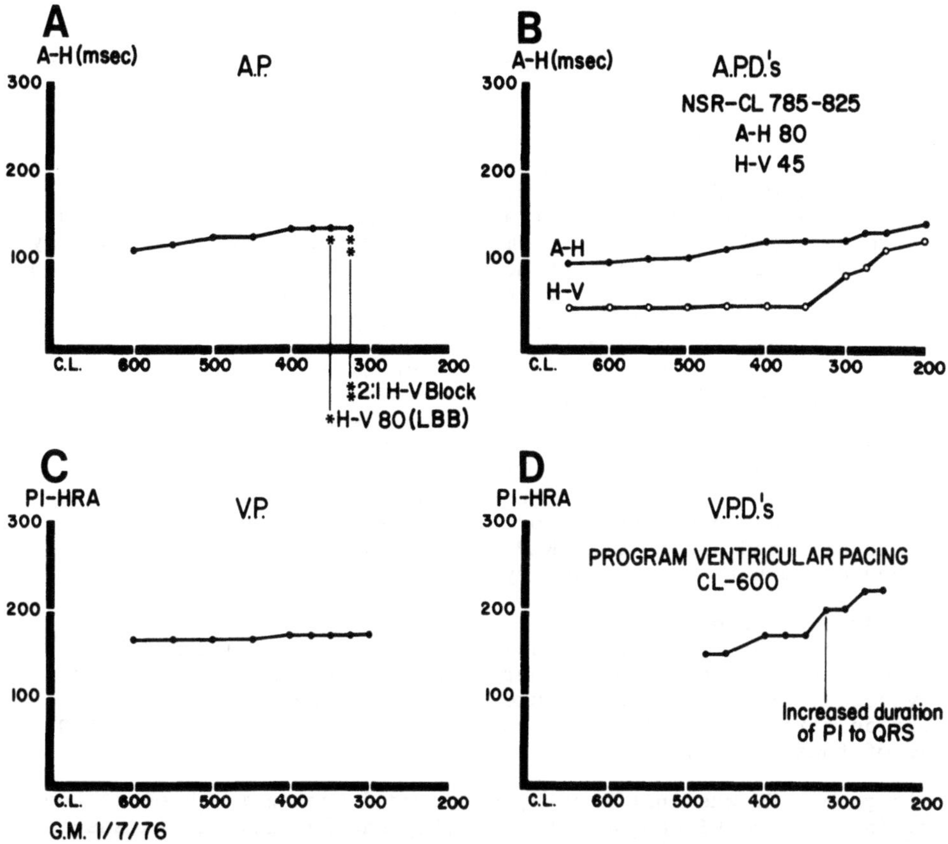

Fig. 8 A-D. Pt. G.M.: Complete ANAP and depressed H-V conduction.
(A) As the CL of atrial pacing was shortened, there was no significant increase in A-H time. However, at a CL of 350 ms, there was lengthening of the H-V time and left bundle branch block (*LBBB*). At a CL of 325 ms, 2:1 H-V block had developed.
(B) Atrial premature depolarizations (*APDs*) with CLs as short as 200 ms were associated with only a minimal increase in the A-H interval, 45 ms. However, APDs of CLs shorter than 350 ms resulted in progressive increase in the H-V interval.
(C) During ventricular pacing (*VP*) at progressively shorter CLs up to 300 ms, there was no significant increase in ventriculoatrial conduction times.
(D) Ventriculoatrial conduction times remained relatively constant as the CL of ventricular premature depolarizations (*VPDs*), during VP, were progressively shortened.
However, the PI to HRA time increased mostly due to latency of ventricular conduction. There was an increase in th PI to QRS onset time. Ventriculoatrial conduction time was not measured because it is not possible with reasonable certainty to determine the true onset of ventricular activation from the three surface ECG leads recorded.

Although the A-H time of 80 ms during NSR is normal, the constancy of A-H and ventriculoatrial (*PI-HRA*) conduction times is consistent with an antegrade and retrograde accessory A-V pathway. In addition, the normal and lengthened H-V times during atrial pacing are indicative of an antegrade complete ANAP.

PT. G.M. was the only one of the cases with a complete ANAP in whom the atria were not paced at a CL of 300 ms. This was not done because in this case at an atrial-paced CL of 325 ms 2:1 H-V block had occurred heart could be completely captured, not only by ventricular, but also by atrial pacing at CLs of 345 ms or less (the intrinsic CL of this patient's VT was 360 ms). These observations suggest PFs for the site of origin of these VTs.

In two cases, M.S. (Figs. 1-4) and R.R.J., the critical symptoms which had been ascribed to paroxysms of VT were observed to occur during SVTs. M.S. was described above. In R.R.J., who had a complete ANAP, an SVT was initiated by atrial pacing and terminated by atrial premature depolarizations. The termination of the SVT was followed by a prolonged period of cardiac standstill. The SVT and its termination were associated with severe chest pain, profound hypotension, and near syncope. Because of these symptoms, the preoperative electrophysiologic study was terminated prematurely. Electrocardiograms showing the reported VTs prior to admission to our institution for this patient, who had a noninfarcted normal ventricle and severe three-vessel disease, were not obtainable. The symptoms previously described were identical to those which occurred during the electrophysiologic study. Therefore, it appeared reasonable to ascribe this patient's ominous symptoms to recurrent SVTs and sinoatrial dysfunction in the presence of severe coronary artery disease. In one case, A.B., who also had a complete ANAP, a tachycardia was never observed by us and could not be initiated by pacing.

Medical Group (Table 6)
By the criteria described previously, two of the six patients had complete ANAPs. In both cases, there was bidirectional accelerated atrioventricular conduction. Figure 8 exhibits the antegrade and retrograde atrioventricular conduction times obtained during pacing in one of these cases.

In this group, VT was initiated by programmed pacing in three of the cases. In two, the VT was self-terminating and in one, it was sustained. In the latter, the site of origin of the tachycardia appeared to be a PF (the heart was completely captured by pacing, but the VT was not terminated). Figure 9 shows ECGs recorded from one of these three patients, G.M., during a clinical episode of VT and normal sinus rhythm (NSR). In this patient, programmed pacing resulted in the initiation of three electrophysiologically different TAs, including VT (Figs. 10 and 11). The mode of initiation of this VT suggested the possibility of BH – bundle branch reentry (see legend, Fig. 10) [16, 31].

In H.P., SVTs with a wide QRS (tachycardia-dependent intraventricular conduction defect) was repeatedly initiated by programmed atrial pacing and terminated by atrial premature depolarizations. The ECG recorded during the SVTs was identical to that obtained during his bout of reported "VT".

In two patients of this group, TAs could not be initiated by pacing.

Therapy and Clinical Course
There was no mortality or lasting morbidity in the surgical group. Table 3 presents the surgical procedures performed in these six patients. In one, M.S., aside from aneurysmectomy and revascularization, a complete AVAP was cut and a pacemaker removed; in another, R.K., the BH was cut and a pacemaker implanted. In the former case, there has been no return of ventricular preexcitation (Fig. 4); however, in the latter 1:1 A-V conduction returned 2 weeks postoperatively. In patient R.R.J., postoperative electrophysiologic study showed normalization of sinus node function. Sinoatrial conduction and sinus node recovery times were found to be normal.

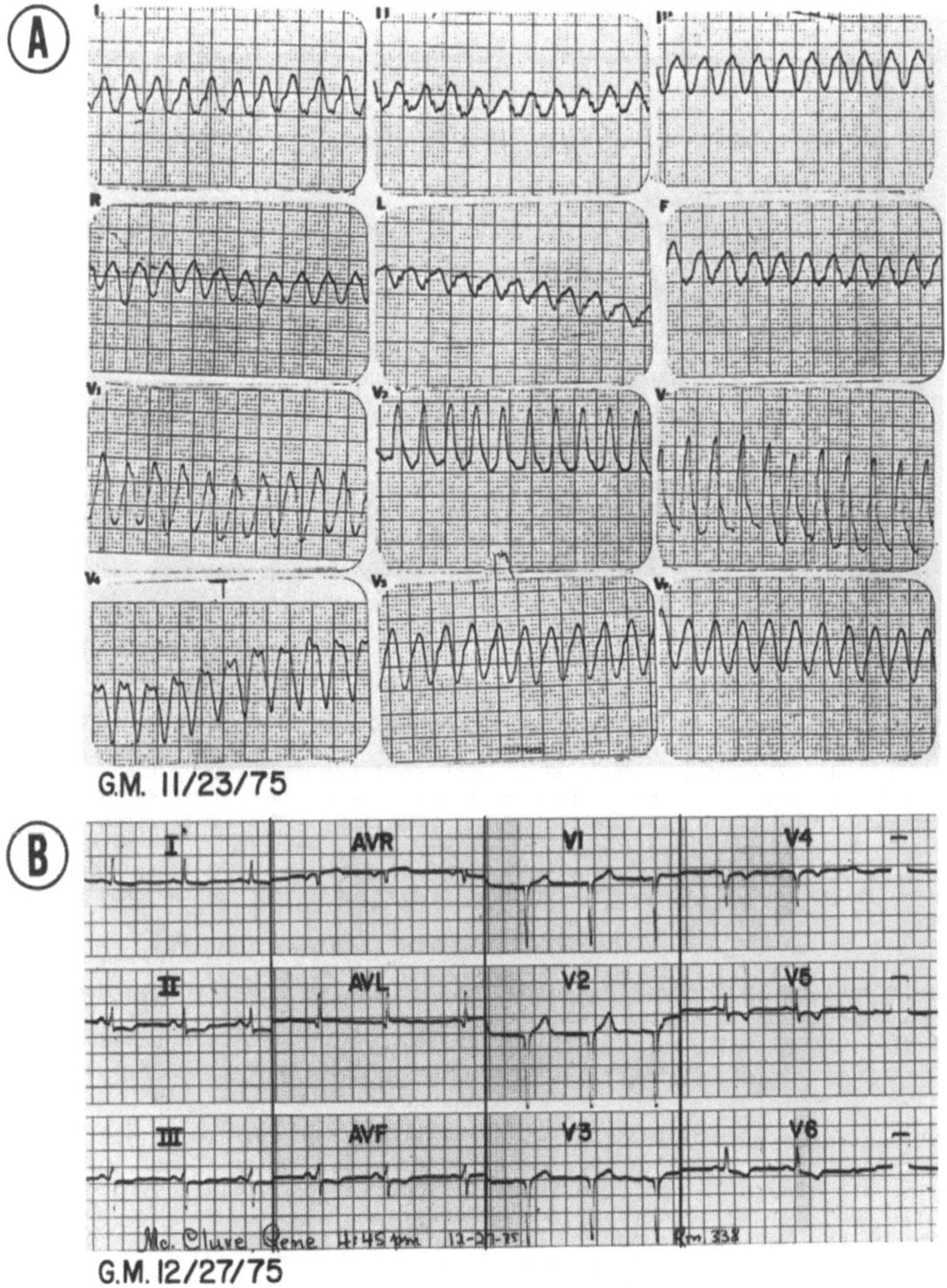

Fig. 9 A and B. Pt. G.M.: 12-lead ECGs during TA and NSR. (A) VT at 240/min. This tachycardia was tolerated surprisingly well. (B) Normal sinus rhythm with an anteroseptal myocardial infarction and elevated ST segments consistent with a ventricular aneurysm

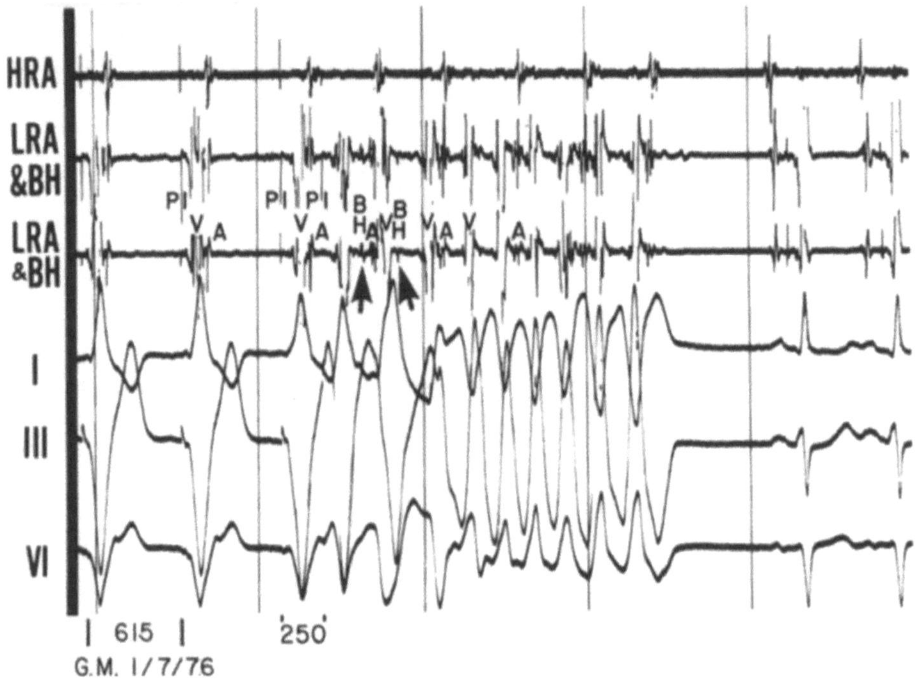

Fig. 10. Pt. G.M.: Initiation of VT.
A VPD at an interval of 250 ms during programmed VP initiated paroxysms of VT. BH deflections (*arrows*) are seen after each of the first two beats of the VT. These deflections represent retrograde BH activation and suggest BH-bundle branch reentry. The beats subsequent to the first beat of the VT have a different QRS configuration than the originating beat. Short paroxysms of VT could be repeatedly precipitated by pacing and always the same sequence of ventricular and BH activation as described above was associated with the initiation of the tachycardia. The rate and QRS configuration of the VT shown is similar to, but not the same as that shown in Fig. 9 A

Each patient in the medical group has continued under active medical management and is being treated with various combinations of the following drugs: digoxin, quinidine, procaineamide, di-isopyramide, and propranolol. When available, serum drug levels were used as a guide for therapy.

All patients were contacted in the last week of February, 1978. During an average follow-up period of 27.6 months, none of the surgical patients (Table 3) had experienced a recurrence of their symptomatic TAs, and, during an average follow-up period of 14.3 months, only one of the medical group (Table 6) had had a symptomatic bout of TA requiring specific therapy. This single case was treated as an outpatient by DC countershock.

Five of the six surgical patients have continued to exhibit premature ventricular beats and all are receiving antiarrhythmic drugs. As noted above, the medical patients continue to receive intensive pharmacologic therapy. Comparison of the post- and pre-hospitalization dose level of medications shows that post-hospital, the surgical group is taking less and the medical group significantly greater amounts of antiarrhythmic agents.

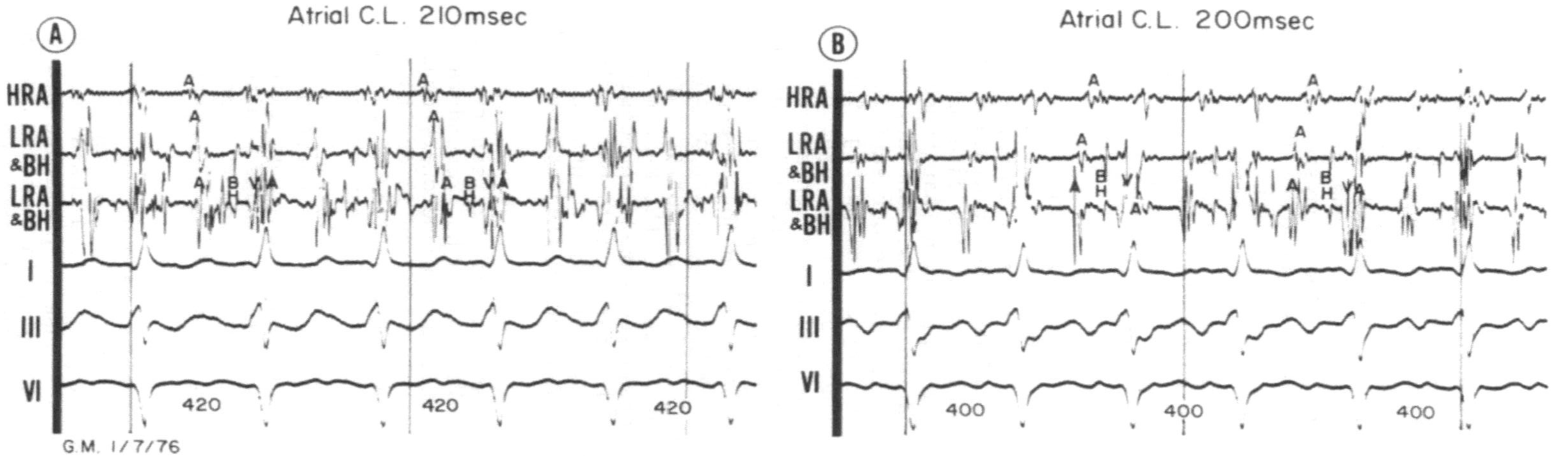

Fig. 11 A and B. Pt. G.M.: Two different SVTs. This patient, who has a complete ANAP, exhibited three electrophysiologically different TAs (Fig. 10). In both (A) and (B) the tachycardia was initiated by a single APD during programmed atrial pacing and terminated by rapid atrial pacing. In both instances, the atrial CL is similar [in (A) 210 ms, and in (B) 200 ms], there is 2:1 A-H block, and there is aberrant ventricular conduction (see Fig. 9 B). However, in (A) the HRA is activated prior to the LRA, while in (B) the LRA is activated prior to the HRA. In both (A) and (B), the atrial rate suggests that the probable reentrant pathway is solely relegated to the atria, or in (A) involves only a small segment of the sinus node and in (B) a small segment of the A-V node

Discussion

In patients with ischemic heart disease, with or without ventricular aneurysms, TAs causing life-threatening symptoms are not necessarily VT [32], and a comprehensive electrophysiologic and functional anatomic evaluation should be done. Three of our 12 patients were shown to have been suffering from SVTs, rather than the presumed VTs (Tables 5 and 6). Only in one of these cases, M.S., (Figs. 1 and 2) was it possible to arrive at this conclusion without electrophysiologic study. Also, unexpectedly seven of our patients had AVAPs (Tables 5 and 6). In one, old ECGs prior to pacemaker implantation showed a delta wave (Fig. 2). In the other six, there was no electrocardiographic evidence of AVAPs. In the group with complete ANAPs all had either prolonged intra-atrial and/or H-V conduction times. In the patient with the AVN-BHAP, the absence of a delta wave on the ECG is best explained by the distal end of the accessory pathway terminating in the BH, prior to its bifurcation.

Recently VT and VF has been reported to occur in patients with ANAPs (Lown-Ganong-Levine syndrome) and no significant heart disease [26]. Therefore, it is to be expected that in patients with AVAPs, the superimposition of ischemic or other significant heart disease will result in placing this group in an unusually high risk category. In the seven patients with AVAPs, it was our impression that these pathways were a contributing cause to the patients' TAs. However, only in one case, R.R.J., were we able to relate the two to our satisfaction. The SVTs could be initiated and terminated by atrial pacing. The termination of the SVT exposed ischemia-induced sinoatrial dysfunction [33] (Table 5), which was corrected by revascularization surgery. In the other six with AVAPs, and unequivocal cause and relationship between the AVAPs and TAs could not be established. In the case of WPW syndrome, it was shown that the complete AVAP could not be a part of the reentrant pathway, because there was A-V dissociation during the SVT (Fig. 1). Nevertheless, the KB was localized and cut at surgery to avoid possible future problems. In the case with the Mahaim fiber bypass tract, the elelctrophysiologic study suggested the possibility that the BH was a contributing cause in initiating this patient's bouts of VT and VF (Table 5). Therefore, at surgery, an unsuccessful attempt at creating permanent complete A-V block by transection of the BH was done.

There are three recognized possible mechanisms for VT: reentry, automaticity, and triggering (after potentials) [34]. The preponderance of evidence suggests that most VTs in patients with coronary heart disease, ventricular aneurysms, and remote infarction is due to reentry [15,16,35-40]. Especially, the recent observations of El-Sherif et al. [36-38] and Josephson et al. [39,40] strongly support this contention: the former, in dogs 3-7 days post-infarction, using composite electrodes mapped the epicardial surface of the heart during VT and recorded continuous electrical activity, which they believed to be generated in reentry pathways; the latter in humans, using catheters, recorded continuous electrical activity from the endocardial surface, which they also believed to be coming from reentrant pathways.

Criteria, as previously described for reentry, were not met in our nine patients with VT. Nevertheless, it is probable that these VTs were due to a reentrant mechanism. In six patients, a sustained VT could not be initiated. Therefore, the response to premature beats and pacing could not be tested. The inability to initiate sustained VT in patients who have experienced this tachycardia has been previously reported [15], and does not negate a reentry mechanism. The three instances of PFs may have been because the pacing sites were too distant from the site of origin of the VT [16]. The inability of RV and BH pacing to terminate the VTs may suggest the originating site of the VTs to be in the left ventricle relatively far from the pacing site, rather than the arrhythmia not being due to reentry.

The combination of TA and ventricular aneurysm does not necessarily mean that the TA originates in or near the aneurysm. The TA may be supraventricular [32] or ventricular, and in the latter cases, the tachycardia may arise in the ventricle in an area remote from the aneurysm [41]. Since in our cases of VT, we did not attempt to record from the expected originating ventricular site, the left ventricle, our aim was to eliminate the BH and bundle branches as a site of origin, and to localize the originating focus to the left ventricle. The QRS configuration on the electrocardiogram during VT cannot be reliably used to determine the site of origin of the tachycardia [39]. In our three cases with a PF, the originating site of the VT was localized to the left ventricle (see above). A BH-bundle branch reentry was highly improbable because of BH pacing and in one case (O.R.), atrial pacing with capture of the ventricles did not result in termination of the VTs. However, in three of our patients R.K. (see above), G.M., and G.F. (Tables 5 and 6) electrophysiologic study suggested that proximal BH-bundle branch reentry may have played a role in their VTs [16,31]. An effort was made to create permanent complete A-V block in R.K.; in the case of G.M., who had a well-defined ventricular aneurysm, it was decided not to submit him to surgery because of the electrophysiologic findings and his ability to tolerate his VT quite well; G.F. had no anatomic surgical lesions and therefore surgery was not a consideration.

At surgery, the ventricles were not mapped in order to localize the site of origin of the VTs. Although there are several reports in the literature of localization of the foci of VTs by epicardial mapping and their successful obliteration [13,43-49], epicardial mapping does not appear to be reliable [8,22,41,50]. It has been shown for VTs which originate in the subendocardial His-Purkinje system, the initial point of epicardial breakthrough of the impulse may be several centimeters from the focus [22,50]. In an effort to make mapping at surgery more reliable, Wittig and Boineau [41] performed transmural, epicardial, and endocardial mapping in three patients. In all three, they were able to localize the focus of origin of the VTs and successfully excise them. However, preoperative endocardial mapping as recently described by Josephson et al. appears to hold the most promise. Up to the present, neither mapping at surgery, nor endocardial mapping in the cardiac catheterization laboratory has proven to be reliable. They have not yet been time-tested.

The goals of our electrophysiologic studies were: (1) to define the rhythm disturbance which was causing symptoms, (2) to determine the presence or absence of AVAPs, and (3) in those cases in the surgical group who had VT, to localize the site of origin of the VT to one ventricle or another and to evaluate the probability of BH-bundle branch reciprocation [13,14,51]. Although by today's standards our studies were incomplete, in most cases they yielded the sought-after information.

Taking into consideration that aneurysmectomy and myocardial revascularization up to the present have not yielded uniformly good results [1-8] we used the following criteria for selecting patients for surgery: (1) an anatomically correctable lesion, (2) a high probability that the TAs would be eliminated by correction of the surgically remedial lesions, and (3) life-threatening symptoms, and/or uncontrollable TAs.

The critical difference between the medical group with coronary artery disease and the surgical group was their ventricular function, as was reflected in the severity of symptoms. The surgical patients had significantly poorer ventricular function than did the medical patients. At present, all patients are alive and well. None in the surgical group and only one in the medical group had recurrence of their symptomatic TA. In the medical group, an increase in the intensity of arrhythmia therapy has had a salutary effect. However, at the present state of the art of pharmacologic antiarrhythmic therapy their future remains uncertain. Although thus far our surgical results have been good, as of this communication, the overall results of surgery for VT do not warrant an aggressive surgical approach [1-8,50]. In the future, should endocardial mapping [16,39,40] prove reliable in localizing the site of origin of VTs, the surgical results should improve and surgery may be more aggressively pursued in this high risk group of patients.

Acknowledgements
We wish to acknowledge the assistance of the following Miami Heart Institute personnel: Mr. Stanley Dzwonkowski, Miss Frances Ann Blair, Miss Mary R. Gosset, and Mrs. Linda Hudson (Cardiopulmonary Laboratory), as well as, Dr. Minor Duggan, Mr. Rand Johns, and Mrs. Klara Soos (Medical Illustration and Publications Department).

References

1. Magidson, O.: Resection of postmyocardial infarction ventricular aneurysms for cardiac arrhythmias. Dis. Chest *56*, 211 (1969)
2. Thind, G.S., Blakemore, W.S., Zinsser, H.F.: Ventricular aneurysmectomy for the treatment of recurrent ventricular tachyarrhythmia. Am. J. Cardiol. *27*, 690, (1971)
3. Kenaan, G., Mendez, M., Zubiate, P., et al: Surgery for ventricular tachycardia unresponsive to medical treatment. Chest *64*, 574 (1973)
4. Giacchino, R., Moran, J.F., Schreiber, R., et al: The problem of recurrent ventricular tachycardia in the presence of angiographically proven coronary artery disease. Circulation *51-52*, II-110 (1975) (Abs. # 430)
5. Winkle, R.A., Alderman, E.L., Fitzgerald, J.W., et al: Treatment of recurrent symptomatic ventricular tachycardia. Ann. Intern. Med. *85*, 1 (1976)
6. Yashar, J., Yashar, J.J., Witoszka, M., et al: The treatment of patients with recurrent ventricular fibrillation. Am. J. Surg. *133*, 453 (1977)
7. Ricks, W.B., Winkle, R.A., Shumway, N.E., et al: Surgical management of life-threatening ventricular arrhythmias in patients with coronary artery disease. Circulation *56*, 38 (1977)
8. Gallagher, J.J.: Surgical treatment of arrhythmias: Current status and future directions. Am. J. Cardiol. *41*, 1035 (1978)
9. Steinberg, M.: Das chronische partielle Herzaneurysma. Vienna: 1914
10. Parade, G.W.: Aneurysmatische Elongation des Herzens. Med. Klin. *30*, 1357 (1934)
11. Parkinson, J., Bedford, D.E., Thomson, W.A.R.: Cardiac aneurysm. Q. J. Med. *7*, 455 (1938)
12. Narula, O.S., Scherlag, B.J., Samet, P.: Pervenous pacing of the specialized conducting system in man. His bundle and A-V nodal stimulation. Circulation *41*, 77 (1970)
13. Spurrell, R.A.J., Sowton, E., Deuchar, D.C.: Ventricular tachycardia in 4 patients evaluated by programmed electrical stimulation of heart and treated in 2 patients by surgical division of anterior radiation of left bundle-branch. Br. Heart J. *35*, 1014 (1973)

14. Wellens, H.J.J., Lie, K.I., Durrer, D.: Further observations on ventricular tachycardia as studied by electrical stimulation of the heart. Chronic recurrent ventricular tacyhcardia and ventricular tachycardia during acute myocardial infarction. Circulation *49*, 647 (1974)
15. Denes, P., Wu, D., Dhingra, R.C., et al: Electrophysiological studies in patients with chronic recurrent ventricular tachycardia. Circulation *54*, 229 (1976)
16. Josephson, M.E., Horowitz, L.N., Farshidi, A., et al: Recurrent sustained ventricular tachycardia. 1. Mechanisms. Circulation *57*, 431 (1978)
17. Lister, J.W., Worthington, F.X. (Jr.), Gentsch, T.O., et al: Preexcitation and tachycardias in Wolff-Parkinson-White syndrome, type B. A case report. Circulation *45*, 1081 (1972)
18. Moore, E.N., Hoffman, B.F., Patterson, D.F., et al: Electrocardiographic changes due to delayed activation of the wall of the right ventricle. Am. Heart J. *68*, 347 (1964)
19. Gallagher, J.J., Gilbert, M., Svenson, R.H., et al: Wolff-Parkinson-White syndrome. The problem, evaluation, and surgical correction. Circulation *51*, 767 (1975)
20. Kupersmith, J.: Electrophysiologic mapping during open heart surgery. Prog. Cardiovasc. Dis. *19*, 167 (1976)
21. Harrison, L., Gallagher, J.J., Kasell, J., et al: Cryosurgical ablation of the A-V node, His bundle. A new method for producing A-V block. Circulation *55*, 463 (1977)
22. Spielman, S.R., Michelson, E.L., Horowitz, L.N., et al: The limitations of epicardial mapping as a guide to the surgical therapy of ventricular tachycardia. Circulation *57*, 666 (1978)
23. Mandel, W.J., Laks, M., Obayashi, K.: Atrioventricular nodal reentry in the Wolff-Parkinson-White snydrome. Chest *68*, 321 (1975)
24. Williams, D.O., Scherlag, B.J., Hope, R.R., et al: Selective versus non selective His bundle pacing. Cardiovasc. Res. *10*, 91 (1976)
25. Mendoza, I.J., Sung, R.J., Mallon, S.M., et al: Multiple intracardiac recordings in evaluation of patterns occurring during attempted His bundle pacing in man. Am. J. Cardiol. *41*, 1068 (1978)
26. Benditt, D.G., Pritchett, E.L.C., Smith, W.M., et al: Characteristics of atrioventricular conduction and the spectrum of arrhythmias in Lown-Ganong-Levine syndrome. Circulation *57*, 454 (1978)
27. Iannone, L.A.: Electrophysiology of atrial pacing in patients with short PR interval, normal QRS complex. Am. Heart J. *89*, 74 (1975)
28. Caracta, A.R., Damato, A.N., Gallagher, J.J., et al: Electrophysiologic studies in the syndrome of short P-R interval, normal QRS complex. Am. J. Cardiol. *31*, 245 (1973)
29. Narula, O.S.: Retrograde pre-excitation. Comparison of antegrade and retrograde conduction intervals in man. Circulation *50*, 1129 (1974)
30. Lister, J.W., Gosselin, A.J., Sayfie, E.J., et al: Arrhythmia Analysis by Intracardiac Electrocardiography. pp. 263-268. Springfield (Ill.): Thomas 1976
31. Akhtar, M., Damato, A.N., Ruskin, J.N., et al: Characteristics and coexistence of two forms of ventricular echo phenomena. Am. Heart J. *92*, 174 (1976)
32. Basta, L.L., Takeshita, A., Theilen, E.O., et al: Aneurysmectomy in treatment of ventricular and supraventricular tachyarrhythmias in patients with postinfarction and traumatic ventricular aneurysms. Am. J. Cardiol. *32*, 693 (1973)
33. Jordan, J., Yamaguchi, I., Mandel, W.J.: Characteristics of sinoatrial conduction in patients with coronary artery disease. Circulation *55*, 569 (1977)
34. Wit, A.L., Cranefield, P.F.: Triggered activity in cardiac muscle fibers of the simian mitral valve. Circ. Res. *38*, 85 (1976)
35. Wellens, H.J.J., Duren, D.R., Lie, K.I.: Observations on mechanisms of ventricular tachycardia in man. Circulation *54*, 237 (1976)
36. El-Sherif, N., Scherlag, B.J., Lazzara, R., et al: Re-entrant ventricular arrhythmias in the late myocardial infarction period. 1. Conduction characteristics in the infarction zone. Circulation *55*, 686 (1977)
37. El-Sherif, N., Hope, R.R., Scherlag, B.J., et al: Re-entrant ventricular arrhythmias in the late myocardial infarction period. 2. Patterns of initiation and termination of re-entry. Circulation *55*, 702 (1977)

38. El-Sherif, N., Lazzara, R., Hope, R.R., et al: Re-entrant ventricular arrhythmias in the late myocardial infarction period. 3. Manifest and concealed extrasystolic grouping. Circulation *56*, 225 (1977)
39. Jospehson, M.E., Horowitz, L.N., Farshidi, A., et al: Recurrent sustained ventricular tachycardia. 2. Endocardial mapping. Circulation *57*, 440 (1978)
40. Josephson, M.E., Horowitz, L.N., Farshidi, A.: Continuous local electrical activity. A mechanism of recurrent ventricular tachycardia. Circulation *57*, 659 (1978)
41. Wittig, J.H., Boineau, J.P.: Surgical treatment of ventricular arrhythmias using epicardial, transmural, and endocardial mapping. Ann. Thorac. Surg. *20*, 117 (1975)
42. Gallagher, J.J., Oldham, H.N., Wallace, A.G., et al: Ventricular aneurysm with ventricular tachycardia. Report of a case with epicardial mapping and successful resection. Am. J. Cardiol. *35*, 696 (1975)
43. Moran, J.M., Talano, J.V., Euler, D., et al: Refractory ventricular arrhythmia: the role of intraoperative electrophysiological study. Surgery *82*, 809 (1977)
44. Fontaine, G., Guiraudon, G., Frank, R. et al: Epicardial mapping and surgical treatment in six cases of resistant ventricular tachycardia not related to coronary artery disease. In: The conduction system of the heart. Wellens, H.J.J., Lie, K.I., Janse, M.J. et al (edts.), pp. 545-563. Leiden: Stenfert Kroese 1976
45. Guiraudon, G., Fontaine, G., Frank, R., et al: Traitment de la tachycardie ventriculaire orientee par cartographie epicardique. A propos de 22 cas. Arch. Mal. Coeur (in press) (1978)
46. Spurrell, R.A.J., Yates, S.K., Thornburn, C.W., et al: Surgical treatment of ventricular tachycardia after epicardial mapping studies. Br. Heart J. *37*, 115 (1975)
47. Spurrell, R.A.J.: Surgery for ventricular tachycardia. In: Cardiac Arrhythmias. Goodwin, J.F. (ed.), pp. 195-207. Philadelphia: Saunders 1975
48. Gallagher, J.J., Anderson, R.W., Kasell, J., et al: Cryoablation of drug-resistant ventricular tachycardia in a patient with a variant of scleroderma. Circulation *57*, 190 (1978)
49. Petitier, H., Polu, J., Dodinot, B., et al: Tachycardie ventriculaire irreductible traitment par electrocoagulation apres localisation du foyer. Arch. Mal. Coeur *64*, 331 (1971)
50. Fontaine, G., Guiraudon, G., Frank, R., et al: Stimulation studies and epicardial mapping in ventricular tachycardia: study of mechanisms and selection for surgery. In: Reentrant arrhythmias. Kulbertus, H.E. (ed.), pp. 334-350. Lancaster: MTP 1977
51. Guerat, C.L., Vateri, P.A., Castello-Fenoy, A., et al: Tachycardia per reentri de branche a branche. Arch. Mal. Coeur *67*, 1 (1975)
52. Barold, S.S., Linhart, J.W., Samet, P., et al: Supraventricular tachycardia initiated and terminated by a single electrical stimulus. Am. J. Cardiol. *24*, 37 (1969)

Does Aneurysmectomy Reduce Life-Threatening Ventricular Arrhythmias?

H. Klein, P. R. Lichtlen, and H. G. Borst

Ventricular arrhythmia frequently complicates ventricular aneurysm in coronary heart disease [1,2]. The poor prognosis of recurrent ventricular tachycardia refractory to medical treatment is well known. Since the first clinical report [3] of successful control of recurrent ventricular tachycardia by resection of a left ventricular aneurysm, surgical treatment is considered to be indicated to abolish ventricular arrhythmia refractory to medical therapy.

It has been reported (4-8) that patients with coronary artery disease showed a higher incidence of premature ventricular contractions in cases of depressed left ventricular function, ventricular akinesis, and ventricular aneurysms than in cases of normal left ventricular function or without ventricular aneurysms. Therefore, it is of interest to know whether resection of a left ventricular aneurysm can abolish or reduce ventricular ectopic activity. The present study is concerned with the behavior of ventricular arrhythmia before and after aneurysmectomy.

Patients and Methods

Eighty-one patients underwent left ventricular aneurysmectomy between 1969 and 1976. The average age was 51 years (range 30-67). Of this group 69 were men and 12 were women. All patients had a previous myocardial infarction between 2 months and 8 years (average 20 months) before resection of a left ventricular aneurysm. The indication for surgery was severe congestive heart failure with or without angina pectoris in 68 patients, recurrent ventricular tachyarrhythmia refractory to medical treatment in 11 patients, and two patients underwent aneurysmectomy because of thromboembolic complications. Twenty-seven patients underwent concomitant coronary artery bypass grafting and four patients had mitral valve replacement because of mitral regurgitation resulting from papillary muscle dysfunction. Until the follow-up study, 68 patients were alive, six patients died before leaving the hospital (early mortality 7%), and seven patients died between 4 and 35 months following discharge. Sixty-six patients gave consent for the follow-up study and three patients refused re-examination. Follow-up ranged from 12 to 95 months (average 21 months). All patients were given a physical examination, chest roentgenogram, standard 12-lead ECG, and 10-h ambulatory monitoring. Fifty-nine patients had an exercise stress test and 27 patients were reinvestigated with left ventriculography and coronary angiography.

Results

In 66 patients, 10-h ambulatory ECGs were obtained and ventricular ectopic activity was graded quantitatively and qualitatively. The quantitative grading system analyzed the average number of ventricular premature contractions (VPC) per hour. The qualitative classification was done according to the grading system described by Lown [9] (class 0 - no VPC; class I - less than 30 VPC/h; class III - multiform VPC; class IV - repetitive ventricular responses as couplets or ventricular tachycardia). In only 30% of patients no ventricular premature contractions (VPC) were recorded after aneurysmectomy; in 35% occasional VPC were registered and 35% showed frequent VPC. According to the Lown classification 24% (16 patients) were found to be in class III and class IV; that means they had multifocal VPC, couplets, or short runs of ventricular tachycardia (Fig. 1). Of the 66 patients, 21 underwent concomitant coronary bypass grafting (16 single vessel grafting, 5 double vessel grafting). Only two patients were found to be free from ventricular arrhythmias after aneurysmectomy, ten patients demonstrated few unifocal ventricular premature contractions and were classified Lown class I, yet nine patients had to be classified Lown class II, III, and IV.

Ventricular arrhythmias after aneurysmectomy n = 66

VPC/h	Patients n	Patients %
0	20	30
1-10	23	35
11-100	17	26
>100	6	9

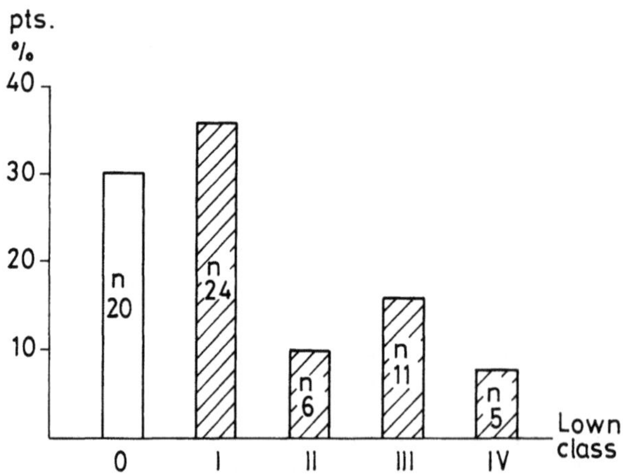

Fig. 1. Incidence of ventricular premature contractions (*VPC*) after aneurysmectomy. Quantitative and qualitative analysis of 10-h ambulatory monitoring in 66 patients

Table 1. Incidence of ventricular premature contractions (*VPC*) during ambulatory monitoring (Holter) and during cycle exercise test (x-test)

Lown-class	Holter	X-test
	n-patients	
O + I	39 (66%)	4 (7%)
II	5 (9%)	O
III + IV	15 (25%)	11 (19%)
Total	59	15

7 patients had no X-test

Table 2. Ejection fraction (EF) before and after aneurysmectomy of the two groups of Lown class. Statistical analysis of the data was carried out using the Student *t* test

	EF (%)		
Lown-class	pre.-op.	post-op.	
O - I	36.4 ± 14.3	52.7 ± 10.8	<0.0025
II - IV	40.3 ± 14.2	44.6 ± 10.4	n.s.
	n.s.	<0.05	p

Fifty-nine patients underwent exercise testing using cycle ergometry after aneurysmectomy. In seven patients exercise testing was not performed because of poor left heart function. Twenty-five percent of all patients showed VPC during exercise test. Among these there was a prevalence of Lown class III and IV (11 of 15 patients). As far as the more favorable Lown class I and II is concerned, ambulatory monitoring more often detected ventricular arrhythmias than exercise testing. Yet it could be assessed that the incidence of ventricular ectopic beats of Lown class III-IV during cycle exercise testing was almost equal to the incidence of VPC during ambulatory monitoring (Table 1).

We tried to find out if cases with postoperatively improved left ventricular function showed a decrease of ventricular ectopic activity. Patients were grouped in Lown class O-I and Lown class II-IV. (Table 2). It was noted that in patients of Lown class O-I ejection fraction after aneurysmectomy was significantly increased when compared with preoperative ejection fraction. Patients of Lown class II-IV showed no significant improvement of ejection fraction after resection of the aneurysm. When postoperative ejection fraction of Lown class II-IV was compared with postoperative ejection fraction of Lown class O-I, it could be noted that ejection fraction of patients found in Lown class II-IV was significantly lower. When left ventricular end-diastolic pressure and cardiac output were related to the two groups, no significant difference between pre- and postoperative situation was found neither in Lown class O-I or in Lown class II-IV. After aneurysmectomy, left ventricular end-diastolic pressure and cardiac output showed no significant difference between patients of Lown class II-IV and patients of Lown class O-I.

In 25 patients ambulatory monitoring was performed before and after aneurysmectomy (Fig. 2). It was noted that the incidence of ventricular premature contractions showed no significant difference before and after aneurysmectomy, neither in the group of patients with few ventricular premature beats nor in the group of severe ventricular arrhythmia. Only seven patients showed an improvement in Lown classification after resection of the aneurysm. Five patients were found to be improved by one class and two patients – preoperatively in class IV – became free from ventricular arrhythmia. Ten patients remained in the same class, while eight patients worsened postoperatively and moved to an unfavorable class. Four of the latter did not even have arrhythmias preoperatively.

Patients who were reinvestigated with left ventriculography and coronary angiography were grouped with those who worsened or remained in the same Lown class and those who improved (Table 3). It was noted that patients who postoperatively moved to a better Lown class showed a significant increase of cardiac output and a significant decrease of left ventricular end-diastolic pressure in comparison to the group of worsened or unchanged Lown class. There was a trend to a more increased ejection fraction in the improved group; however, the difference was not significant.

In 11 of 81 patients recurrent ventricular tachyarrhythmia refractory to medical treatment was the main indication for aneurysmectomy (Fig. 3). Three patients died in the early postoperative period 4 days to

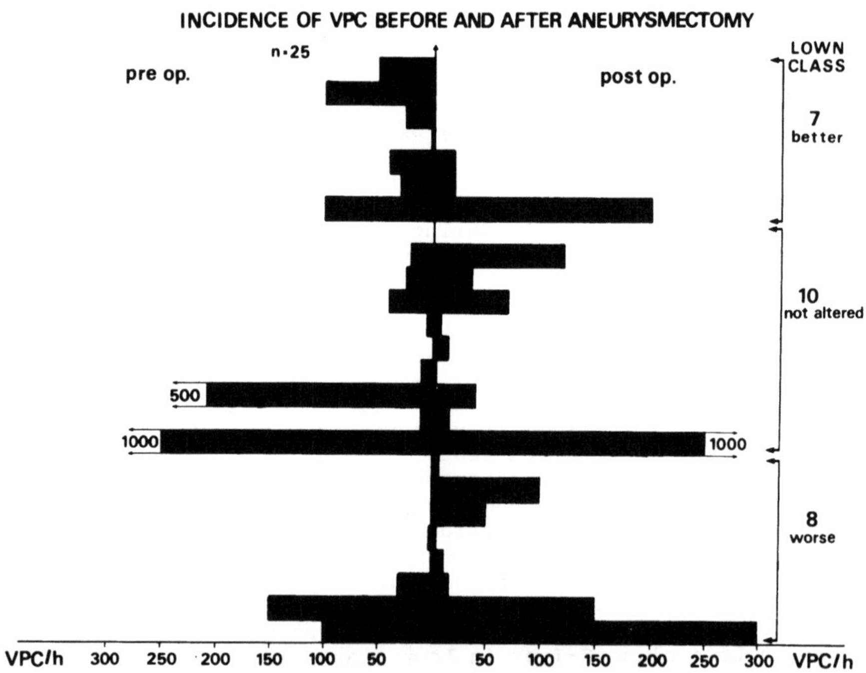

Fig. 2. Incidence of ventricular premature contractions (*VPC*) before (left) and after (right) aneurysmectomy. *Abscissa* indicates VPC per hour in each of the 25 patients

Table 3. Alteration of Lown class (above) in comparison to alteration of hemodynamics (below). ΔCI, ΔLVEDP, and ΔEF indicate the difference between pre- and postoperative hemodynamic data. $\Delta\bar{X}$, $\Delta\bar{Y}$ are the mean values

ALTERATION OF LOWN-CLASS VERSUS ALTERATION OF HEMODYNAMICS

LOWN CLASS	worse				not altered				$\Delta\bar{X}$	better			$\Delta\bar{Y}$	2P
PRE	0	0	0	I	III	II	II	I		IV	IV	I		
POST	I	II	III	III	III	II	II	I		0	0	0		
ΔCI (l/min/m²)	-0.3	-0.4	0.2	-0.7	-0.3	0.5	-0.4	-0.6	-0.25	0.4	1.3	0.1	0.6	<0.025
Δ LVEDP (mmHg)	-5	10	1	-10	22	3	1	0	2.7	-12	-16	-8	-12	<0.05
Δ EF (%)	48	-2	25	17	-11	6	-9	11	10.6	-1	54	32	28.3	n.s.

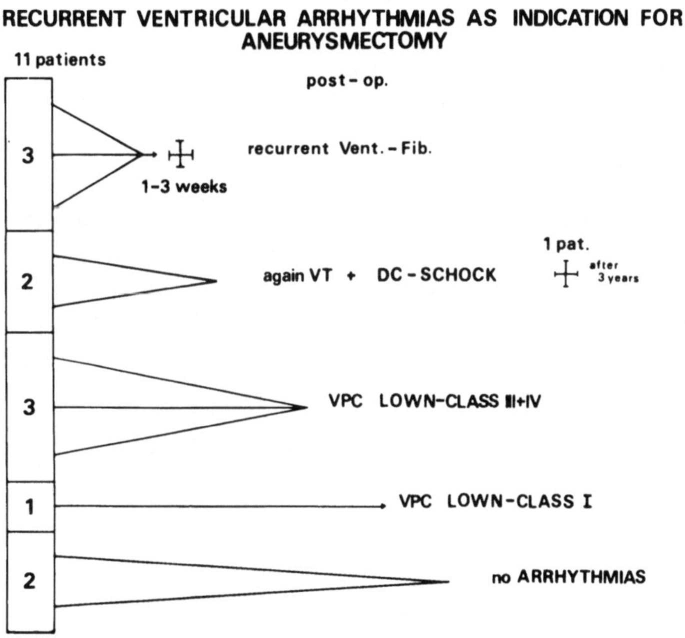

Fig. 3. Follow-up of 11 patients operated for recurrent ventricular tachyarrhythmia

3 weeks after resection of the aneurysm due to recurrent ventricular fibrillation and unseccessful resuscitation. The remaining eight patients survived to leave the hospital. Two patients again developed episodes of ventricular tachycardia or ventricular fibrillation and required multiple direct current cardioversions. One patient is still alive,the other died suddenly 3 years after aneurysmectomy. Three pa-

tients developed frequent multifocal ventricular premature contractions and were found in Lown class III and IV, one patient had few unifocal ventricular premature beats during abulatory monitoring, and only 2 of 11 patients were asymptomatic and showed no ventricular ectopic activity.

Discussion

To better gather information about the behavior of ventricular ectopic activity after resection of a left ventricular aneurysm in patients with coronary heart disease, a long-term follow-up was performed. The present study revealed that ventricular arrhythmia could be found in a high incidence after aneurysmectomy. In cases in which pre- and postoperative ambulatory monitoring was performed, it could be demonstrated that ventricular premature contractions persisted or became even worse in more than 50%. The results of aneurysmectomy for recurrent ventricular tachycardia are rather poor. Only 2 of 11 operated for life-threatening ventricular arrhythmia became free from ectopic activity. The relationship between depressed left ventricular function and incidence of ventricular premature contractions was studied by some authors [4,5,7]. They reported a striking correlation between ventricular ectopic activity and low ejection fraction, increased left ventricular end-diastolic pressure, and low cardiac output. Our study demonstrated that patients who showed a significant improvement of ejection fraction after resection of an aneurysm had no or only few ventricular premature beats. Patients in whom ejection fraction was not improved by aneurysmectomy postoperatively were found in Lown class II-IV. When postoperative ventricular ectopic activity was compared with the preoperative situation, it could be assessed that patients with improvement in Lown classification showed a significant increase in cardiac output and a significant decrease of left ventricular end-diastolic pressure in comparison to patients who postoperatively were found in the same Lown class or even moved to a more unfavorable Lown class.

There are reports [10,12] indicating the effectiveness of coronary bypass grafting to control recurrent ventricular tachyarrhythmia. Yet in our series, 50% of all patients who underwent aneurysmectomy in combination with bypass grafting postoperatively showed ventricular premature beats of Lown class II-IV.

An increasing number of reports confirm the successful surgical treatment of medically refractory recurrent ventricular arrhythmias [13-21]. But long-term follow-up studies [20,22-26] demonstrate persistence of ventricular ectopic activity in a high percent. There was high mortality when resection of the aneurysm was performed within 4 weeks after acute myocardial infarction [21,23], but good postoperative results and long-term survival were obtained when aneurysmectomy was done more than 1 months after acute infarction. In our series all patients underwent surgery later than 2 months after infarction. Early in-hospital mortality for those operated for ventricular arrhythmia was 27%. All patients, including the one who died 3 years after aneurysmectomy, died because of sudden unseccessfully treated ventricular tachyarrhythmias.

Although there is some indication that ventricular arrhythmias in the late phase after myocardial infarction may originate in the surviving subendocardial Purkinje system [27,28] adjacent to the infarcted area, the mechanism of ventricular arrhythmias is still unclear. The reason why ventricular ectopic activity often persists after aneurysmectomy

and surgical treatment of life-threatening ventricular arrhythmia is less effective may well be the fact that total resection of the scar is often impossible because of operating techniques or because the dyskinetic area is not clearly defined. If the irritable ventricular focus is not excised or interruption of a re-entry pathway is unsuccessful, ventricular ectopic activity will persist.
The development of epicardial and endocardial mapping techniques during open heart surgery [28-31] made it possible to locate the irritable focus more precisely so that the anatomic margin for the surgical resection can be delineated or direct surgical excision of the area of irritability will be feasible.

The present follow-up study indicates that long-term survival is better in patients operated for ventricular aneurysm in comparison to those not operated [39], but it could be demonstrated that removal of a scar eliminates premature ventricular contractions only in a small percent. We conclude that antiarrhythmic therapy should not be discontinued after aneurysmectomy in most patients.

Summary

Incidence and type of premature ventricular contractions were studied by ambulatory monitoring in 66 patients at the average 20 months after left ventricular aneurysmectomy. In 25 of these patients, monitoring was obtained before and after surgical intervention. After aneurysmectomy only 30% of all patients showed no ventricular premature contractions (VPC); 35% had few VPC and 35% demonstrated frequent VPC. In 16 patients (24%) VPC of Lown class III and IV were found. Only 7 of 25 patients of the group analyzed before and after aneurysmectomy improved by one or more Lown classes; ten patients remained in the same class and eight patients worsened. In 11 patients ventricular arrhythmia refractory to medical treatment was the indication for aneurysmectomy. There were three in-hospital deaths. Of the remaining eight patients, only two became free from ventricular ectopic activity, six continued to have multifocal VPC, two of them required repeat DC cardioversions and one died 3 years after aneurysmectomy because of sudden cardiac death. It is concluded that only a small percent of patients with left ventricular aneurysm become free from ventricular ectopic activity after aneurysmectomy. Result of aneurysmectomy for intractable ventricular arrhythmia is unpredictable.

References

1. Parkinson, J., Bedford, D.E., Thompson, W.A.R.: Cardiac aneurysm. Q. J. Med. *7*, 455 (1938)
2. Davis, R.W., Ebert, P.A.: Ventricular aneurysm. A clinica-pathologic correlation. Am. J. Cardiol. *29*, 1 (1972)
3. Couch, O.A.: Cardiac aneurysm with ventricular tachycardia and subsequent excision of aneurysm. Circulation *20*, 251 (1959)
4. Sharma, S.D., Ballantyne, F., Goldstein, S.: The relationship of ventricular asynergy in coronary artery disease to ventricular premature beats. Chest *66*, 358 (1974)
5. Schulze, R.A., Rouleau, J., Rigo, P., Bowers, S., Strauss, H.W., Pitt, B.: Ventricular arrhythmias in the late hospital phase of acute myocardial infarction. Relation to left ventricular function detected by gated cardiac blood pool scanning. Circulation *52*, 1006 (1975)

6. Schulze, R.A., Humphries, J.O., Griffith, L.S.C., Ducci, H., Achuff, S., Baird, M.G., Mellits, E.D., Pitt, B.: Left ventricular and coronary angiography anatomy. Relationship to ventricular irritability in the late hospital phase of acute myocardial infarction. Circulation *55*, 839 (1977)
7. Bethge, K.P., Bethge, H.C., Graf, A., van den Berg, E., Lichtlen, P.: Kammer-Arrhythmien bei chronisch koronarer Herzkrankheit. Z. Kardiol. *66*, 1 (1977)
8. Calvert, A., Lown, B., Gorlin, R.: Ventricular premature beats and anatomically defined coronary heart disease. Am. J. Cardiol. *39*, 627 (1977)
9. Lown, B., Wolf, M.: Approaches to sudden death from coronary heart disease. Circulation *44*, 130 (1971)
10. Ecker, R.R., Mullins, C.B., Grammer, J.C., Rea, W.J., Atkins, J.M.: Control of untractable ventricular tachycardia by coronary revescularization. Circulation *44*, 666 (1971)
11. Nakhjavan, E.K., Morse, D.P., Nichols, H.T.: Emergency aorto-coronary bypass: treatment of ventricular tachycardia due to ischemic heart disease. J.A.M.A. *216*, 2138 (1971)
12. Graham, A.F., Miller, D.C., Stinson, E.B., Daily, P.O., Fogarty, T.J., Harrison, D.C.: Surgical treatment of refractory life-threatening ventricular tachycardia. Am. J. Cardiol. *32*, 909 (1973)
13. Hunt, D., Sloman, G., Westlake, G.: Ventricular aneurysmectomy for recurrent tachycardia. Br. Heart J. *31*. 264 (1969)
14. Ritter, E.R.: Intractable ventricular tachycardia due to ventricular aneurysm with surgical cure. Ann. Intern. Med. *71*, 1155 (1969)
15. Thind, G.S., Blakemore, W.S., Zinsser, H.F.: Ventricular aneurysmectomy for the treatment of recurrent ventricular tachyarrhythmia. Am. J. Cardiol. *27*, 690 (1971)
16. Wardekar, A., Son, B., Gosaynie, C.D., Bercu, B.: Recurrent ventricular tachycardia successfully treated by excision of ventricular aneurysm. Chest *62*, 505 (1972)
17. Welch, T.G., Fontana, M.E., Vasko, J.S.: Aneurysmectomy for recurrent ventricular tachyarrhythmias. Am. Heart J. *85*, 685 (1973)
18. Kenaan, G., Mendez, A.M., Zubiate, P., Gray, R., Kay, J.H.: Surgery for ventricular tachycardia unresponsive to medical treatment. Chest *64*, 574 (1973)
19. Waxman, M.B., Wald, R.W., Goldman, B.S., Gunstensen, J.: Intractable ventricular tachyarrhythmias postmyocardial infarction. Circulation *51/52*, Suppl. II, 109 (1975)
20. Mundth, E.D., Buckley, M.J., De Sanctis, R.W., Daggett, W.M., Austen, W.G.: Surgical treatment of ventricular irritability. J. Thorac. Cardiovasc. Surg. *66*, 943 (1973)
21. Ricks, W.B., Winkle, R.A., Shumway, N.E., Harrison, D.C.: Surgical management of life-threatening ventricular arrhythmias in patients with coronary artery disease. Circulation *56*, 38 (1977)
22. Winkle, R.A., Alderman, E.L., Fitzgerald, J.W., Harrison, D.C.: Treatment of recurrent symptomatic ventricular tachycardia. Ann. Intern. Med. *85*, 1 (1976)
23. Giacchino, R., Moran, J.F., Schreiber, R., Johnson, S., Gunnar, R.: The problem of recurrent ventricular tachycardia in the presence of angiographically proven coronary artery disease. Circulation *51/52*, Suppl. II, 110 (1975)
24. Hazan, E., Block, G., Rioux, C., Louville, Y., Cirotteau, Y., Mathey, J.: Surgical treatment of aneurysm and segmental dyskinesia of the left ventricular wall after myocardial infarction. Am. J. Cardiol. *31*, 708 (1973)
25. Nitter-Hauge, S., Storstein, O.: Surgical treatment of recurrent ventricular tachycardia. Br. Heart J. *35*, 1132 (1973)
26. Sami, M., Charpin, D., Chabot, M., Bourassa, M.G.: Long-term follow-up of aneurysmectomy for recurrent ventricular tachycardia or fibrillation. Am. J. Cardiol. *39*, 269 (1977)
27. Wit, A.L., Bigger, J.T.: III The electrophysiology of lethal arrhythmias. Possible electrophysiological mechanisms for lethal arrhythmias accompanying myocardial ischemia and infarction. Circulation *51/52*, Suppl. III, 96 (1975)
28. Wittig, J.H., Boineau, J.P.: Surgical treatment of ventricular arrhythmias using epicardial, transmural and endocardial mapping. Ann. Thorac. Surg. *20*, 117 (1975)

29. Gallagher, J.J., Oldham, H.N., Wallace, A.G., Peter, R.H., Kasell, J.: Ventricular aneurysm with ventricular tachycardia. Report of a case with epicardial mapping and successful resection. Am. J. Cardiol. *35*, 292 (1975)
30. Fontaine, G., Frank, R., Guiraudon, G.: Surgical treatment of resistant reentrant ventricular tachycardia by ventriculotomy: a new application of epicardial mapping. Circulation *50*, Suppl. III, III - 82 (1974)
31. Spurrell, R.A.J., Yates, A.K., Thorburn, C.W., Sowton, D.E., Deuchar, D.C.: Surgical treatment of ventricular tachycardia after epicardial mapping studies. Br. Heart J. *37*, 115 (1975)
32. Moran, J.M., Scanlon, P.J., Nemickas, R., Pifarre, R.: Surgical treatment of postinfarction ventricular aneurysm. Ann. Thorac. Surg. *21*, 107 (1976)

Modification of Ventricular Function by Hypercontraction of the Surviving Heart Muscle Following Myocardial Infarction

P. Mathes, W. A. Baxley, A. Neiss, H. Sebening, and H. Blömer

During and after a myocardial infarction, variable amounts of left ventricular muscle are lost through the process of necrosis and replacement by scar tissue. The compensatory mechanisms that follow recovery from the infarct and the success of these mechanisms determines the overall functional status of the ventricle and, to a large part, the symptomatic status of the patient. In reviewing left ventricular cine angiograms of postinfarction patients, it appears that some ventricles exhibit a greater than usual degree of contraction in the noninfarcted portion as a compensation for poor contraction in the scarred portion of the ventricle. The purpose of this study was to further investigate this phenomenon of regional hypercontraction as a compensatory mechanism in postinfarct patients. The objectives were to quantitate the extent of these hypercontracting segments by angiographic techniques, to determine their incidence and significance, and to evaluate the conditions under which they develop.

To accomplish these objectives, angiograms and clinical data were reviewed on a consecutive series of patients with coronary disease. Sixty-nine patients were studied because of persisting symptoms 6-12 months after a single documented transmural infarction. Studies were contrasted with those of a separate group of 25 patients who were studied for chest pain, which turned out to be normal. The patients all had left ventricular cineangiography in right and left anterior oblique projections, with quantitative determination of volumes and ejection fraction as well as regional analysis of wall motion. All had coronary angiography and quantitative determination of stenotic lesions.

Figure 1 shows an example of a normal control left ventriculogram in the right anterior oblique projection. For regional wall motion analysis, a radial reference system was utilized with superimposition of the midpoint of the long axis at enddiastole and endsystole. Segments 180° and 210° were omitted as they reflected primarily the aortic and mitral valve segments. The shaded area in the lower section represents the range of normal motion in terms of mean velocity of radial shortening, consisting of the mean value $\pm$ 1 S.D. derived from the 25 normal controls.

The segments were tabulated as either normal, hypocontractile, or hypercontractile, according to whether they were within, below, or above 1 standard deviation of the mean of the normal control values.

Figure 2 ist an example of a patient demonstrating hypercontraction of the anterior wall following an inferior infarction.

The results of the study revealed that 37 of 69 patients (54%) had hypercontracting segments ranging up to six in number. Thus, over half of the patient population exhibited this phenomenon. All of the patients had hypocontracting segments, as would be expected by their histories of infarction. These ranged up to 18 of the 30° segments,

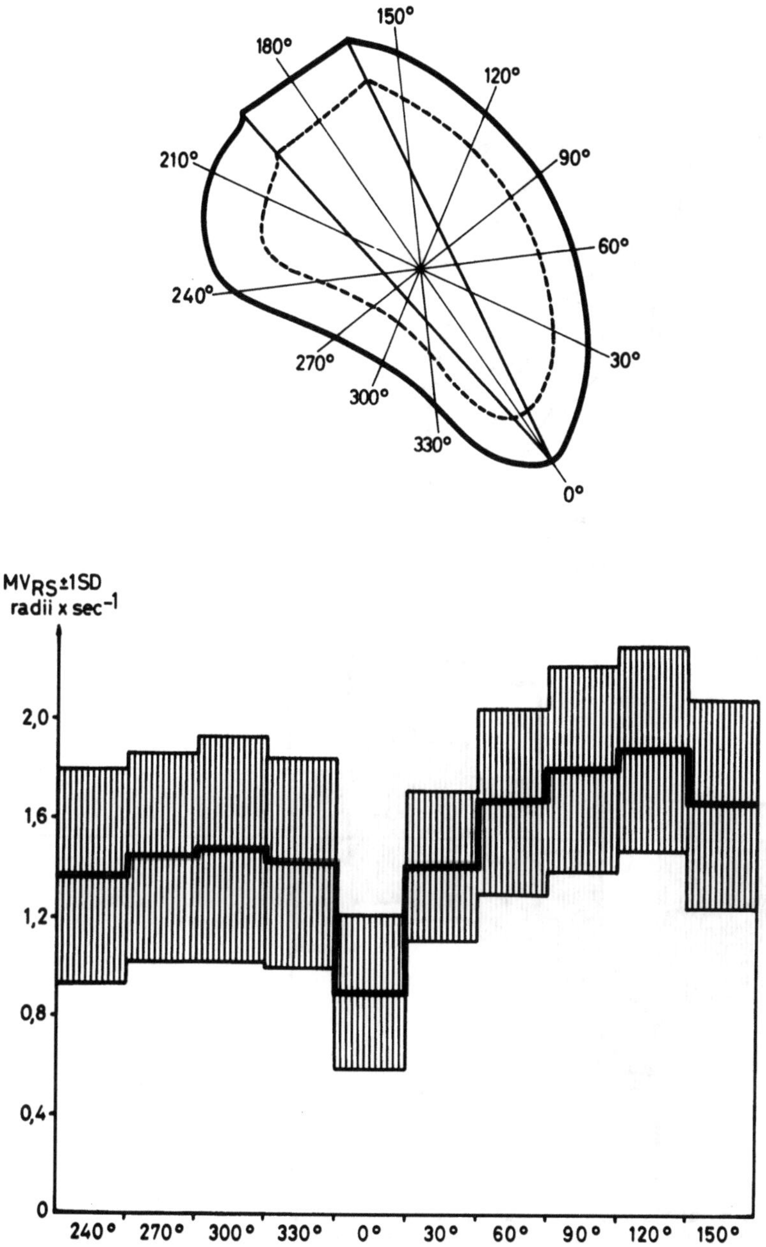

Fig. 1. Schematic drawing of a normal ventricular silhouette, superimposed at the midpoint of the long axis, the 0-reference point of the radial motion analysis. *Shaded area*: the normal range of motion (mean $\pm$ 1 S.D.)

which would represent global hypokinesis. Coronary lesions were tabulated as more or less than 75% stenoses, and by this criterion 16 (23%) of the patients had multivessel disease; the rest single vessel disease.

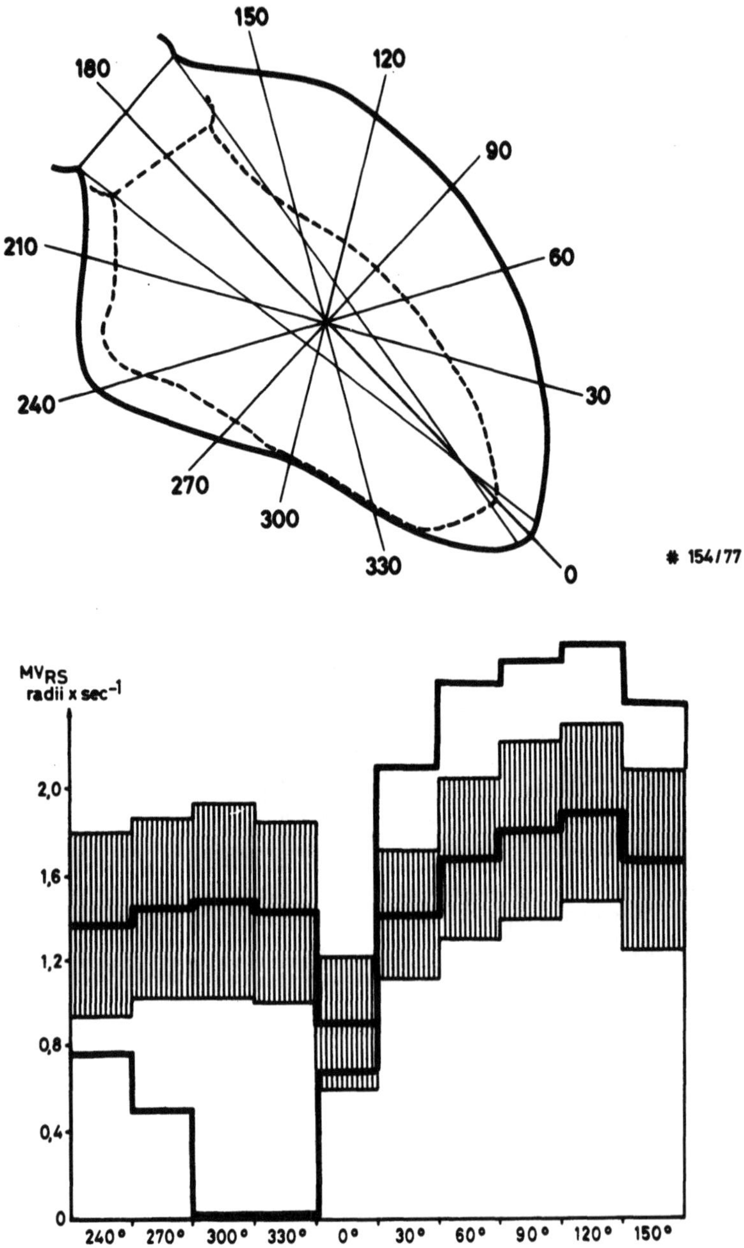

Fig. 2. Example of hypercontraction of the anterior wall following an inferior infarct. Akinesis as well as hyperkinesis are clearly evident in relation to the normal range of motion (*shaded area*)

Of 37 patients with hypercontraction, all but two had ejection fractions above 45%, whereas of the 32 without hypercontraction, 20 (62%) had low ejection fractions. For any given number of poorly contracting segments, those patients with hypercontraction were able to maintain a better ejection fraction than those without. However, none of the patients with more than 12 hypocontractile segments exhibited hypercontraction. Twelve segments represent two-thirds of the ventricular perimeter. One might suspect that when this extent of poor contraction is exceeded, the work load on the remaining myocardium is so great that hypercontraction can not be generated.

The patients without hypercontracting segments tended to have lower ejection fractions and larger enddiastolic volumes than those with hypercontracting segments. The difference in ejection fraction between the two groups was most marked in those patients with enddiastolic volumes greater than 150 ml. Most patients of both types with volumes less than 150 ml had a normal ejection fraction. However, with larger volumes, there was greater scattering of ejection fractions. Of interest is the difference between these two groups of patients with the larger volumes. Thus, of the ten patients with hypercontracting segments with these large volumes, only one had a low ejection fraction. In contrast, of the 21 patients with enlarged volumes, but without hypercontracting segments, 15 (71%) had depressed ejection fractions. Thus, hypercontracting segments appeared to be most important in maintaining ejection fractions in those patients with enlarged enddiastolic volumes.

Summary

Sixty-nine patients had quantitative biplane cine left ventriculography and coronary angiography 6-12 months post myocardial infarction, to investigate the phenomenon of regional hypercontraction. This hyperfunction was found to occur commonly, that is in 54% of late postinfarct patients. It occurs primarily in the absence of coronary disease to the surviving myocardium, if less than 2/3 of the ventricle is hypokinetic. Finally, regional hypercontraction is an important compensatory mechanism in maintaining overall ventricular function, particularly in the setting of left ventricular enlargement.

Factors Influencing Results in Surgery of Postinfarction Ventricular Aneurysms

R. Rivera and J. L. Delcan

Our knowledge of the physiopathology of postinfarction ventricular aneurysm and akinesis has progressed markedly in recent years as a result of the experience gained from the study of patients before and after surgery, and also as a result of a better understanding of the mechanism and metabolism of normal and abnormal cardiac contraction. As a consequence, the results of surgery have improved both in terms of operative mortality and postoperative long-term survival and from the point of view of postoperative ventricular performance.

In this paper we have surveyed a series of 66 consecutive patients operated on for postinfarction ventricular aneurysms. Factors influencing the progressive decline of mortality from 33% before 1975 to 3.2% in the last 31 patients and the reduction of postoperative ventricular volumes to near normal values were also considered.

Material and Methods

From 1973 through April 1977, 66 patients underwent resection of left ventricular aneurysm in our unit. Indications for surgery were based in part on preoperative symptoms, as well as, on pathologic anatomy. Angina pectoris and congestive heart failure were the most common preoperative symptoms, and either singly or combined were found in more than 88% of our cases. Three patients had ventricular arrhythmias and four had suffered previous embolic episodes. In 57% of the patients in this series ventriculography had disclosed the presence of thrombus in the left ventricular cavity. In one patient a partial rupture of the ventricular wall was demonstrated with the development of a false aneurysm in pericardium.

Location of the aneurysm is shown in Table 1: In 97% of the cases the aneurysm was localized in the anteroseptal wall of the ventricle, but in nine patients the septum was not involved: In one case there was isolated involvement of the septum, and in another the aneurysms was localized in the posterolateral wall. This means that in 84% of our patients there was involvement of the septum[1].

Myocardial Protection

To accomplish aneurysmectomy, we used cardiopulmonary bypass and crossclamping of the aorta under conventional hypothermia in the initial 11 patients. Later, in 197 patients we realized simultaneously the importance of improving myocardial protection and that the protection afforded by aortic crossclamping to avoid the hazard of

[1] Since this review was completed, of 5 additional patients we operated on, 2 had aneurysm located in the posterodiaphragmatic wall of the left ventricle.

Table 1. Location and extension

		No.	%
Anterolateral wall		64	96.9
A) Alone	9		
B) With septum	45[a]		
C) With septum and RV	10[a]		
Septum (alone)		1[a]	1.5
Posterolateral		1	1.5

[a]Septal involvement = 56 cases (84.8%)

emboli, was more theoretical than practical, because with the aortic valve closed, the exit of thrombi to the aortic root is more difficult than with the aortic valve open after crossclamping the aorta. Thus, through 1975 and 1976 we operated under general hypothermia at 24°C and deep local hypothermia induced by the method of Shumway [1]. Cold saline at 4°C was poured into and aspirated from the pericardial well, maintaining a continuous flow during the performance of the aneurysmectomy and the period of cardiac ischemia. Aortic crossclamping was used only in cases of associated revascularization in order to provide a better exposure of the left coronary artery branches to perform distal graft anastomoses. More recently, in 1977, we have induced cardiac hypothermia by perfusing the aortic root with 1000 cc of cold Ringer-lactate at 4°C after crossclamping the aorta.

Associated Revascularization

In all patients we tried to revascularize the arteries with significant stenosis by establishing coronary artery bypass grafts (CABG) using saphenous vein, with the exception of the artery involved in the production of the aneurysm. In anteroseptal aneurysms no particular care was taken to preserve the distal portion of the left anterior descending coronary artery (LAD) which after aneurysmectomy, was usually included within the suture line. However, in cases of apical aneurysm in which the basal zone of the septum was not involved, the LAD was grafted in order to revascularize septal and diagonal branches not involved in the aneurysmectomy. In the common cases, we paid special attention to revascularize the lateral wall of the left ventricle by grafting diagonal branches and branches of the circumflex artery.

In 28 cases we performed 2 triple grafts, 7 double grafts and 19 single grafts. The right coronary artery was grafted in 14 cases, the circumflex branches in 14 cases, the diagonal in 4 cases, and the LAD only in 7 cases.

Surgical Technique

After the report from Stoney et al. [2] in 1973 describing the technique of exclusion of the septum in the treatment of ventricular aneurysms, we tried to adapt ventricular resection to the extension and location of the akinetic area.

To excise anteroseptal aneurysms a longitudinal ventriculotomy is made 1 cm to the left of the LAD. In the usual situation, when the aneurysm involves the anterolateral wall of the ventricle and the anterior portion of the septum (Fig. 1) the ventriculotomy is closed using three rows of sutures reinforced with teflon strips advancing the lateral edge of the myocardium down to the junction of the scar

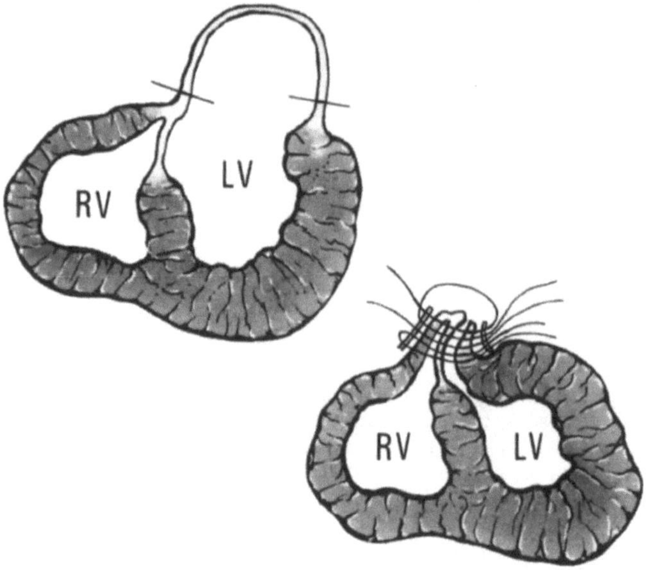

Fig. 1. Aneurismatic resection and ventricular reconstruction in cases in which the aneurysm involves the anterolateral wall of the left ventricle and the anterior portion of the intraventricular septum

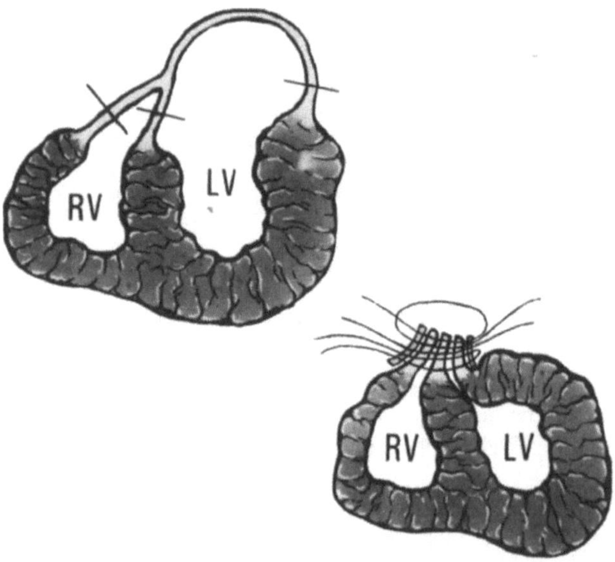

Fig. 2. Aneurismatic resection and ventricular reconstruction in cases in which the aneurysm involves the anterolateral wall of the left ventricle, the anterior portion of the septum, and the anterior wall of the right ventricle

and the normal myocardial tissue in the septum. In this manner, the diseased portion of the septum is included in the closure and excluded from the left ventricular cavity.

When the anterior wall of the right ventricle is also involved (Fig. 2), the resection of the aneurysm implies the opening of both ventricles. The anterior portion of the septum can be excised and the repair is completed by joining the edges of these three structures: right ventricle, septum, and left ventricle.

In the rare instances in which the aneurysm and mural thrombus are limited to the interventricular septum (Fig. 3), it is not neccessary to excise any portion of the free ventricular wall of the left ventricle. The thrombus is then removed, as completely as possible, through a longitudinal left ventriculotomy. Closure is accomplished through suturing the left edge of the ventricular wall down to the junction of the scar and the healthy muscle in the septum with the technique previously described.

In cases of inferior ventricular aneurysms (Fig. 4) surgery is performed as in the anteroseptal aneurysms, but in the posterior wall of the heart, which is rotated superiorly. A longitudinal ventriculotomy is made parallel and to the left of the interventricular posterior coronary artery (IVP) and the resection is extended to the left with the posterior papillary muscle as the lateral limit. In a similar way, closure is effected by suturing the border of the left ventricle to the junction of the posterior scar and the anterior healthy muscle of the septum.

Conventional aneurysmectomy is reserved for cases of true anterolateral, lateral, or posterobasal aneurysms in which the diseased myocardium is confined to the free wall of the left ventricle (Fig. 5). In such cases the LAD is preserved and can be revascularized if necessary.

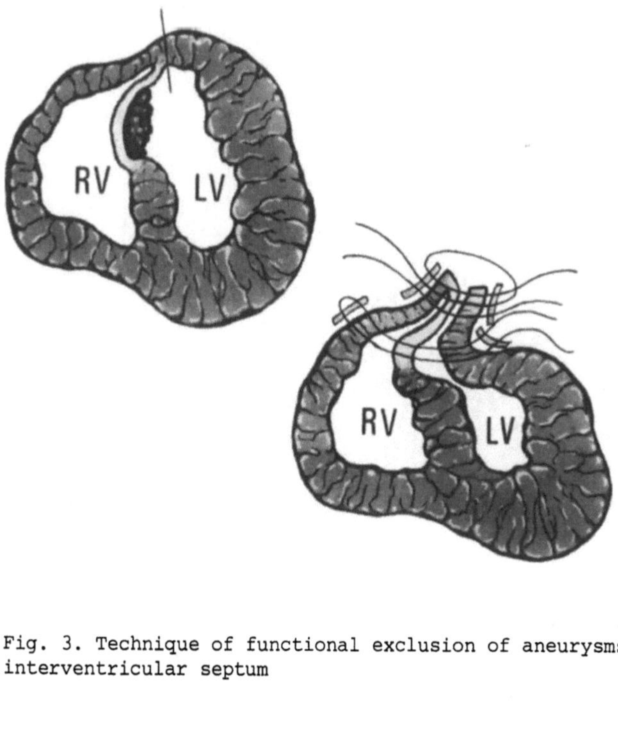

Fig. 3. Technique of functional exclusion of aneurysms located exclusively in the interventricular septum

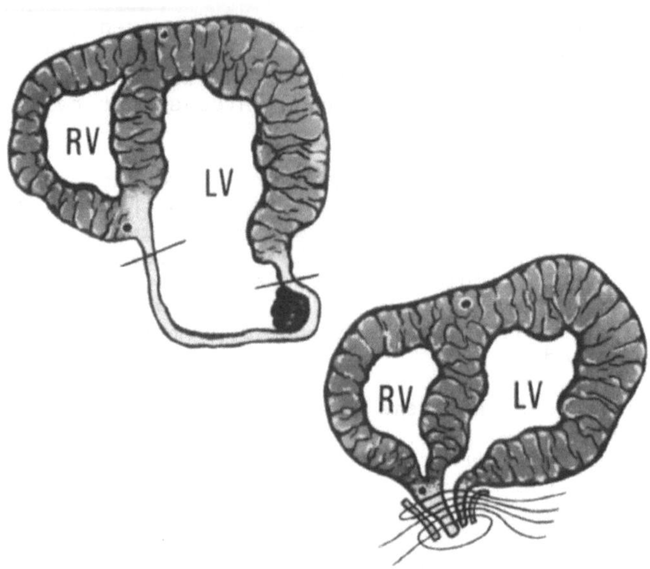

Fig. 4. Technique of resection and ventricular reconstruction in cases in which the aneurysm involves the diaphragmatic wall of the left ventricle and the posterior portion of the septum

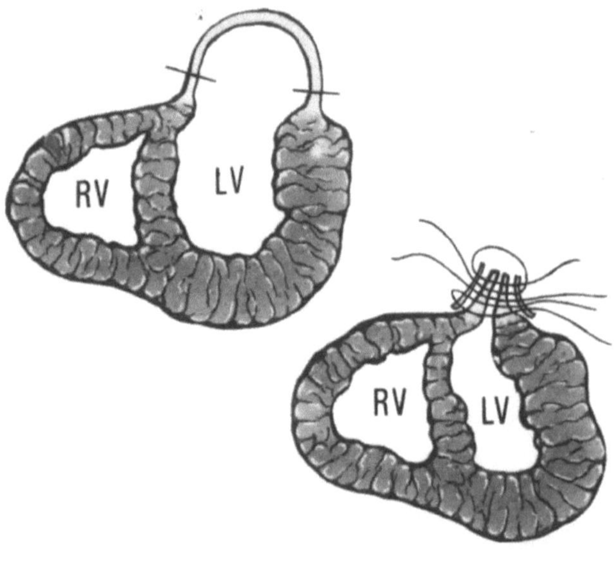

Fig. 5. Aneurismatic resection and reconstruction of the left ventricle in cases in which the septum is not involved

Catheterization Studies

We performed preoperative cardiac catheterization in all patients and postoperatively we studied, at the time in which this report was prepared, 36 cases. The average interval between operation and the second catheterization was 3.6 months.

Pre- and postoperative ventriculograms were compared. Each ventriculogram in RAO projection was evaluated by tracing a superimposed systolic and diastolic frame from 35 mm cinefilm projected in a Tagarno projector. The surfaces of the pre- and postoperative enddiastolic and endsystolic tracings were measured and the pre- and postoperative enddiastolic and endsystolic volumes were calculated by the Dodge method. The contractile area and volume of the left ventricle were also estimated and compared with the area and volume determined after the operation. Ejection fraction was also calculated preoperatively for the whole left ventricular cavity and for its contractile zone and compared with that which was calculated postoperatively.

Results

Hospital mortality in our series was 12% (8 patients). A chronological analysis of this mortality (Table 2) shows a progressive reduction from 50% and 30% in 1973 and 1974 to 5% in 1976 and 1977. We believe that this improvement resulted from two main factors: namely, better myocardial protection during the procedure and associated myocardial revascularization by coronary artery bypass graft.

The influence of the method of myocardial protection in the operative mortality rate is shown in Table 3. In the group of 11 patients in which the aorta was crossclamped under conventional hypothermia (28°C), five died (four from low cardiac output). In the group of 55 patients operated under deep local hypothermia in which aortic crossclamping was used only to perform distal graft anastomosis to the left coronary branches, the mortality rate was only 5% (P <0.01).

Table 2. Hospital mortality (0-30 days)

Year	Cases	Mortality
1973	2	1 = 50%
1974	13	4 = 30%
1975	20	2 = 10%
1976	20	1 = 5%
1977	11	0
Total	66	8 = 12%

Table 3. Myocardial protection vs mortality

Method	Cases	Mortality
Aortic clamping under gral. hypothermia (28°C)	11 (1[a])	5 = 45%
Deep local hypothermia with or without aortic clamping	55 (27[a])	3 = 5%

[a]Cases with coronary artery bypass graft P <0.01.

Table 4. Revascularization vs mortality

	Cases	Mortality
Aneurysmectomy only	38	8 = 21%
Aneurysmectomy + CABG[a]	28	0
CABG x 3 = 2 cases		
CABG x 2 = 7 cases		
CABG x 1 = 19 cases		

[a]Coronary artery bypass graft $P < 0.025$.

Table 5. Pre- and postaneurysmectomy left ventricular volumes[a]

	Preop	Postop	Reduction	Normal
Enddiastolic volume	282 ± 124	190 ± 54	92 = 33%	175
Endsystolic volume	179 ± 111	91 ± 41	88 = 50%	75
Ejection fraction	0.38 ± 11	0.53 ± 10		

[a]Mean values of 36 cases in ml.

The influence of associated revascularization on the mortality rate is shown in Table 4. There was no mortality in the group of cases in which coronary artery bypass grafting was associated with aneurysmectomy. The total mortality of eight cases was encountered in the group of patients in which aneurysmectomy was not complimented by myocardial revascularization ($P < 0.025$).

Table 5 shows the results of the catheterization studies in 36 cases. There is a mean reduction of 27% in enddiastolic area (from 138 ± 36 cm^2 to 101 ± 18 cm^2) and of 38% in the endsystolic area (from 105 ± 35 cm^2 to 66 ± 19 cm^2). Aneurysmectomy reduced mean enddiastolic volume 33% (from 282 ± 124 cc to 190 ± 54 cc) and mean endsystolic volume was reduced 49% (from 179 ± 111 cc to 91 ± 41 cc).

These postoperative values are very close to the upper level of normality in our laboratory (175 cc and 75 cc) for enddiastolic and endsystolic left ventricular volumes.

The ejection fraction increased after aneurysmectomy from 38 ± 11 to a practically normal mean value of 53 ± 10 postoperatively.

In general there is a good correlation between the postoperative values of area, volume, and ejection fraction and the estimate made preoperatively of the contractile zone of the left ventricle (Fig. 6).

The left ventricular enddiastolic pressure was obtained before and after repair in 36 patients. A reduction was noted in 18 patients and no changes or a slight increase was recorded in 18 cases. The mean enddiastolic left ventricular pressure was 17.8 mmHg preoperatively and 20.5 mmHg postoperatively.

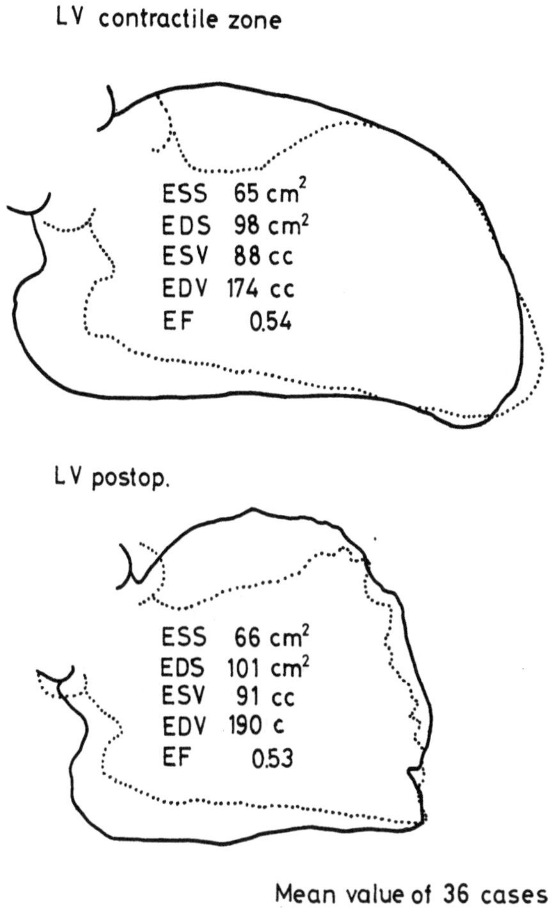

Fig. 6. Systolic (*dotted line*) and diastolic (*continuous line*) tracings of pre- and postoperative ventriculograms in RAO projections. There is a great similarity between the mean values for the preoperative contractile zone, shown above, and the postoperative whole left ventricular cavity, shown below

Discussion

Formerly, paradoxical movement of the left ventricular wall was considered the main factor causing impaired left ventricular performance. At present, experimental and clinical studies have shown that in the area of the myocardium where wall motion is absent, insufficient tension is developed to accomplish fiber shortening, with the result that fiber shortening and tension development in the remaining areas of the ventricle must increase to maintain an adequate stroke volume. When 20%-25% of the left ventricular wall becomes akinetic, ventricular dilatation must ensue if the limits of fiber shortening of the healthy muscle are not to be exceeded.

When ventricular dilatation occurs, as a consequence of the former mechanism, the physiopathology of the left ventricular function can be explained purely on mechanical basis by Laplace's law of membranes. Thus, for a ventricle twice as big as another, four times as much tension must be developed within its wall to maintain the same pressure [3].

This additional requirement in wall tension is reflected in additional myocardial oxygen requirement which impaired coronary circulation may not be able to meet. Surgical excision permits the maintenance of the intraventricular pressure with less wall tension and, at the same time, improves ventricular performance and relieves angina. Adequate revascularization of the rest of the ventricle, when needed, must logically ensure a better prognosis in terms of control of angina and recovery of cardiac function.

According to these principles, the surgical treatment of postinfarction ventricular aneurysm and akinesis should realize the maximal reduction of the different radii of the left ventricular cavity, by excision or exclusion of all akinetic areas. Conventional anterior aneurysmectomy confined excision to the diseased myocardium in the free wall of the left ventricle. However, in most anterior aneurysms of the left ventricle the septum is involved, so it becomes necessary to admit that this conventional procedure realizes only a partial aneurysmectomy (Fig. 7).

Anatomically, the performance of total aneurysmectomy with a technique adapted to the location and the extension of the aneurysms seems justified. From the standpoint of the physiopathology of postinfarction ventricular aneurysm, the excision or the exclusion of the whole fibrous scar solves the problem if we admit the mechanism of the akinesis, as well as if we consider the mechanism of the paradoxical pulsation. The operation eliminates the nonelastic sac and reduces the size of the ventricular cavity, thus decreasing the dissipation of energy. As less wall tension is needed to generate the same amount of intracavitary pressure, oxygen consumption is reduced and myocardial metabolism is improved.

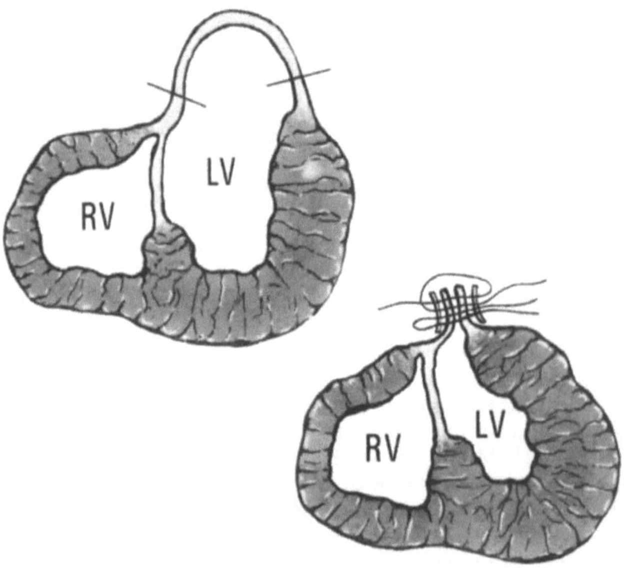

Fig. 7. Conventional technique of aneurysmectomy. In anteroseptal aneurysms the excision is confined to the free wall of the left ventricle leaving in place the involved portion of the septum. (*RV* Right ventricle. *LV* Left ventricle)

In any case, since the availability of aortocoronary bypass graft surgery, its simultaneous employment in association with ventricular aneurysm resection seems justified in order, to revascularize coronary arteries not directly involved in the aneurysm formation and to improve the contractility of zones of chronically ischemic, but viable myocardium, around the area of totally infarcted and fibrotic muscle.

Conclusions

In surgery of postinfarction ventricular aneurysms, in order to obtain adequate functional results, it is necessary to adapt the technique of aneurysmectomy to the anatomic location and to the extension of the fibrotic scar. That implies that in most of the patients (in which there is septal involvement) it is necessary to exclude functionally the akinetic zone of the septum.

Surgical mortality will be improved if adequate myocardial protection is used and revascularization with CABG is associated.

The myocardial revascularization of the residual left ventricular walls and the restoration of near normal left ventricular volumes make it possible to expect in these patients a healthier and longer survival than in those, in which only conventional aneurysmectomy was performed, and associated revascularization was not accomplished.

References

1. Hurley, E.J., Lower, R.R., Dong, E.Jr., Pillsbury, R.C., Shumway, N.E.: Clinical experience with local hypothermia in elective cardias arrest. J. Thorac. Cardiovasc. Surg. *47*, 51 (1964)
2. Stoney, W.S., Alford, W.C., Burrus, G.R., Thomas, C.S.: Repair of anteroseptal ventricular aneurysm. Ann. Thorac. Surg. *15*, 394 (1973)
3. Ellis, F.H.: Surgery for chronic asynergy of the left ventricle: A current appraisal. Surgery *70*, 801 (1971)

Functional Analysis of the Left Ventricle with Postinfarction Aneurysm

K. L. Neuhaus, K. Bornikoel, and H. J. Schrage

During the past 20 years, thousands of postinfarction aneurysms have been resected. Nevertheless, indication for surgery and the effects of aneurysmectomy still remain a matter of controversy [3,4,5]. A problem which contributes greatly to this debate is the functional analysis of the left ventricle with aneurysms [2].

Enddiastolic volume, ejection fraction, and the velocity of circumferential fiber shortening have been shown to adequately describe ventricular function in the normally shaped ventricle. In the left ventricle with aneurysm, however, these parameters are only loosely correlated to ventricular function, because they are strongly dependent on the relative size of the aneurysm. That means, a large enddiastolic volume and a low ejection fraction in most cases indicate a large aneurysm and not a poor ventricular function.

Enddiastolic pressure and cardiac output are not directly related to ventricular dimensions, therefore, the validity of these parameters for the assessment of ventricular function is not affected by the aneurysm. Furthermore, in contrast to ventricular volume and ejection fraction, filling pressures and cardiac output can be measured easily during exercise.

Overall function of the left ventricle with aneurysm primarily depends on the functional state of the contracting myocardium. The contractile area, which has been used in the analysis of the left ventricle with aneurysm, is defined as the relation between contracting and noncontracting parts of the ventricle, that means, it is an expression of the relative size of the aneurysm and not an index of myocardial function.

The ejection fraction of the contracting part is certainly a very good parameter of its myocardial function [5]. However, we have found that this ejection fraction can be determined accurately only in ventricles with an aneurysm of the saccular type. If the aneurysm presents more as a large akinesis, it can be defined accurately only during systole. Therefore, we have decided to measure only the diameters of the contracting ventricle and calculate the corresponding velocity of circumferential fiber shortening V_{CF}. From these diameters, wall thickness and ventricular pressure wall stress can be calculated as an stimate of myocardial load conditions [2].

Fifty-seven patients with a left ventricular aneurysm were investigated. As to the clinical signs of heart failure, 19 patients were in NYHA class I or II, 29 were in class III, and 9 patients in class IV. Enddiastolic volumes in class II and III were almost identical, only the patients in class IV had significantly larger volumes (Fig. 1). The same was found for the ejection fraction and V_{CF}, there was no difference between classes II and III, and significantly lower values for ejection fraction and V_{CF} were only found in class IV. A statistically significant difference between functional classes II and III

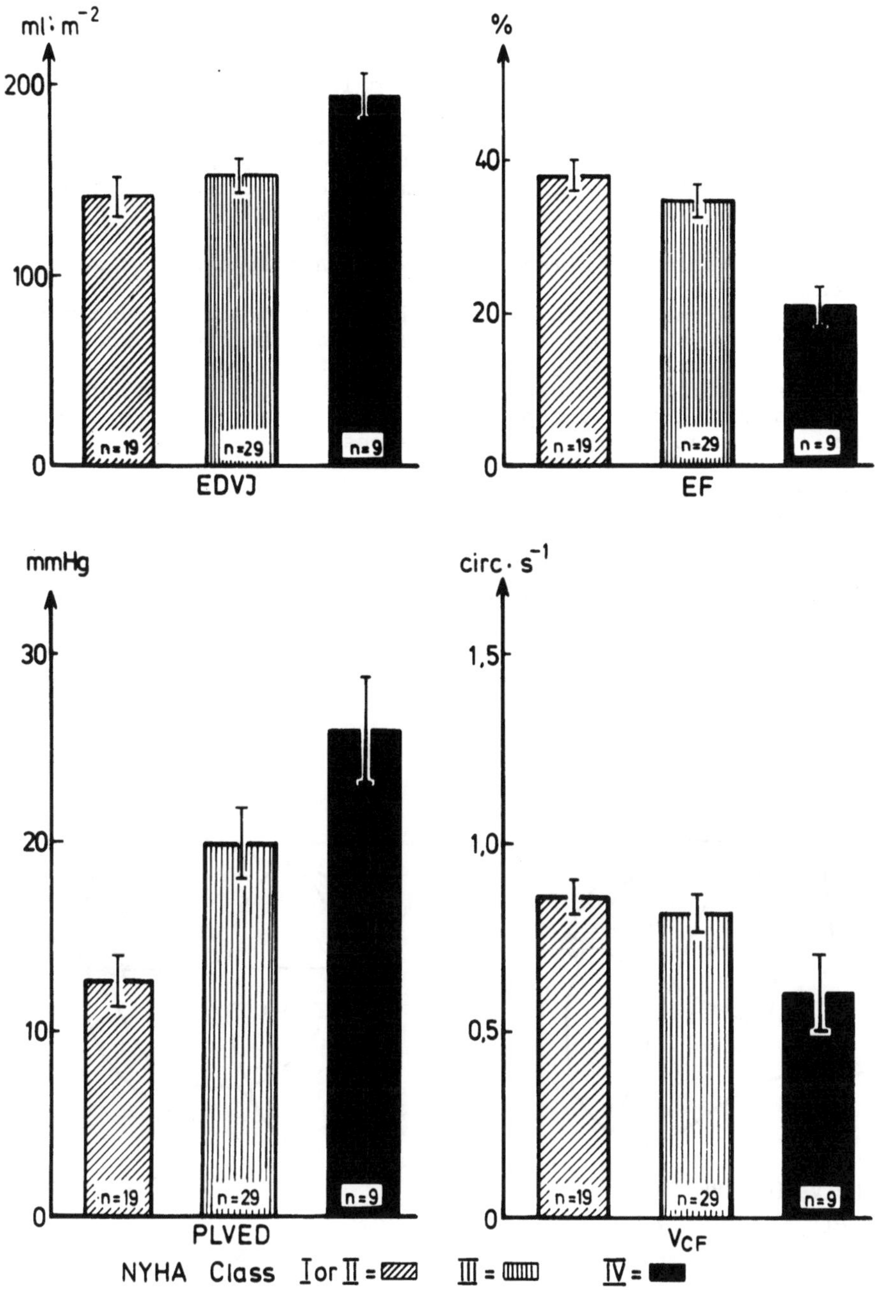

Fig. 1. Left ventricular function and clinical classification of heart failure in 57 patients with aneurysm. *EDV* enddiastolic volume; *EF* ejection fraction (biplane); *PLVED* enddiastolic pressure; *VCF* mean velocity of fiber shortening in the contracting part of the left ventricle. *Vertical bars* ± SEM

was only found for left ventricular filling pressure; all parameters which were related to dimensions were significantly different only in class IV.

In 21 of these patients a more detailed functional analysis was performed by calculations of wall stress.
The typical contours of a ventricle with aneurysm of the anterior wall are shown in Fig. 2. Wall stress was calculated frame by frame during one cardiac cycle from the mean diameter of the contracting part, thickness of the posterior wall, and ventricular pressure, which was measured simultaneously. From these diameters V_{CF} was calculated also. Wall stress in the aneurysm was calculated in a similar way, using wall thickness of the lateral free wall.

In Fig. 3 the variation of stress during the cardiac cycle is shown in a typical example.
The variation of stress during ejection in the contracting myocardium is quite similar in shape as it is in the normal ventricle. Peak stress is reached early during ejection, then falls rapidly with decreasing diameters and increasing wall thickness. In the aneurysm, wall stress is much higher and parallels ventricular pressure, because there is almost no change in dimensions.

Mean values of stress in 21 patients are presented in Fig. 4. At enddiastole, wall stress in the contracting myocardium on the average is moderately elevated, systolic stress both early and late during ejection are in the normal range. That means, myocardial afterload in the contracting segments is usually normal. At least in the resting state, the aneurysm does not lead to a myocardial overload in terms of stress.

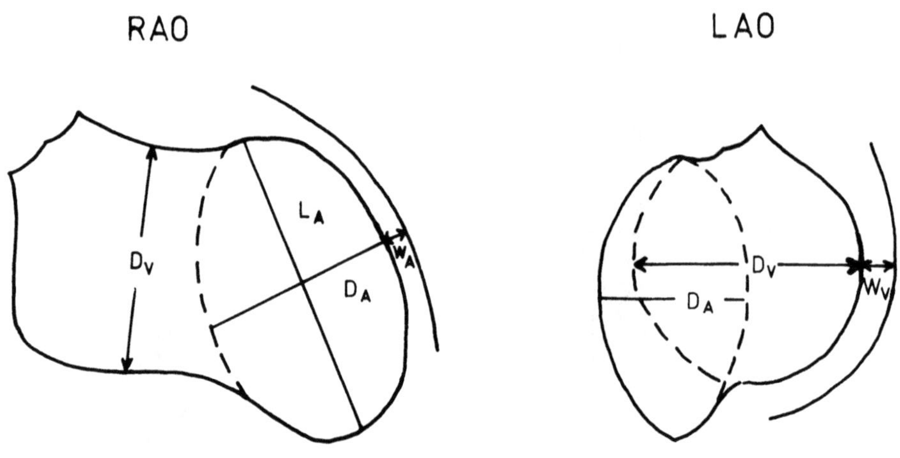

$$\sigma_V = f(PLV, \bar{D}_V, W_V)$$
$$\sigma_A = f(PLV, \bar{D}_A, L_A, W_A)$$

Fig. 2. Dimensions and calculations of stress in the contracting part (σV) and the aneurysmal wall (σA); $\bar{D}v$ mean diameter of the contracting part in RAO and LAO projection; *WV* the lateral free wall (aneurysm); *DA* and *LA* short and long axis of the aneurysm; *PLV* left ventricular pressure. Explanation see text

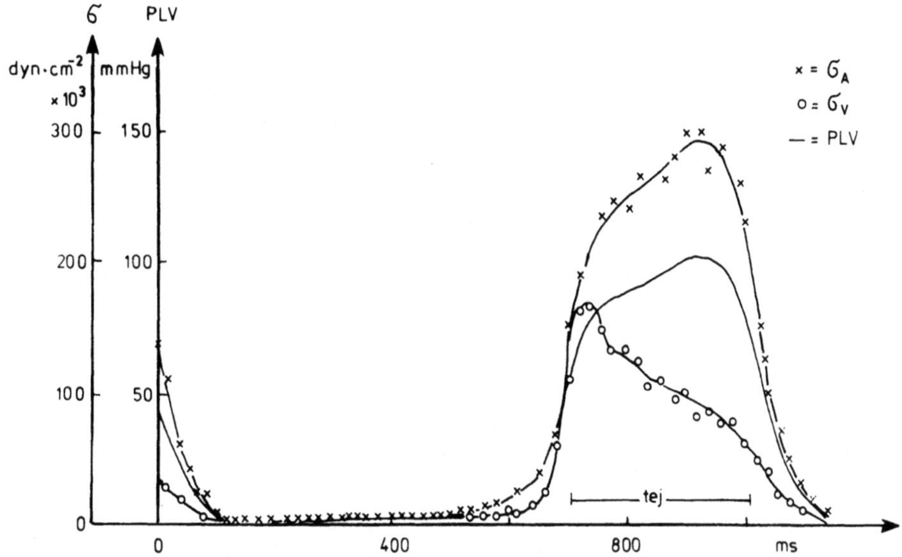

Fig. 3. Wall stress in the contracting myocardium (*o*) and in the aneurysm (*x*) during the cardiac cycle. *tej* ejection time. Explanation see text

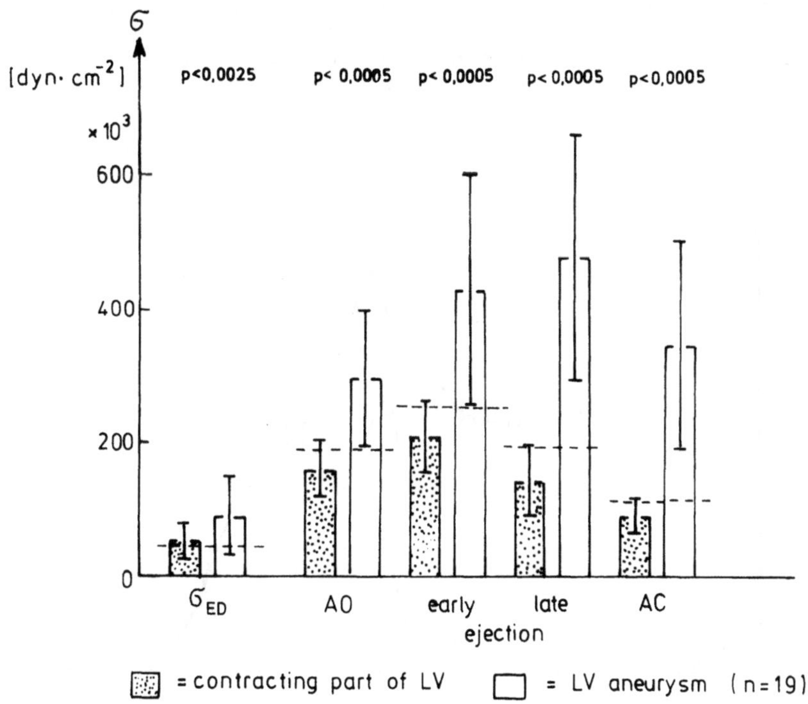

Fig. 4. Mean values of stress in 19 patients with left ventricular aneurysm (*x*). *Vertical bars* ± 1 S.D.; *horizontal broken lines* upper limit of normal range. At enddiastole (σ_{ed}), aortic valve opening (*AO*), early and late ejection, and at aortic valve closure (*AC*)

In the aneurysmal wall, stress is consistantly higher throughout the cardiac cycle, and it is extremely high during systole. It must be mentioned that these are not stresses in the thin wall of an aneurysm of the saccular type. These stresses are measured in aneurysms which present as a large akinesis. Quite the same pattern of wall stress has been found in the akinetic anterior wall due to acute myocardial infarction.
This systolic overload probably contributes to the definite loss of function, and may be to the enlargement of necrosis in the early stages of myocardial infarction.
Further analysis of myocardial function has been done as follows: From the curves in Fig. 5, myocardial preload can be estimated from enddiastolic stress, myocardial afterload from systolic stress, and velocity of fiber shortening from the diameter curve [2].

From mean stress during ejection and mean velocity of diameter shortening, an estimate of systolic myocardial power can be derived. Myocardial functional state can be defined by plotting mean systolic power versus diastolic stress (Fig. 6).

The normal ventricle works at low enddiastolic stress and systolic power; that is at the lower left. Most of the patients in class I or II had normal myocardial preload and afterload at rest, thus falling into the normal range.
These patients probably should not be operated because the aneurysm apparently does not significantly stress the contracting myocardium. The patients at the upper left were also in clinical class II. Already at rest an increased myocardial power is developed which can be maintained only by a corresponding increase in preload. In these cases the aneurysm should be resected to avoid a progressive deterioration of myocardial function by the chronic overload.

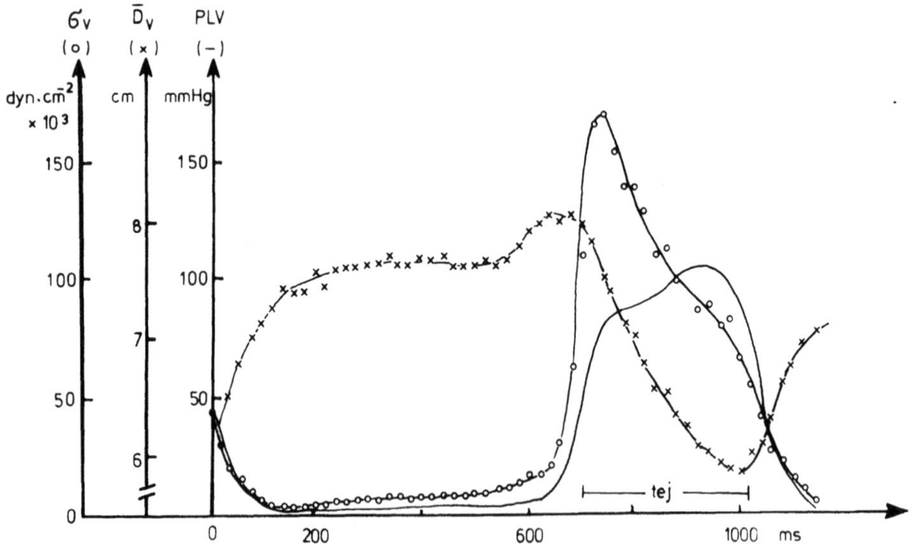

Fig. 5. Variation of stress in the contracting myocardium (σV), mean diameter of the contracting part of the left ventricle ($\bar{D}v$), and ventricular pressure during the cardiac cycle

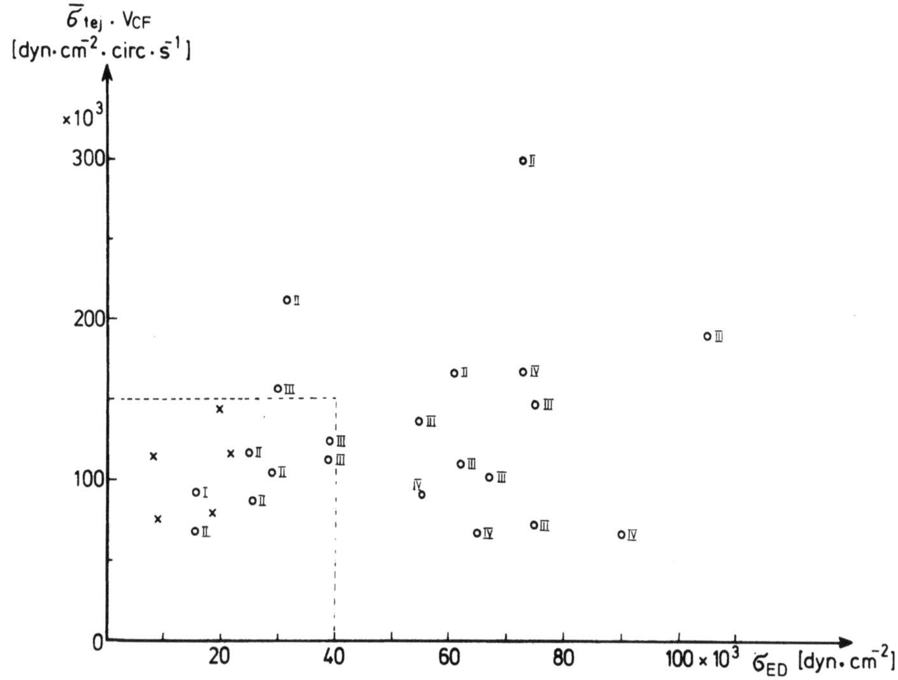

Fig. 6. Myocardial function of the contracting part of the left ventricle and classification of failure (NYHA) σ_{tej} mean stress during ejection; *VcF* mean velocity of fiber shortening in the contracting part; σ_{tej} x *VcF* estimate of systolic myocardial power; σ_{ed} enddiastolic stress. *Crosses* normal left ventricle; *circles* ventricles with aneurysm. *I-IV* NYHA classification of heart failure; *broken lines* limits of the normal range. Explanation see text

Patients with heart failure at reast usually have very high filling pressures, accordingly, enddiastolic stress in the contracting myocaridum is consistantly elevated, while systolic power is normal or even reduced; myocardial function is severely depressed.
In these cases, favorable results of aneurysmectomy may not be expected, because resection per se will not improve myocardial function.
Good clinical results have been observed in patients with normal or slightly increased systolic power and elevated preload.

As far as it can be said from the first ten of these patients, who meanwhile have been operated, such a detailed analysis of myocardial function allows for an improved prediction of the surgical result. In some cases, however, the clinical results have been unexpected; they might have been influenced by the amount of contracting myocardium which was left by incomplete resection or unknown geometrical reasons. These questions deserve further study, including measurements of overall and regional LV function during exercise, before we can predict which patient will benefit from aneurysmectomy.

References

1. Kitamura, S., Echevarria, M., Kay, J.H., Krohn, B.G., Redington, J.V., Mendez, A., Zubiate, P., Dünne, E.F.: Left ventricular performance before and after removal of non contractile area. Circulation *45*, 1005 (1972)
2. Neuhaus, K.L., Bornikoel, K., Rönsberg, D., Schrage, F.-J., Loogen, F.: Funktionsanalyse des linken Ventrikels mit Aneurysma. Cardiology *67*, 335 (1978)
3. Schäfer, G.E., Kober, G., Becker, H.-J., Guldner, N., Kaltenbach, M.: Die Resektion von Ventrikelwand-Aneurysmen. Dtsch. Med. Wochenschr. *101*, 734 (1976)
4. Schönbeck, M., Senning, A., Rutishauser, W., Lichtlen, P., Krayenbühl, H.P., Maier, W., Müller, M., Wellauer, J.: Der Einfluß der Aneurysmektomie auf die linksventrikuläre Funktion. Dtsch. Med. Wochenschr. *100*, 77 (1975)
5. Trieb, G., Schmidt, H., Sigwart, U., Mertens, H.M., Gleichmann, U., Borst, H.G.: Einfluß der Aneurysmektomie auf die linksventrikuläre Belastungshämodynamik. Herz/Kreisl. *9*, 511 (1977)

4. Anesthesia and Myocardial Protection in Coronary Heart Surgery

Primary Importance of Myocardial Blood Flow in Determining the Survival of Ischemic Myocardium

E. S. Kirk, H. O. Hirzel, and E. H. Sonnenblick

In Fig. 1, the distribution of myocardial necrosis 24 h after acute coronary ligation is shown. Corresponding blood flow measurements are shown in the lower part of the diagram. Collateral flow has been redistributed when compared to just after occlusion, increasing in the epicardial layers which have survived, while decreasing in the endocardial layers which have gone on to necrosis [4]. Subendocardial necrosis extends uniformly from the center of the infarction to the lateral borders. The irregular interdigitating margins create peninsulas of ischemic tissue extending into normal areas and vice versa [5]. Of importance: (1) the infarct is limited laterally to the zone made ischemic by the ligation, i.e., to the area at risk, and (2) the transmural extent of necroses is the same in the center as it is throughout the lateral extent of the infarct [3]. Variability of infarct size within the area at risk does not occur at the lateral margins. These lateral edges are fixed by the distribution of the vasculature. However, the transmural extent of infarction is variable, as a function of collateral blood flow. From these observations, a simplified model of infarction evolves.

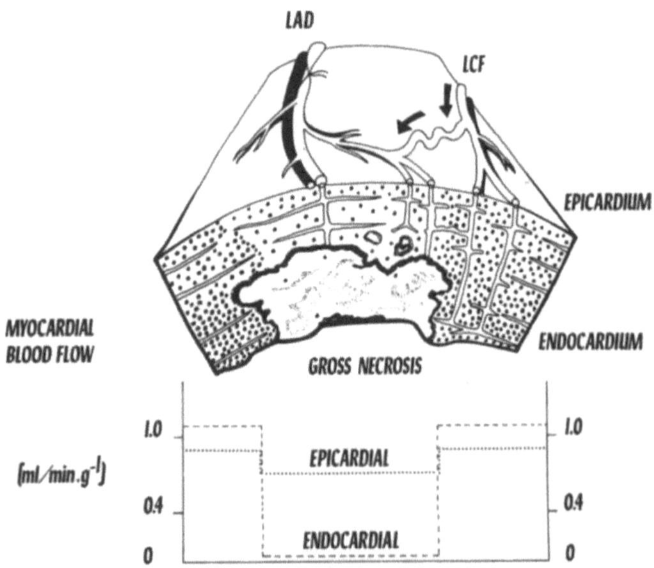

Fig. 1. Development of myocardial infarction and blood flow distribution 24 h after acute coronary artery ligation

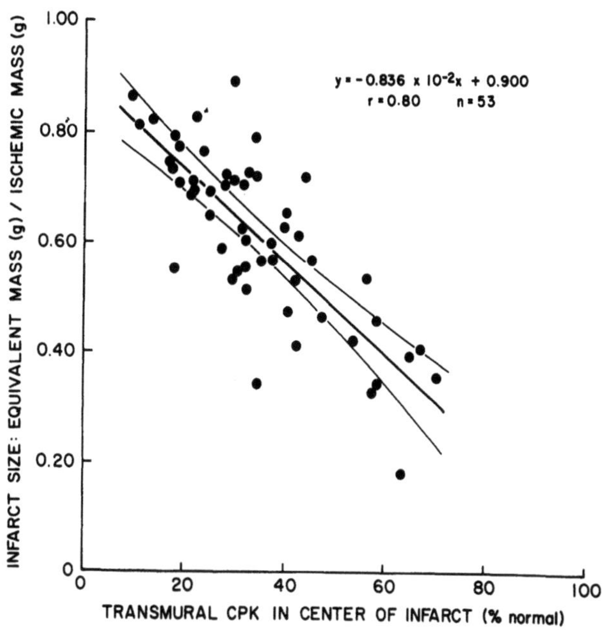

Fig. 2. Relationship between transmural CPK and normalized infarct size

In Fig. 2, the infarct size, measured as the total CPK loss from the tissue, has been normalized by the mass of the tissue at risk [3]. Creatine phosphokinase activity in the tissue has been used as an index of tissue viability. On the ordinant, the volume of tissue infarcted, measured by total CPK loss, has been divided by the CPK level of the entire area at risk. On the abscissa, the CPK level of a transmural biopsy in the center of the infarction is given. Thus, results for infarcts in the ischemic zone ranging from 5 to 35 g are expressed as relative necrosis within each zone. A value of 1.00 on the ordinant denotes 100% necrosis of the ischemic area. As noted, the central biopsy provides a good measure of the relative degree of necrosis in the total area at risk. Hence the central biopsy essentially provides a normalization of infarct size.

Once myocardial blood flow and thus oxygen delivery are inadequate to meet oxygen demands, ischemia develops. If the ischemia is sustained, necrosis ensues. The following data supports the view that ultimate survival of myocardiaum is largely dependent on residual collateral blood flow in the area of myocardium at risk. Essential to this concept is a new model of an acute myocardial infarction in which myocardium at risk is determined by anatomic vascular features and extent of infarction is determined transmurally by collateral blood flow and its distribution [1-3].

In Fig. 3, the general effects of an acute coronary occlusion are shown. The data derives from experiments in dogs but parallels the phenomenon of an acute coronary occlusion in man. Immediately following an acute coronary ligation, myocardial blood flow is reduced in the segment of the heart wall fed by this artery. This segment varies widely depending on the vascular anatomy. The diagram shows our findings on blood flow distribution measured with radioactive microspheres. The density of the dots corresponds to local blood flow. Representative values are shown below in the graph. We have found

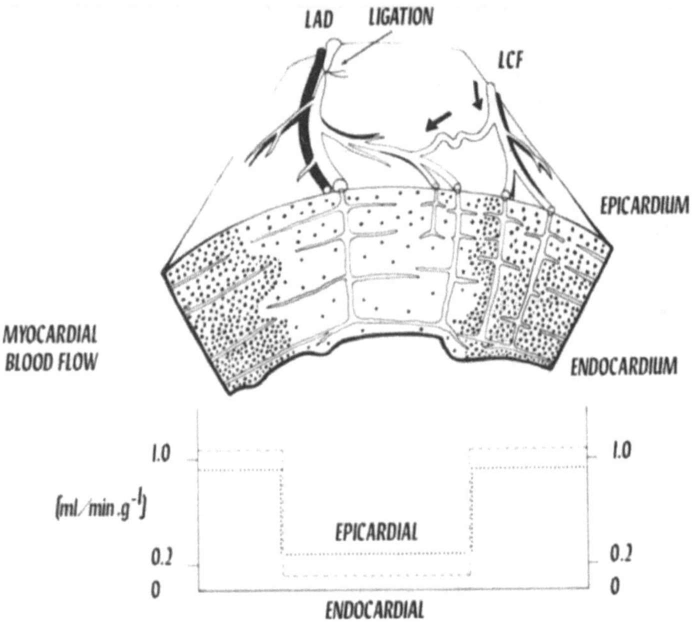

Fig. 3. Blood flow distribution after acute coronary artery ligation

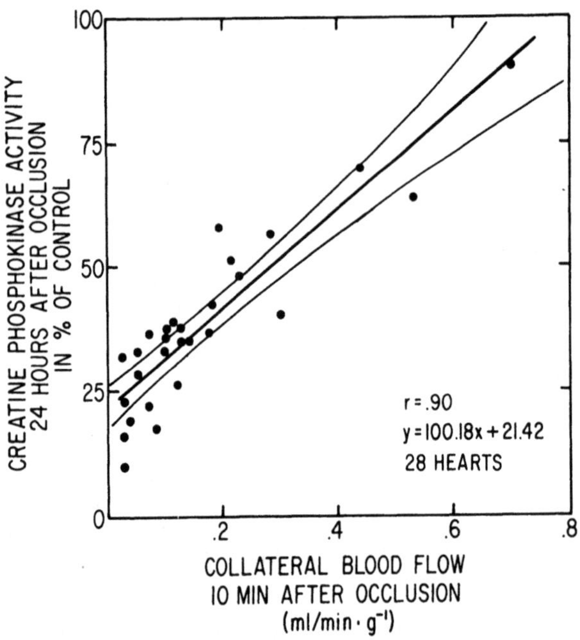

Fig. 4. Relationship between collateral blood flow and infarct size in untreated dogs

that coronary collateral blood flow is distributed throughout the ischemic zone so that the tissue near the center is perfused, as well as, the tissue near the lateral boundaries. Of note, the border between the ischemic and normal tissue is sharp, although quite irregular [1-3]. Levels of intermediate reduction of flow at the lateral borders of the ischemic area at risk have been shown to be due to admixture of normally perfused tissue and tissue perfused by collaterals entering the distal portions of the occluded vessel. Within the region of myocardium at risk, myocardial blood flow supplied by collaterals is greatly, but variably reduced. The reduction is greatest in endocardial layers and least in the epicardial layers of the wall. We have evaluated this area at risk by multiple means in our laboratory, using special microsphere techniques [3], and have found it to vary from 5 to 35 g in a series of animals with similar ligations of the left anterior coronary artery. This is true because the lateral borders of the region at risk and the subsequent infarction are fixed, and the extent of necrosis is determined by the extent of uniform transmural ischemia as related to collateral blood flow.

In Fig. 4, an index of the normalized infarct size is plotted on the ordinant versus the transmural collateral flow observed in 10 min following a coronary occlusion. Both measurements are derived from a biopsy from the center of the infarct and are representative of the tissue throughout the infarct. Thus, the graph is independent of the size of the ischemic area since partial infarction of the area at risk is occurring transmurally and these events extend between lateral borders. The major conclusion derived is that the extent of infarction is strongly dependent on collateral blood flow. A large range of collateral coronary blood flow is present immediately after occlusion in these randomly selected dogs with lesions in the same area of the artery. This indicates the heterogeneity of pre-existing collateral function in this species as is observed in man. Some animals have collaterals that virtually prevent necrosis following occlusion. With intermediate levels of collateral flow, subendocardial infarction ensues. Other animals have little collateral flow and transmural infarction occurs.

The relation shown in Fig. 4 permits delineation of factors that may alter the extent of transmural infarction. For example, an intervention which alters collateral flow would either increase or decrease the extent of infarction by moving along the same line. Were an intervention to reduce the extent of infarction by other means, such as altering metabolic requirements, points would lie above the line as an indication that the extent of infarction was reduced for any level of initial collateral blood flow. It is clear that alterations in infarct size require consideration of the individual variations in coronary collateral blood flow.

In Fig. 5, the results of studies [6] in 14 dogs treated for 3 h with intravenous isoproterenol (4 μg/min) are shown. The regression line and its limits of confidence for the control data of Fig. 4 are shown by the shaded area. Isoproterenol was started just after these measurements were made. One notes that isoproterenol significantly alters the relation between collateral blood flow and tissue CPK. The slope of the regression line differs from control at the $P < 0.001$ level. These data indicate that isoproterenol increases the extent of necrosis. However, this detrimental effect is only seen in animals with higher than average levels of collateral blood flow. At low collateral flows (<0.2 ml/min/g), the extent of infarction was not altered, i.e., a transmural infarction is fixed, and does not extend laterally.

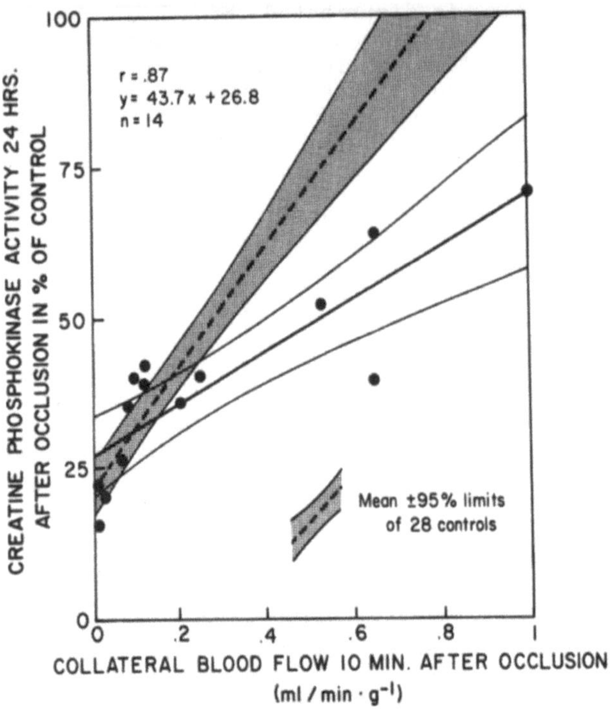

Fig. 5. Relationship between collateral blood flow and infarct size in isoproterenol treated dogs

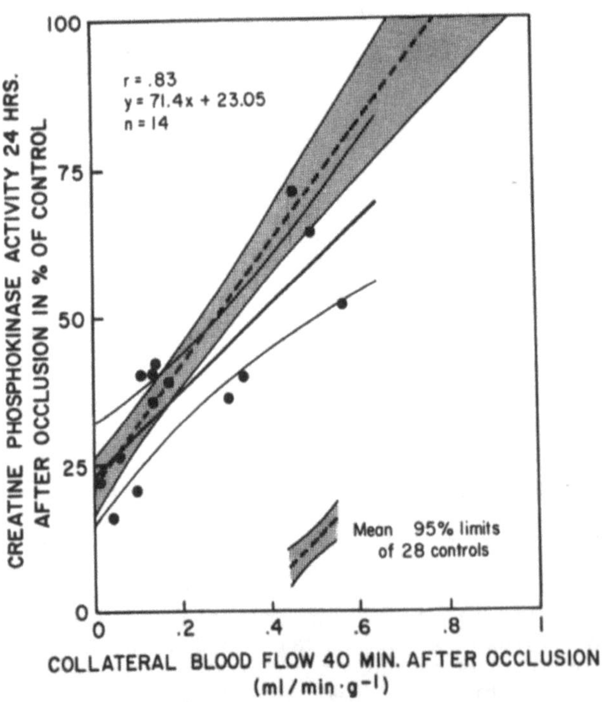

Fig. 6. Relationship between collateral blood flow and infarct size in isoproterenol treated dogs

Measurements of collateral blood flow shown in Fig. 5 reflect that which existed before the isoproterenol infusion. They may not represent collateral flow during the infusion, since isoproterenol may produce tachycardia and some degree of hypotension. Both of these changes can greatly reduce collateral flow. In Fig. 6, coronary collateral flow has been measured *after* the isoproterenol was begun. The graph is similar to Fig. 5 and the CPK values are for the same animals. Of note, several animals which had high levels of collateral blood flow before the isoproterenol infusion now have markedly reduced flows. Indeed, the level of flows obtained, now predict CPK levels similar to control animals and the regression lines are not significantly different. The infarct sizes that evolve in isoproterenol treated animals correspond to that which would be expected in control animals having collateral blood flows equal to the flows measured during the isoproterenol infusion. The detrimental effectt of isoproterenol can be explained largely by its actions to produce a tachycardia and hypotension, both of which reduce collateral flow. Of interest, no other detrimental metabolic effect of isoproterenol could be shown in these experiments.

In summary, we have provided evidence for a new model of myocardial ischemia and infarction following acute coronary occlusion. In this model, derived from animal experiments, the area at risk is strictly defined by the primary vasculature. The lateral borders of this area are sharp, but irregular. Collateral blood flow enters the area via relatively large arterial connections. Thus, collateral blood flow is distributed uniformly from lateral to lateral border, but least in the endocardium. Over several hours, collateral blood flow is redistributed to favor the epicardium at the expense of the endocardium. Transmural survival of myocardium is a variable determined largely by the amount of collateral flow remaining in the region. Isoproterenol increases transmural infarct size, but only in animals with well developed collaterals. Severe transmural infarcts are not affected. The primary mechanism by which isoproterenol is detrimental is by reducing collateral blood flow by increasing heart rate and reducing diastolic blood pressure. Since most of the detrimental effects are ascribed to a change in collateral blood flow, detrimental metabolic effects are not apparent. The findings suggest that a concern for blood flow in treating ischemic tissue plays a dominant role in the pathophysiology of ischemia, and thus, in concepts of therapy.

References

1. Fischl, S.J., Sonnenblick, E.H., Kirk, E.S.: Absence of a border ischemic zone following acute coronary occlusion. Circulation *50*, 680 (1974)
2. Kirk, E.S., Sonnenblick, E.H.: Topography of ischemia and necrosis following coronary occlusion: Pathophysiology of the border zone. U.S.-U.S.S.R. 3rd Joint Symposium on Myocardial Metabolism. Williamsburg (Virginia) 9-11 May 1977
3. Hirzel, H.O., Sonnenblick, E.H., Kirk, E.S.: Absence of a lateral border zone of intermediate creatine phosphokinase depletion surrounding a central infarct 24 h after acute coronary occlusion in the dog. Circ. Res. *41*, 673-683 (1977)
4. Hirzel, H.O., Nelson, G.R., Sonnenblick, E.H., Kirk, E.S.: Redistribution of collateral blood flow from necrotic to surviving myocardium following coronary occlusion. Circ. Res. *39*, 214-222 (1976)
5. Factor, S.M., Sonnenblick, E.H., Kirk, E.S.: The histological border zone of acute myocardial infarction: islands or peninsulas? Am. J. Pathol. (in press) (1978)
6. Kirk, E.S., Hirzel, H.O., Sonnenblick, E.H.: The relative role of supply and demand in the effect of isoproterenol on infarct size. Circulation *56*, 571 (1977)

Myocardial Protection by Cardioplegic Solutions

N. Bleese

The aim of myocardial protection in coronary bypass surgery is to guarantee the functional and structural integrity of the whole myocardium which should be independent of the preoperative myocardial and coronary conditions and the number of grafted coronary arteries. The evidence of perioperative myocardial infarctions occurring within a zone of myocardium supplied by an ungrafted artery or myocardial infarctions occurring in regions supplied by arteries, which are grafted from patent veins, demonstrates that none of the methods of intraoperative myocardial protection in coronary bypass surgery until now was fully able to guarantee this.

In certain circumstances, apart from the technical problems involved, performing distal bypass anastomoses on a beating or fibrillating heart can lead to regional myocardial ischemia, especially in those areas that are supplied by the grafted arteries. Methods that do not involve coronary perfusion allow surgery on the arrested heart emptied of blood. The disadvantage, however, is that the ischemic tolerance cannot be accurately assessed, since the energy requirement of the ischemically arrested heart even in hypothermia cannot be calculated under operating conditions.

Table 1. Schema of myocardial function during a period of ischemia

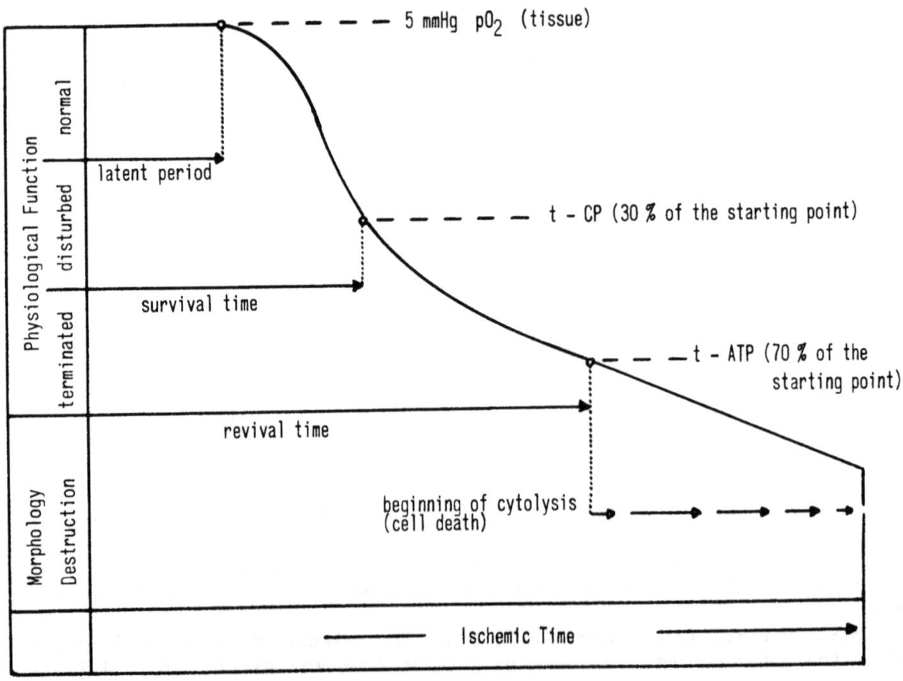

Table 1 shows a diagram of the biochemical and structural course after the coronary blood supply is cut off. After a short period - the so-called latent period - the pO_2 of the tissue drops below 5 mmHg. This period lasts approximately 6-8 heart beats. Subsequently the period of disturbed function begins: arrhythmias occur, the heart starts fluttering or fibrillating. The phosphocreatine which is usually metabolized to ATP drops drastically. If the phosphocreatine of the myocardium reaches 30% of the initial value the heart will stop. In the following period constant loss of ATP is seen, because the anaerobic metabolism is incapable of resynthesizing ATP sufficiently. However, if the intracellular content of ATP drops below 70% of the initial value the first irreversible structural damages occur, which lead to permanently decreased function after reanimation.

According to Bretschneider this is the limit of the practical survival time or the so-called t-ATP. In normothermia t-ATP is reached after only 10 min of cardiac arrest induced by plain ischemia. This is because the ischemically induced cardiac arrest is brought about by the initial loss of ATP and the further splitting of ATP during the arrest due to membrane ATPase activities (Table 2).

Table 2. Cardiac arrest induced by plain ischemia

Principle:	cardiac arrest by loss of energy (ATP ↓; CP ↓)
Disadvantage:	*delayed* cardiac arrest (beating → fibrillating → arresting)

Table 3. Induced cardiac arrest by cardioplegic solution

Principle:	Immediate cardiac arrest due to 1) stabilization of the cell membrane and 2) uncoupling of excitation-contraction
	(The cardiac arrest occurs with normal levels of energy-rich phosphate-compounds)

Table 4. Compounds of cardioplegic solutions

		Kirsch[a]	Bretschneider[b]
Sodium	(Na^+)	--	10
Potassium	(K^+)	--	7-10
Calcium	(Ca^{++})	--	--
Magnesium	(Mg^{++})	80	2
Chlorine	(Cl^-)	--	30
Procaine		11	7

Arrest due to [a]Magnesium-aspartate-procaine.
[b]withdrawal of sodium and application of procaine.

On the other hand, cardiac arrest induced by cardioplegia results in excitation-contraction uncoupling, so that the stores of energy rich phosphate compounds remain undepleted (Table 3). Furthermore, membrane stabilizing cardioplegic solutions additionally stabilize the membrane potential during the arrest, thus inhibiting membrane ATPases. Depolarizing cardioplegic solutions, for instance potassium, induce immediate arrest, but cannot sufficiently reduce the ATP splitting during the arrest in normothermia, since they have no membrane stabilizing effect. It is often forgotten that the maintenance of the membrane resting potential and the cellular structure during cardiac arrest requires a high energy supply.

Clinically proven cardioplegic solutions with a membrane stabilizing effect were introduced by Bretschneider (sodium and calcium depletion, procaine) and be Kirsch (magnesium and procaine) in the 1960s in Europe (Table 4).

The cardioplegic solution according to Kirsch contains procaine, which stabilizes the cell membranes by inhibiting sodium permeation, thus preventing action potentials (Table 5). In addition the solution is free of sodium and calcium, so that not only action potentials are prevented, but also excitation-contraction is uncoupled. The high concentration of magnesium in the Kirsch solution enhances these effects, so that a rapid cardiac arrest can be induced, while during the arrest the membranes remain polarized.

In animal experiments this method was combined with hypothermia (Table 6). The actual survival time could be considerably prolonged, so that t-ATP at 15°C was reached only after 250-280 min.

It is suggested by the results of the animal experiments that cardioplegic solutions combined with deep hypothermia of the heart provide the ideal way of protecting the myocardium during arrest, as it makes it possible to operate on an arrested, relaxed, and empty heart for a sufficiently long period while still guaranteeing safe reanimation for all areas of the myocardium (Table 7).

Table 5. Acting mechanisms of magnesium-aspartate-procaine (Cardioplegin^{R}) (Kirsch)

Mg^{++}	1) inhibits the influx of Ca^{++}ions thus inhibiting actomyosin-ATPase
	2) inhibits the influx of Na^{+}ions thus inhibiting membrane potentials
	3) inhibits Na^{+}-K^{+} ATPase
Na^{+}	withdrawal - prevents membrane potentials
Ca^{++}	withdrawal causes excitation-contraction uncoupling
Procaine	inhibits Na^{+} carrier-system thus stabilizing the polarized cell membrane

The saving of energy is due to

1) *immediate* cardiac arrest
2) reduction of the membrane ATPase activity of the arrested heart muscle

Table 6. Practical survival time = 30% ATP - splitting

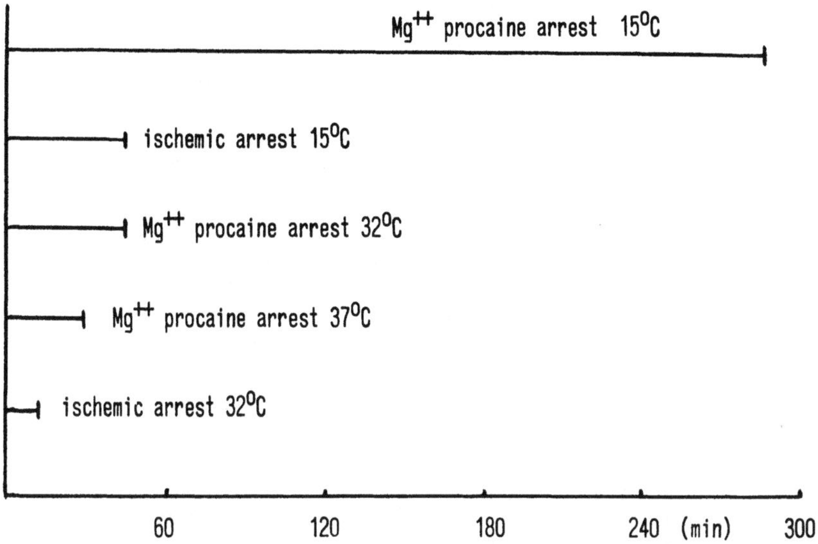

Table 7. Principles of an ideal protection of the myocardium

1) Cardiac arrest induced by cardioplegic solution (thus saving the physiological content of energy-rich phosphate-compounds)
2) Reduction of the metabolic rate during arrest by cardioplegic solution in hypothermia (15-20°C)

Table 8. Cardioplegic solution for coronary perfusion

I. Cardioplegic	by procaine	4 mM	
	Na^+	50 mM	
	Mg^{++}	2 mM	
II. Oxidative metabolism	by pO_2	600 mmHg	
	glucose	10 mM	
III. Protection against edema of the tissue			
by	colloid osmotic pressure	46 cm H_2O (6% HES)	
	osmolarity	320 mosmol/l	
	and 250 mg 6-methylprednisolon/l		

Under operating conditions, however, noncoronary blood supplies can wash out the cardioplegic solution and rewarm the heart. The rate of energy-consuming metabolism during the resulting ischemic phase therefore largely depends on the temperature of the myocardium and/or the activity of the remaining cardioplegia. It is important therefore to lower the temperature of the heart and to keep it lowered cardioplegically.

Since the only way of rapidly and effectively reducing the temperature of the whole myocardium in the operating room is by perfusion, we developed a cardioplegic solution for coronary perfusion, which is suitable for intermittent, as well as, continuous perfusion (Table 8).

Using this cardioplegic coronary perfusate we can cool the myocardium down to 15°-20°C without loss of energy rich phosphate compounds and without causing structural damage.

The solution contains no red blood cells (Table 9). Its cardioplegic effect is the result of its procaine content and the low level of sodium. The oxydative metabolism of a heart cardioplegically perfused in this way can be fully maintained by the amount of oxygen dissolved physically and its glucose content. Another important factor, apart from a slightly raised osmolarity, is the presence of colloidal components in the perfusion mixture. Only the oncotically active substances in an erythrocyte free solution can prevent edema in a perfused and arrested heart. Due to 6% hydroxyethyl starch our solution has an oncotic pressure of about 32 mmHg. This makes it suitable for continuous coronary perfusion as long as the perfusion pressure does not exceed the oncotic pressure in the solution.

To summarize (Table 10) methods of intraoperative myocardial protection should be applied as follows:

Introduction and continuation of cardiac arrest cardioplegically,
Guaranteeing myocardial hypothermia,
Intermittently restoring cardioplegia and oxidative metabolism,
Thereby washing out lactate and blood.

Under these conditions the period of cardiac arrest can be extended to over 120 min.

Should the heart warm up faster than expected during the period of ischemia, or should mechanical activity begin, cardioplegic coronary perfusion can and should be resumed at any stage and carried out either continuously or intermittently. However, in each case we perform a short cardioplegic coronary reperfusion of 3-4 min after 50-60 min of cardioplegic arrest, to wash out lactate and blood and to restore cardioplegia.

Table 9. Cardioplegic solution for perfusion

6% hydroxyethyl starch		
2 mM magnesium aspartate		
4 mM procaine · HCl		
0,5 mM $CaCl_2$		
5 mM KCl		
25 mM $NaHCO_3$		
10 mM glucose		
200 mM mannitol		
250 mg 6-methyl prednisolone/l		
Total Na^+-content:		50 mM
Osmolarity:		320 mosmol
Colloid osmotic pressure:		46 cm H_2O
pH: 7,40	pO_2:	>600 mmHg

Table 10. Myocardial protection by cardioplegia and hypothermia (Hamburg)

Principles
Cardiac arrest induced by Magnesium-Procaine-Cardioplegia
followed by
aerobic, hypothermic Cardioplegic Coronary Perfusion
and
topical cooling

Table 11. Myocardial protection by cardioplegia and hypothermia (Hamburg). Myocardial cooling by cardioplegic coronary perfusion

Procedure	No[a]	Perfusion rate[b] (ml/min)	Perfusion time (min)	Septal temperature (°C)
Valve replacement	195	120 ± 30	8 ± 3	16 ± 2
ACVB surgery	152	87 ± 24	8 ± 4	17 ± 3

[a]Number of measurements.

[b]Maximum perfusion pressure: 30 mmHg.

The flow rates and the time needed to lower the temperature of the heart are seen in Table 11. Neither coronary stenosis nor myocardial hypertrophy are limiting factors for an effective core cooling. In the coronary group the average flow rate at a perfusion pressure of 30 mmHg is about 90 ml/min and the myocardium is cooled down to less than 20°C within 8 min.

We examined biochemical parameters in intraoperatively taken human myocardium (Fig. 1). In accordance with our clinical results the concentration of energy rich phosphate compounds (two upper curves) and the content of lactate and the pH value (two lower curves) demonstrate that only after 120 min the actual survival time is reached. This is the time span of arrest after which the heart can be resuscitated without functional losses.

We used this method of cardioplegia on 292 patients who underwent coronary bypass surgery (Table 12). In 35 cases one, in 100 cases two and in 124 cases more than two coronary arteries were grafted. In 33 cases an additional ventricular aneurysmectomy was performed. In all cases aortic vein anastomoses without extracorporal circulation were first established. After starting total bypass, cardiac arrest and cardioplegic coronary perfusion were carried out. The peripheral anastomoses were performed during a single period of cardiac arrest.

The overall hospital mortality rate was 3.1%. In only one case death was due to insufficient protection of the myocardium. In this case an unnoticed and unforeseen rapid rewarming of the myocardium occurred due to noncoronary blood supply.

The frequency of perioperative infarctions - not due to technical errors - counts for a measure of quality of intraoperative myocardial protection (Table 13). The table shows that the rate of perioperative myocardial infarctions defined by accepted parameters totals 1.4% in the coronary group and is unrelated to the length of aortic crossclamping time or the number of coronary bypasses performed.

In conclusion, we believe that cardioplegia in hypothermia seems to be the best method for coronary bypass surgery and the method of choice in borderline cases with multiple-vessel diseases, left ventricle, and/or other lesions.

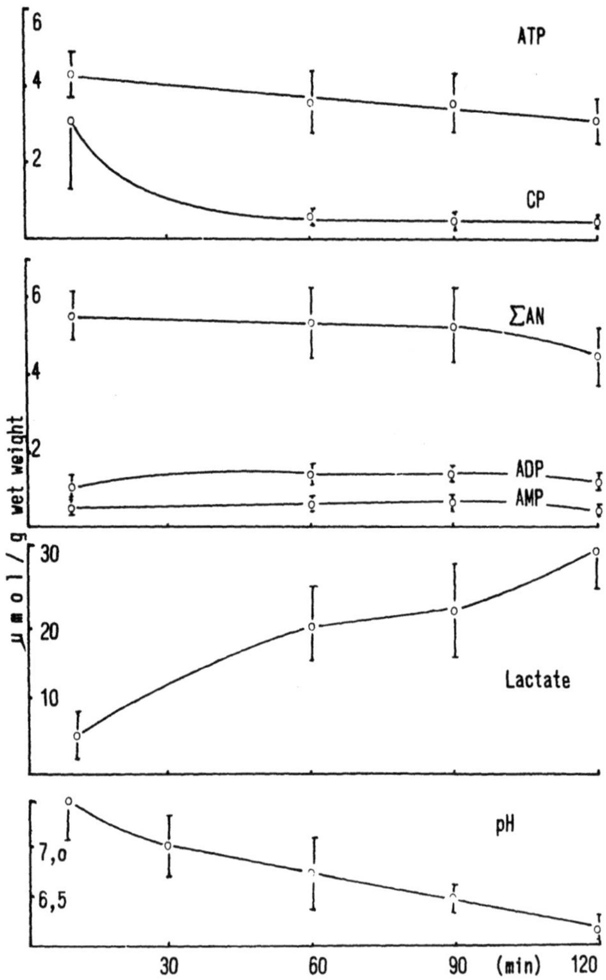

Fig. 1. Time course of myocardial content of energy rich phosphate compounds and lactate as well as epicardial pH-level during an ischemia in hypothermia (20°C) and cardioplegia (human myocardium, n=10)

Table 12. Myocardial protection by cardioplegia and hypothermia (Hamburg). Aorto-coronary bypass-group

Procedure	n	Hospital mortality	
Single	35	0	(- %)
Double	100	3	(3.0%)
Triple	124	4	(3.2%)
ACVB + aneurysmectomy	33	2	(6.1%)
Total	292	9	(3.1%)

Causes of death

2 x Myocardial infarction pre-ECG
2 x Unknown (1-2 weeks postoperative)
4 x Myocardial infarction due to technical errors
1 x Insufficiency of myocardial protection

Table 13. Coronary heart disease rate of perioperative myocardial infarction of survivors

Surgical procedure	n	Aortic crossclamping time (min)	Infarctions n	%
ACVB single	35	55 ± 25	-	-
double	97	79 ± 16	2	2.1
triple, quadruple, quintuple	120	106 ± 22	2	1.7
combined with aneurysmectomy	31	85 ± 38	-	-
Total	283		4	1.4

References

1. Assad-Morell, J.L., Frye, R.L., Connolly, D.C., Gau, G.T., Pluth, J.R., Barnhorst, D.A., Wallace, R.B., Davis, G.D., Elveback, L.R., Danielson, G.K.: Relation of intraoperative or early postoperative transmural myocardial infarction to patency of aortocoronary bypass grafts and to diseases ungrafted coronary arteries. Am. J. Cardiol. *35*, 767 (1975)
2. Bleese, N., Döring, V., Gercken, G., Pokar, H., Rodewald, G.: Long-time cardiac arrest by cardioplegic perfusion. 10th Congress of the European Society for Experimental Surgery. Paris, 6.-9. April 1975
3. Bleese, N., Döring, V., Gercken, G., Kalmar, P., Lierse, W., Pokar, H., Polonius, M.-J., Steiner, D., Rodewald, G.: Langzeitherzstillstand durch cardioplegische Coronarperfusion. Thoraxchirurgie *24*, 468 (1976)
4. Bretschneider, H.J.: Überlebenszeit und Wiederbelebungszeit des Herzens bei Normo- und Hypothermie. Verh. Dtsch. Kreislaufforsch. *30*, 11 (1964)
5. Döring, V., Gercken, G., Bleese, N., Pokar, H., Rodewald, G.: Long time cardiac arrest by cardioplegic coronary perfusion. Pflügers Arch. *355* [Suppl.] R 10 (1975)
6. Döring, V., Baumgarten, H.G., Pokar, H., Gercken, G.: Metabolism and fine structure of the Mg^{++}-procaine arrested perfused heart. Basic Res. Cardiol. *70*, 186 (1975)
7. Döring, V., Baumgarten, H.G., Bleese, N., Kalmar, P., Pokar, H., Gercken, G.: Metabolism and structure of the magnesium aspartate-procaine arrested ischemic heart of rabbit and man. Basic Res. Cardiol. *71*, 119 (1976)
8. Gay, W.A. (Jr.), Ebert, P.A.: Functional, metabolic and morphological effects of potassium-induced cardioplegia. Surgery *74*, 284 (1973)
9. Hottenrott, C.E., Maloney, J.V., Buckberg, G.: Studies of the effects of ventricular fibrillation on the adequacy of regional myocardial blood flow. J. Thorac. Cardiovasc. Surg. *68*, 615 (1974)
10. Kalmar, P., Bleese, N., Kirsch, U., Lutz, G., Pokar, H., Rodewald, G.: Kombination von Kardioplegie und Coronarperfusion bei Herzoperationen in Normothermie. Thoraxchirurgie *20*, 427 (1972)
11. Kalmar, P., Bleese, N., Döring, V., Gercken, G., Kirsch, U., Lierse, W., Pokar, H., Polonius, M.-J., Rodewald, G.: Induced ischemic arrest. Clinical and experimental results with magnesium aspartate procaine solution (carоplegin[R]). J. Cardiovasc. Surg. *16*, 470 (1975)
12. Kirsch, U., Rodewald, G., Kalmar, P.: Induced ischemic arrest. Clinical experience with cardioplegia in open heart surgery. J. Thorax. Cardiovasc. Surg. *63*, 121 (1972)
13. Kolff, W.J., Effler, D.B., Groves, L.K., Peereboom, G., Maraca, P.P., Aoyama, S., Sones, F.M.: Elective cardiac arrest by the Melrose technic: Potassium asystole for experimental cardiac surgery. Clev. Clin. Q. *23*, 98 (1956)
14. Melrose, D.G., Dreyer, B., Bentall, H.H., Baker, J.B.: Elective cardiac arrest: Preliminary communication. Lancet *1955/II*, 21

15. Shumway, N.E., Lower, R.TR., Stofer, R.C.: Selective hypothermia of the heart in anoxic cardiac arrest. Surg. Gynecol. Obstet. *109*, 750 (1959)
16. Søndergaard, T., Senn, A.: Klinische Erfahrungen mit der Kardioplegie nach Bretschneider. Langenbecks Arch. Klin. Chir. *319*, 661 (1967)
17. Steiner, D., Bleese, N., Döring, V., Roesner, K.: Prevention of edema during coronary perfusion with cardioplegic solution. Thoraxchirurgie *25*, 235 (1977)
18. Stemmer, E.A., McCart, P., Stanton, W.W., Thibault, W., Dearden, L.S., Conolly, J.E.: Functional and structural alterations in the myocardium during aortic crossclamping. J. Thorac. Cardiovasc. Surg. *70*, 666 (1975)
19. Wukasch, D.C., Reul, G.J., Milam, J.D., Halman, G.L., Cooley, D.A.: The "stone-heart" syndrom. Surgery *72*, 1071 (1972)

Myocardial Protection by Pulsatile Flow - Clinical Experience

D. Bregman

Summary

Until now, it has not been possible to use counterpulsation routinely during open heart surgery. A new pulsatile assist device (PAD) has been developed to convert roller pump flow to pulsatile flow. In addition, the PAD can be used as an arterial counterpulsator before and after cardiopulmonary bypass (CPB).

The PAD is inserted in the arterial line close to the aortic root. The device consists of a flexible valveless balloon through which the arterial blood flows. The balloon is contained within a rigid plastic housing which is connected to a standard intra-aortic balloon pump, thereby enabling the blood filled balloon to be squeezed.

The PAD was employed in 400 adult patients undergoing open heart surgery for coronary artery and/or valvular heart disease from 1975-1978. Of these patients, 72% were NYHA Class III or IV or had ejection fractions of <0.3. The device functioned as a hemodynamically effective counterpulsator before and after CPB. Urinary outputs during CPB were more than doubled on the PAD when compared to a control group. In addition, coronary graft blood flow (CBF) increased an average of 21.4% with the PAD during CPB. Free plasma hemoglobins after CPB were not elevated. Only eight patients (2%) had a perioperative myocardial infarction and three of these patients were successfully treated with IABP. Total mortality in this series was eight patients (2%).

It is suggested that the PAD is a simple and reliable device for both intraoperative counterpulsation and for the creation of pulsatile CPB. More significantly, use of the PAD may decrease both the incidence of perioperative myocardial infarction and the need for postoperative IABP.

The recent development of modern direct techniques for coronary revascularization has resulted in a multitude of critically ill patients requiring open heart surgery. In an effort to deal with the increasing numbers of patients requiring urgent open heart surgery and presenting complicated patterns of coronary artery and/or valvular heart disease, a spectrum of cardiac assist measures ranging from simple pharmacologic maneuvers to a variety of mechanical cardiac assist techniques have been developed. Those temporary mechanical cardiac assist devices which employ the principle of arterial counterpulsation have met with the most consistent clinical success [1-5]. It is the purpose of this paper to summarize our clinical experience with a new pulsatile assist device (PAD) in patients requiring open heart surgery at the Columbia-Presbyterian Medical Center.

Pulsatile Cardiopulmonary Bypass

The potential importance of pulsatile cardiopulmonary bypass (CPB) has been recognized for several years by investigators in the field [6-26].

The advantages of pulsatile flow during clinical CPB include:

1) Better capillary perfusion
2) Less metabolic acidosis
3) Increased oxygen consumption
4) Lower peripheral arterial resistance
5) Better renal perfusion
6) Improved cerebral perfusion
7) Less hepatocellular injury
8) Better myocardial perfusion
   (Especially in the subendocardium)
9) Less elevation of coronary sinus lactate

Basically these categories suggest an improvement in both peripheral and organ perfusion. With specific reference to the heart, it has been found that pulsatile flow results in better perfusion of the subendocardium during ventricular fibrillation [27], even in the presence of a critical coronary stenosis [28,29]. Pulsatile CPB has not been utilized clinically on a routine basis because of the lack of simple technology to create the pulsations.

Development of Pulsatile Cardiopulmonary Bypass
Although the earliest heart-lung machines could create pulsatile flow, this feature was not used routinely because of excessive hemolysis.

There have been several subsequent pump consoles capable of pulsation and counterpulsation, but the ability to combine both features has generally been unsuccessful, and either the complexity or the hemolysis generated by the equipment precluded long-term or routine use [12,24,29-33].

Berger [34] and Pappas [35,36] first called attention to the use of IABP to create clinical pulsatile CPB. They observed that when patients were taken to the operating room on IABP, the balloon could create pulsatile CPB with no blood trauma. Pappas' data [35,36] suggest that pulsatile CPB improves myocardial metabolism and function and results in less hepatocellular injury (postoperative SGOT levels). In addition, there was better overall tissue perfusion (total LDH), a lower incidence of perioperative myocardial infarctions, and possible improvement in late myocardial function. Postoperative renal failure was rare in comparison with a study of Abel et al [37], who found that 27% of their patients had mild to severe renal failure which correlated with the duration of the operation.

Although use of the balloon is associated with low morbidity [2,38], its use cannot be justified for the routine creation of pulsatile cardiopulmonary bypass, because of additional surgery and the possible high risk associated with peripheral balloon insertion [39].

The Pulsatile Assist Device (PAD[1])
In an effort to broaden the applicability of the principles of intra-aortic balloon pumping, a new pulsatile assist device (PAD) was de-

[1]Registered trademark of the Datascope Corporation, Paramus, New Jersey.

veloped [2,40-43] which is employed *externally* in the cardiopulmonary bypass circuit, and which in all respects simulated the action of an intraoperative intra-aortic balloon.

The PAD[2] is a plastic disposable device inserted in the arterial line during cardiopulmonary bypass. The device can be used with either aortic or femoral artery perfusion (Fig. 1). The PAD consists

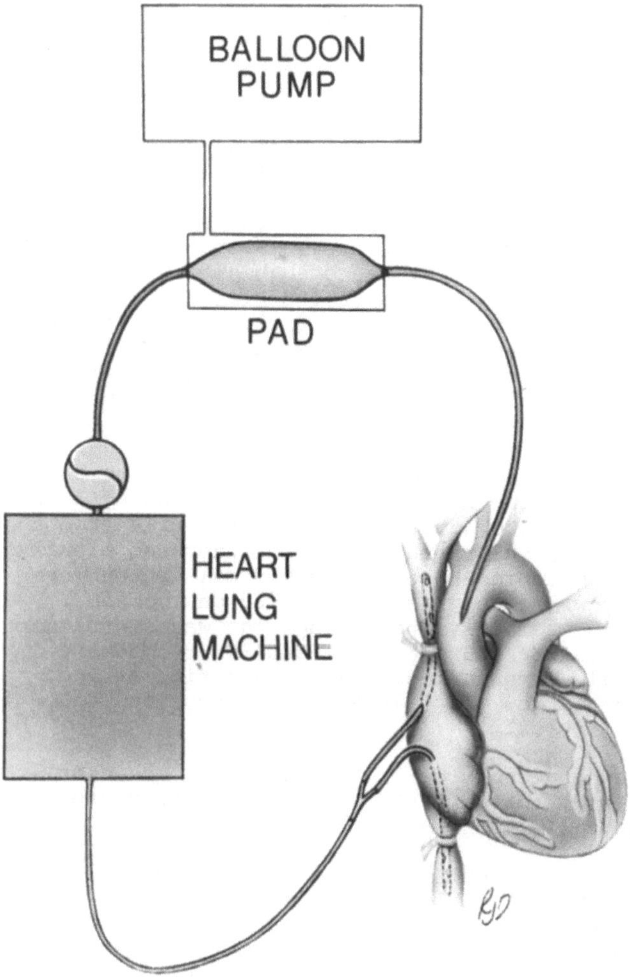

Fig. 1. Schematic of Pulsatile Assist Device (PAD) in cardiopulmonary bypass circuit. Oxygenated blood flows through the valveless balloon within the PAD, and then into the aorta. The balloon pump pneumatically squeezes the PAD balloon to effect either synchronous counterpulsation or pulsatile cardiopulmonary bypass

of a flexible, valveless polyurethane balloon with 3/8 in. ends through which the arterial blood flows. The balloon is contained within a rigid plastic housing which is connected, via an air hose, to a standard System 80 Intra-Aortic Balloon Pump Console[1]. As soon as the arterial perfusion cannula is inserted but before bypass is

[2]Manufactured by the Datascope Corporation, Paramus, New Jersey.

instituted, a tubing clamp is placed between the roller pump and the PAD in order to maximize its central hemodynamic efficacy, and arterio-arterial counterpulsation can be instituted. When cardiopulmonary bypass begins, the clamp is removed and the PAD is pulsed synchronously with the ECG in diastole to create pulsatile cardiopulmonary bypass. During ventricular fibrillation or aortic crossclamping, an internal trigger of 80 beats/min is used. Each time the heart is defibrillated, synchronous ECG triggered pulsatile bypass is resumed. While weaning the patient from bypass, the PAD is again utilized as a counterpulsator, and when bypass is terminated, counterpulsation can continue until protamine is administered. While counterpulsating after bypass, the tubing clamp is again placed between the roller pump and the PAD. This clamp can be removed intermittently as blood is returned in increments from the heart-lung machine. Counterpulsation is continuous, as this blood is reinfused, and weaning from the PAD can be accomplished in a manner similar to IABP [44].

Aside from its pneumatic connection to the PAD in the sterile operative field, the only other mandatory input to the System 80 console for PAD use is the electrocardiogram. Pressure acquisition is optional, but is necessary for PAD counterpulsation timing. The PAD and air hose are kept sterile in the operative field so that the PAD can be as close to the arterial tree as possible to maximize its effectiveness as a counterpulsator [45]. In addition, this position facilitates excision of the PAD in the event of a device failure.

PAD - Clinical Experience

After its initial evaluation in the laboratory [41,42,46], the clinical PAD was first employed during a 27 month period beginning 4 November 1975. During this time, 400 adult patients, primarily from the group with impaired left ventricular function, who underwent elective open heart surgery at the Columbia-Presbyterian Medical Center were assisted intra-operatively with the pulsatile assist device [40]. There were 299 males and 101 females. The average age was 59 (range 29-82) years. Two hundred thirty-four patients underwent coronary artery bypass only, 102 valve replacement only, 8 ventricular aneurism only, 41 combined coronaries and valves, and 15 combined coronaries and ventricular aneurysms.

Two hundred ninety of these patients were NYHA Class III or IV or had ejection fractions of <0.3 or an LVEDP ≥ 18 mmHg on their preoperative catheterization.

Most of the bypasses were carried out with the Bentley Temptrol Q200A[3] disposable bubble oxygenator using a clear fluid prime. More recently the new Bentley Spiraflow BOS-10 oxygenator has been employed. Our clinical experience has been primarily with ascending aortic perfusion utilizing a #24 Bardic[4] arterial perfusion catheter with a short arterial inlet.

Our technique of coronary bypass surgery with the PAD is as follows: counterpulsation with the PAD begins as soon as the aortic (or femoral) artery cannula is inserted. If a long tipped arterial perfusion cannula is employed, it is directed distally at the beginning of the operation. However, while weaning the patient from bypass at the conclusion of the operation, the cannula tip can be pointed toward the aortic valve, as this direction will maximize the counterpulsation effect from the PAD. As the venous cannulae are being inserted, the

---

[3]Bentley Laboratories, Irvine, California.

[4]U.S. Catheter Corporation. Glens Falls, New York.

console is turned to 1:2, since atrial arrhythmias are frequent at this stage. If one wishes, one or more vein grafts can be sutured to the ascending aorta, while the patient is being counterpulsated 1:1 even before bypass is instituted. Whenever a partial occlusion clamp or an aortic crossclamp is applied to or removed from the ascending aorta, the PAD is always momentarily switched off. When bypass commences, the PAD is turned off for a few minutes until total bypass is established. Our technique of coronary bypass surgery employs the sequence of an aortic anastomosis first (with the heart beating) and a coronary anastomosis second, usually with a short period of cross-clamping. Venting is not routine. Aortic valve surgery is carried out either with coronary perfusion (with the heart beating) or with local topical hypothermia with iced saline. Cardioplegia was employed in the last 80 patients in conjunction with the PAD.

The PAD functioned as a hemodynamically effective arterial counterpulsator before and after cardiopulmonary bypass. During bypass, pulse pressures of 40-50 mmHg were readily obtained without altering our usual average mean arterial perfusion pressures of 80-90 mmHg. There were no device-related complications. During bypass, the urinary outputs of the PAD patients were more than twice the values seen in control patients (9.18 ± 0.68 cc/min versus 3.90 ± 0.35 cc/min). In addition, intraoperative coronary graft blood flow determinations[5] in coronary patients off and on the PAD revealed an increase in coronary graft blood flow of 21.4% with the pusatile bypass.

Three patients required IABP for weaning from CPB. One of these who had an intraoperative infarct, died on the third postoperative day. A total of eight patients (2%) experienced a perioperative myocardial infarction as defined by new Q waves. Three of these patients required postoperative IABP and all survived. There were five other postoperative deaths. Three patients died from arrhythmias, two at 10 days and one at 3 weeks. One patient died from an anaphylactic drug reaction in the recovery room and one patient died during re-exploration for postoperative bleeding.

Conclusions based upon this experience are:

1) The PAD is an effective arterial counterpulsator.
2) The PAD safely creates atraumatic pulsatile CPB.
3) The increase in CBF with the PAD appears to afford greater intraoperative myocardial protection.
4) Renal failure, hepatic failure and CVAs have been minimal (<1%) with pulsatile CPB.
5) The PAD is a simple, non-invasive alternative to the elective use of IABP in many high risk situations (e.g. left main coronary stenosis).
6) Use of the PAD has markedly reduced the need for perioperative IABP.

New applications of the PAD are:

1) PAD + IABP
2) As an alternative to IABP
   (a) When balloon insertion is not possible
   (b) For short perioperative periods of counterpulsation (e.g. crescendo angina)
3) PAD for PA counterpulsation

---

[5] Carolina Medical Electronics, King, North Carolina.

4) To improve reperfusion of a donor heart during cardiac transplantation
5) As an intraoperative therapeutic trial of counterpulsation prior to balloon insertion (especially in pediatric patients)
6) To test for the hemodynamic significance of AI intraoperatively
7) As an aid in simultaneous carotid artery-coronary artery surgery
8) As a perioperative aid in patients requiring a valved conduit for restoration of RA or RV-PA continuity
9) To create pulsatile right or left heart bypass
10) As a possible therapeutic aid in patients with massive pulmonary emboli

Discussion

The potential importance of pulsatile CPB has been recognized for many years. Although it appeared to have several physiological advantages, it has not been routinely employed primarily due to a lack of simple atraumatic technology to produce the pulsations.

The PAD is the first clinical in-line device which produces atraumatic synchronized pulsatile CPB, and which can also function as an arterial counterpulsator. Of importance is that the routine of the surgical procedure is not significantly altered by the presence of the device.

Our animal experiments [46] have clearly documented the hemodynamic effectiveness of the PAD which has been borne out in our initial clinical trials [2,41-43,45]. In every respect the PAD functions similar to an intra-aortic balloon, without the need for additional surgery. Our clinical experience with the PAD has begun to confirm some of the reported advantages of pulsatile CPB. Certainly greater urinary output indirectly implies better renal perfusion. In addition, the increase in intraoperative myocardial blood flow would appear to offer greater protection to the myocardium during cardiopulmonary bypass. The extremely low incidence of perioperative myocardial infarctions in this series would attest to this fact [47]. Of more interest is that during our initial 27 month clinical utilization of the pulsatile assist device, only three patients have required intraoperative intra-aortic balloon pumping. This is a marked reduction in the requirement for intra-aortic balloon pumping in our institution [2,48].

In conclusion, intra-aortic balloon pumping is currently used primarily to open heart surgery. It is our impression that the use of intra-aortic balloon pumping in selected patients undergoing open heart surgery has led to improved patient survival and has enabled us to operate on high risk patients with greater confidence and with improved clinical results. More significantly, use of the pulsatile assist device will extend the role of counterpulsation in open heart surgery.

It is suggested from these data that the use of the PAD will obviate the need for prophylactic intra-aortic balloon pumping in selected high risk patients and that it will decrease both the incidence of perioperative myocardial infarctions and the need for postoperative intra-aortic balloon pumping.

References

1. Bolooki, H., Williams, W., Thurer, R.J., Vargas, A., Kaiser, G.A., Mack, F., Ghahramani, A.R.: Clinical and hemodynamic criteria for use of intra-aortic balloon pumping (IABP) in cardiac surgery patients. J. Thorac. Cardiovasc. Surg. *72*, 26 (1976)
2. Bregman, D.: Mechanical support of the failing heart: Current problems in surgery. Chicago: Yearbook Medical Publishers 1976
3. Bregman, D., Goetz, R.H.: Clinical experience with a new cardiac assist device, the dual chambered intra-aortic balloon assist. J. Thorac. Cardiovasc. Surg. *62*, 577 (1971)
4. Bregman, D., Goetz, R.H.: A failsafe cardiac assist system for intra-aortic balloon pumping. Trans. Am. Soc. Artif. Intern. Organs *17*, 505 (1972)
5. Goldman, B.S., Gunstensen, J., Gilbert, B.W., Kelly, T.C., Scully, H., Williams, W.G., Adelman, A.G.: Increasing operability and survival with intra-aortic balloon pump assist. Can. J. Surg. *19*, 69 (1976)
6. Boucher, J.K., Rudy, L.W. (Jr.), Edmunds, L.H. (Jr.): Organ blood flow during pulsatile cardiopulmonary bypass. J. Appl. Physiol. *35*, 86 (1974)
7. Dunn, J., Kirsh, M.M., Harness, J., Carroll, M., Starker, J., Sloan, H.: Hemodynamic, metabolic and hematologic effects of pulsatile cardiopulmonary bypass. J. Thorac. Cardiovasc. Surg. *68*, 138 (1974)
8. German, J.C., Chalmers, G.S., Hirai, J., Mukherjie, N.D., Wakabayashi, A., Connolly, J.E.: Comparison of nonpulsatile extracorporeal circulation on renal tissue perfusion. Chest *61*, 65 (1972)
9. Goodman, T.A., Gerard, D.F., Bernstein, E.F., Dilley, R.B.: The effects of pulseless perfusion on the distribution of renal cortical blood flow and on renin release. Surgery *80*, 31 (1976)
10. Harken, A.H.: The influence of pulsatile perfusion on oxygen uptake by isolated canine hind limb. J. Thorac. Cardiovasc. Surg. *70*, 237 (1975)
11. Hewitt, R.L., Weichert, R.F.: Diastolic augmentation during heart bypass. J. Thorac. Cardiovasc. Surg. *60*, 123 (1973)
12. Jacobs, L.A., Klopp, E.H., Seamone, W., Topaz, S.R., Gott, V.L.: Improved organ function during cardiac bypass with a roller pump modified to deliver pulsatile flow. J. Thorac. Cardiovasc. Surg. *58*, 703 (1969)
13. Mandelbaum, I., Berry, J., Silbert, M., Burns, W.H., Rother, C.: Regional blood flow during pulsatile and nonpulsatile perfusion. Arch. Surg. *91*, 771 (1965)
14. Mandelbaum, I., Burns, W.H.: Pulsatile and nonpulsatile blood flow. JAMA *191*, 657 (1965)
15. Many, M., Soroff, H.S., Birtwell, W.C., Wise, H.M., Deterling, R.A.: The physiologic role of pulsatile and nonpulsatile blood flow. Arch. Surg. *97*, 917 (1968)
16. Matsumoto, T., Wolferth, C.C., Perlman, M.H.: Effects of pulsatile and nonpulsatile perfusion upon cerebral and conjunctive microcirculation in dogs. Am. Surg. *37*, 61 (1971)
17. Milnor, W.R.: Pulsatile blood flow. Physiology in medicine. N. Engl. J. Med. *287*, 27-34 (1972)
18. Morkin, E.: Analysis of pulsatile blood flow and its clinical implications. N. Engl. J. Med. *277*, 139-146 (1967)
19. Mukherjie, N.D., Beran, A.V., Herai, J., Wakabayashi, A., Sperling, D.R., Taylor, W.F., Connolly, J.E.: In vivo determination of renal tissue oxygenation during pulsatile and nonpulsatile left heart bypass. Ann. Thorac. Surg. *15*, 354 (1973)
20. Nakayama, K., Tamiya, T., Yamamoto, K., Izumi, T., Akimoto, S., Hashizume, S., Iimori, T., Odaka, M., Yazawa, C.: High-amplitude pulsatile pump in extracorporeal circulation with particle reference to hemodynamics. Surgery *54*, 798 (1963)
21. Paquet, K.J.: Hemodynamic studies in normothermic perfusion of the isolated pig kidney with pulsatile and nonpulsatile flows. J. Cardiovasc. Surg. *1*, 45 (1969)
22. Shepard, R.B., Kirklin, J.W.: Relation of pulsatile flow to oxygen consumption and other variables during cardiopulmonary bypass. J. Thorac. Cardiovasc. Surg. *58*, 694 (1969)

23. Trinkle, J.K., Helton, N.E., Bryant, L.R., Griffen, W.O.: Pulsatile cardiopulmonary bypass: clinical evaluation. Surgery *68*, 1074 (1970)
24. Trinkle, J.K., Helton, N.E., Wood, R.E., Bryant, L.R.: Metabolic comparison of a new pulsatile pump and a roller pump for cardiopulmonary bypass. J. Thorac. Cardiovasc. Surg. *58*, 562 (1969)
25. Wesolowki, S.A., Sauvage, L.R., Pinc, R.D.: Extracorporeal circulation: role of the pulse in maintenance of systemic circulation during heart-lung by-pass. Surgery *37*, 663-681 (1955)
26. Wright, G., Sanderson, J.M.: Brain damage and mortality in dogs following pulsatile blood flow in extracorporeal circulation. Thorax *27*, 738 (1972)
27. Habal, S.M., Weiss, M.B., Spotnitz, H.M., Parodi, E.N., Wolff, M., Cannon, P.J., Hoffman, B.F., Malm, J.R.: Effects of pulsatile and nonpulsatile coronary perfusion on canine left ventricular performance. J. Thorac. Cardiovasc. Surg. *72*, 742 (1976)
28. Ciardullo, R., Schaff, H.V., Flaherty, H.T., Gott, V.L.: A new method of producing pulsatile flow during cardiopulmonary bypass using a standard roller pump. J. Thorac. Cardiovasc. Surg. *72*, 585 (1976)
29. Ciardullo, R.C., Schaff, H.V., Flaherty, H.T., Gott, V.L.: Myocardial ischemia during cardiopulmonary bypass. The hazards of ventricular fibrillation in the presence of a critical coronary stenosis. J. Thorac. Cardiovasc. Surg. *73*, 746 (1977)
30. Philips, P.A., Bregman, D.: Intraoperative application of intra-aortic balloon pulsation determined by clinical monitoring of the endocardial viability ratio. Ann. Thorac. Surg. *23*, 45 (1977)
31. Sanderson, J.M., Morton, P.G., Tolloczko, T.S., Vennart, T., Wright, G.: The Morton-Keele pump, a hydraulically activated pulsatile pump for use in extracorporeal circulation. Med. Biol. Eng. *11*, 182-190 (1973)
32. Tamari, Y., Frantz, S.L., Beil, Ar. (Jr.), Degnan, T.J., Siedman, S., Garfinkle, T.J., Newman, J.D., Kaplitt, M.J.: Clinical application of intraoperative counterpulsation without balloon pumping. Cardiovasc. Dis. *2*, 405 (1975)
33. Verbiski, N., Beckett, F., Jerabek, O., Kolff, W.J.: Pulsatile flow blood pump based on the principle of the Wankel engine. J. Thorac. Cardiovasc. Surg. *57*, 753 (1969)
34. Berger, R.L., Saini, F.K.: Conversion of nonpulsatile cardiopulmonary bypass to pulsatile flow by intra-aortic balloon pumping during myocardial revascularization for cardiogenic shock. Circulation *45-46* [Suppl. 2], 130 (1972)
35. Marroux, G., Pappas, G., Jenkins, M., Battock, D., Trow, R., Smith, S.D. (Jr.), Steele, P.: Effect of pulsatile and nonpulsatile flow during cardiopulmonary bypass on left ventricular ejection fraction early after aortocoronary bypass surgery. Am. J. Cardiol. *37*, 1000 (1976)
36. Pappas, G., Winter, S.D., Kopriva, C.J., Steele, P.P.: Improvement of myocardial and other vital organ functions and metabolism with a simple method of pulsatile flow (IABP) during clinical cardiopulmonary bypass. Surgery *77*, 34 (1975)
37. Abel, R.M., Buckley, M.J., Austen, W.G., Barnett, G.O., Beck, C.H. (Jr.), Fisher, J.E.: Etiology, incidence and prognosis of renal failure following cardiac operations. J. Thorac. Cardiovasc. Surg. *71*, 323 (1976)
38. Bregman, D.: Dual chambered intra-aortic balloon counterpulsation. In: Current techniques in extracorporeal surgery. Ionescu, M.I., Wooler, G.H. (eds.), p. 407. London: Butterworth 1976
39. Alpert, J., Bhaktan, E.K., Gielchinsky, I., Gilbert, L., Brener, B.J., Brief, D.K., Parsonnet, V.: Vascular complications of intra-aortic balloon pumping. Arch. Surg. *111*, 1190 (1976)
40. Bregman, D., Bailin, M., Bowman, F.O. (Jr.), Parodi, E.N. Haubert, S.M., Edie, R.N., Spotnitz, H.M., Reemtsma, K., Malm, J.R.: A pulsatile assist device (PAD) for use during cardiopulmonary bypass. Ann. Thorac. Surg. *24*, 574 (1977)
41. Breman, D., Parodi, E.N., Haubert, S.M. Szarnicki, R.N., Spotnitz, H.M., Bowman, F.O. (Jr.), Reemtsma, K., Malm, J.R.: Counterpulsation with a new pulsatile assist device (PAD) in open-heart surgery. Med. Instrum. *10*, 232 (1976)

42. Bregman, D., Parodi, E.N., Haubert, S.M., Szarnicki, R., Edie, R.N., Spotnitz, H.M., Bowman, F.O. (Jr.), Reemtsma, K., Malm, J.R.: Unidirectional intra-aortic balloon pumping and counterpulsation during open heart surgery. In: Mechanical support of the failing heart and lungs. Bregman, D. (ed.). New York: Appleton-Century-Crofts 1977
43. Haubert, S.M., Parodi, E.N., Bregman, D.: Clinical experience with a new pulsatile cardiac assist device. JECT *9*, 22 (1977)
44. Bregman, D.: Management of patients undergoing intra-aortic balloon pumping. Heart Lung *3*, 916 (1974)
45. Furman, S., Whitman, R., Stewart, J., Parker, B., McMullen, M.: Proximity to aortic valve and unidirectionality as prime factors in counterpulsation effectiveness. Trans. Am. Soc. Artif. Intern. Organs *17*, 153 (1971)
46. Habal, S., Parodi, E.N., Hanson, B., Wolvek, S., Bregman, D.: A new pulsatile assist device (PAD) for use in cardiac surgery. ASAIO *5*, 32 (1976) (Abs.)
47. Flemma, R.J., Harjeet, M.S., Tector, A.J., Lepley, D. (Jr.), Gabriel, R.P.: Factors predictive of perioperative myocardial infarction during coronary operations. Ann. Thorac. Surg. *21*, 215 (1976)
48. Bregman, D., Parodi, E.N., Edie, R.N., Bowman, F.O. (Jr.), Reemtsma, K., Malm, J.R.: Intraoperative unidirectional, intra-aortic balloon pumping in the management of left ventricular power failure. J. Thorac. Cardiovasc. Surg. *70*, 1010 (1975)

Comparative Study of Three Methods of Myocardial Protection

R. Rivera, J. L. Cantalapiedra, and C. Trascasas

In coronary artery bypass graft (CABG) surgery there is no doubt that distal anastomoses can be performed with greater ease and precision with the ascending aorta crossclamped. However, we cannot find statistically significant differences in the quality of myocardial protection between the cold ischemic arrest by crossclamping the aorta under general hypothermia and local refrigeration and the technique of local occlusion of the artery to be bypassed while maintaining the perfusion of the rest of the myocardium [1] under general hypothermia at 24°C.

When cardiac arrest is achieved by aortic crossclamping alone the anoxic heart stops when its substrate stores become depleted. The functional consequence of ischemic arrest is depressed postoperative ventricular performance (low cardiac output syndrome). Topical hypothermia lowering myocardial metabolism during aortic crossclamping provides only incomplete protection, because it cannot avoid intramyocardial temperature gradients, nor stop the heart before it expends its substrate. Cold cardioplegic solutions have the advantage of stopping the heart immediately and provide for even myocardial cooling. However, the question has been raised whether these cold cardioplegic solutions are effective by their cardioplegic action or only by providing a better technique of myocardial hypothermia.

The present clinical study was performed in an attempt to clarify this issue by comparing the myocardial protection afforded by: topical hypothermia, cardiac hypothermia by coronary perfusion with cold Ringer-lactate, and cardioplegia with a cold cardioplegic solution.

Material and Methods

Patients

All patients with indication of myocardial revascularization consecutively operated on by one surgeon in our department during the year 1977 and up until the end of February 1978, were divided into two groups (group II and group III), depending on the cold solution (4°C) injected into the root of the aorta immediately after crossclamping. As a control group (group I) we used 42 patients who were operated on between January 1976 and March 1977 by the same surgeon and with the same surgical technique. In this group the myocardial protection during aortic crossclamping was afforded exclusively by topical hypothermia with the method of Shumway [2]; continuous irrigating of the pericardium with cold saline at 4°C. This group of patients was also part of a prospective randomized study, comparing aortic crossclamping with local hypothermia with local occlusion during aortocoronary bypass grafting [1].

The characteristics of the three groups are summarized in Table 1. The patients who received additional procedures such as aneurysmec-

Table 1. Preoperative data of 98 patients

	Group I Topical hypothermia	Group II Cold coronary perfusion	Group III Cold cardioplegia
Number of patients	42	29	27
Mean age	50.2	49.7	51.8
Sex (% male)	95	100	94.5
Stable angina (%)	23	24	26
Unstable angina (%)	40	34	34
Preinfarction angina (%)	33	31	18.5
Postinfarction angina (%)	2	10	18.5

tomy or valve replacement, or suffered from hydatid heart disease were excluded from consideration.

Group I was composed of 42 patients (40 men and 2 women) with an average age of 50.2 years. Surgical indication was established in 10 cases for stable angina, in 17 cases for unstable angina (progressive, recent onset, or Prinzmetal), in 14 cases for preinfarction angina and in one case for postinfarction angina.

Group II was composed of 29 male patients with an average age of 49.7 years. Surgical indication was established in seven cases for stable angina, in ten cases for unstable angina, in nine cases for preinfarction angina and in three cases for postinfarction angina.

Group III was formed by 27 patients (26 men and 1 woman) with an average age of 51.8 years, in which surgery was indicated in seven cases for stable angina, in ten cases for unstable angina, in five cases for preinfarction angina, and in five cases for postinfarction angina.

Operative Technique

In all patients the same anesthetic method, cardiopulmonary bypass (CPB) technique, and postoperative care were used. Cannulation of both venae cavae via the right atrium and cannulation of the ascending aorta, were carried out in standard fashion. The same type of disposable bubble oxygenator* was utilized for CPB, with flow rates adjusted to provide a perfusion pressure between 70-80 mmHg. Decompression of the left ventricle was obtained by gravity with a cannula introduced through the inter-atrial groove and connected with the venous drainage system. Reverse isologous saphenous vein grafts taken from the thigh were utilized in all patients. A continuous suture technique with polipropilene was employed for both proximal and distal anastomoses.

In group I the surgical technique can be summarized as follows: After establishing CPB, the general temperature was reduced to 24°C and the heart fibrillated. The segment of coronary arteries where the vein graft had to be anastomosed were exposed, and then the aorta was crossclamped; at the same time cold saline at 4°C was poured into and aspirated from the pericardial well. A continuous flow of cold saline was maintained over the left ventricle during the whole period of aortic crossclamping. Distal anastomoses were then carried out beginning with the branches of the circumflex coronary artery followed by the diagonal branches, left anterior descending coronary

*Temptrol Q-200 A.

artery, and right coronary artery. During the performance of the distal anastomoses in the circumflex system, the heart was lifted out of the pericardial well and the saline tube was held over the heart to provide a continuous drip of cold saline over the epicardium. General rewarming by activation of the heat exchanger was initiated in this group of patients immediately after crossclamping of the aorta, so that at the time of completing distal anastomoses and unclamping of the aorta, the esophageal temperature was usually 32°-34°C and electrical defibrillation could be effected. With the heart empty, but contracting, the proximal anastomoses were carried out with the aid of a side-biting clamp on the aorta. The mean time of CPB in this group was 99 min and the aortic crossclamping time averaged 27 min.

In group II the surgical technique was the same with the single exception of injecting 1000 ml of cold Ringer-lactate at 4°C in the aortic root immediately after crossclamping the aorta. Local refrigeration and graft anastomoses were carried out as in group I. The mean CPB time in this group was 80.4 min and the aortic crossclamping time averaged 27 min.

In group III the operative technique was identical to the one used in group II, but instead of injecting cold Ringer-lactate, a cold cardioplegic solution was used. This cardioplegic solution was prepared with 1 l of Ringer-lactate, adding potassium chloride until reaching 32 mEq/liter and 4 mEq of sodium bicarbonate to obtain a pH of 7.7 and an osmolarity of 300 mosmol. The mean CPB time in this group was 93.4 min and the aortic crossclamping time averaged 26 min.

In some patients of the three groups the proximal anastomoses were performed before initiating the CPB.

In Table 2 the operative data of the 98 patients of the three groups are summarized. In group I there were 10 single CABG, 20 double CABG, and 12 multiple (3-4) CABG with an average of 2.04 CABG per patient. In group II there were 11 single CABG, 10 double CABG, and 8 with multiple CABG (3-4) with an average of 1.9 CABG per case. In group III there were 5 single CABG, 14 double CABG, and 7 multiple CABG, with an average of 2 CABG per case.

Table 2. Operative data of 98 patients

	Group I Topical hypothermia	Group II Cold coronary perfusion	Group III Cold cardioplegia
Number of patients	42	29	27
1 Vessel grafted	10	11	5
2 Vessel grafted	20	10	14
3-4 Vessels grafted	12	8	7
Number graft/case	2	1.9	2
Pump time (min)	99	80.4	93.4
Perfusion pressure (Torr)	72.5	78.1	75.4
Crossclamping time	27	27	26

Electrocardiograms and Vectocardiograms
Standard 12-lead electrocardiograms were obtained immediately before the operation, every 12 h during the first 3 postoperative days, and on the 8th postoperative day in all patients. In a blind study all electrocardiograms were read by one of the authors without knowledge of the situation of the patient. The criteria for the diagnosis of transmural myocardial infarction were a Q wave, not present preoperatively, of more than 0.04 s duration with or without corresponding ST segment changes in one or more leads and a marked (50%) loss of R-voltage in lead V4 without evidence of conduction block. The development of Q waves adjacent to previously infarcted areas was considered to represent perioperative extension of infarction. Changes in ST segments and T waves were not considered in this analysis.

The criteria for the vectocardiographic diagnosis of myocardial infarction were those of Benchimol and Chov modified for the postoperative period of aortocoronary saphenous vein bypass surgery according to Pischrama.

Enzyme Studies
Blood samples were drawn on the morning of the day of the operation and on the first, second, third, and eighth postoperative days. All the enzyme determinations were carried out in the same laboratory by one of the authors. Serum glutamic oxaloacetic transaminase (SGOT) was determined by the method of Reitman and Frankel. Creatine phosphokinase (CPK) and hydrosybutyric dehydrogenase isoenzyme (HBDH) were also measured. Lactic dehydrogenase (LDH) was determined by the method of Wrobleswsky with conversion of results to international units (IU). The isoenzymes of the lactic dehydrogenase were measured by the electrophoretic method in celulose acetate.

Results

Comparison of Patient Groups
Tables 1 and 2 compare the patients' preoperative and perioperative characteristics in the three groups. The patients in the three groups were comparable in regard to age, sex, and severity of disease and, although there were differences in the CPB time, the number of grafts per case and the aortic crossclamping time were similar.

Mortality Rate
There were three deaths (7.1%) in group I, four (13%) in group II, and one (3.8%) in group III (Table 3). In group I, two of the patients who died were in the preinfarction angina subgroup, and both died from a low cardiac output syndrome. One male patient with three CABG died in the operating room and one female patient with two CABG

Table 3. Results

	Group I Topical hypothermia	Group II Cold coronary perfusion	Group III Cold cardioplegia	P Value
Number of patients	42	29	27	
Mortality	3 (7.1%)	4 (13.7%)	1 (3.7%)	n.s.
Perioperative infarction	1 (2.3%)	1 (3.7%)	---	n.s.

died on the 11th postoperative day. The third patient in group I, a 74 year-old man with three CABG died on the 5th postoperative day as a consequence of a technical mistake in the treatment of a respiratory insufficiency.

In group II there were four deaths: a 68 year-old man with three-vessel disease, previous inferior myocardial infarction, and post-infarction angina died in the operating room as a consequence of a new anterolateral myocardial infarction during the induction of anesthesia. A 51 year-old man with unstable angina and an old inferior myocardial infarction, was operated as an emergency because the coronary angiography disclosed a subtotal obstruction of the main left coronary artery and occlusion of the right coronary artery. After performing two CABG the patient developed an extensive anterolateral myocardial infarction and died in the operating room. A 58 year-old man with unstable angina and three-vessel disease died from renal failure 12 days after myocardial revascularization with four CABG. A 63 year-old man with unstable angina and two vessel disease died 11 days after revascularization with two CABG, having developed postoperatively, a disseminated intravascular coagulation.

In group III one patient died 24 days after a single CABG as a consequence of cerebrovascular insufficiency.

Incidence of Myocardial Infarction
The overall transmural infarction rate was 4% (4 of 98) in the total series. In group I, excluding mortality, there was one transmural myocardial infarction, in group II one, and in group III no myocardial infarction. The differences among the three groups were not statistically significant.

Postoperative Serum Enzyme Studies
Table 4 lists the average values of SGOT, CPK, HBHD, and LDH for the first postoperative day in the three groups of patients. There are no statistically significant differences among them.

Discussion

Myocardial hypothermia induced by topical cooling [2], selective cooling by perfusion of the coronary arteries, or by a combination of these methods has proved to be an effective method for protection of the myocardium during cardiac surgical procedure requiring interruption of normal coronary perfusion. For patients undergoing coronary bypass grafting procedures, selective myocardial hypothermia (15°-18°C) resulting in cardiac arrest over a period of several minutes has been shown to be superior to ventricular fibrillation and

Table 4. Postoperative serum enzyme values[a]

Group	Cases	SGOT	LDH	CPK	HBDH
I - Topical hypothermia	40	96	550	129	143
II - Cold coronary perfusion	27	90	581	165	364
III - Cold cardioplegia	27	111	474	190	259
P Value		n.s.	n.s.	n.s.	n.s.

[a]First postoperative day mean values in i.u.

moderate hypothermia [4]. Hypothermic cardioplegia produced by a cold solution containing potassium has also been shown to be an effective method of myocardial protection, which experimentally results in less depletion and more rapid restoration of myocardial energy stores than anoxic arrest at similar temperatures [4]. In dogs, Nelson [5] has shown that hearts subjected to topical hypothermia plus cardioplegia for 1 h functioned as well as they did before the aortic crossclamping was placed. In contrast, this normal ventricular performance could not be maintained in hearts subjected to either cardioplegia alone (31% depression) or topical hypothermia alone (49% depression).

However, despite the theoretical advantages of hypothermic cardioplegia, few clinical studies, particularly in patients undergoing coronary artery grafting procedure, are available to document the beneficial effects noted in the experimental studies; such as the study of Kouchoukos [6] who showed on two groups of 25 patients that hypothermic cardioplegia does not provide any greater protection of the myocardium than hypothermic ischemic arrest.

The data of our clinical study indicates that these three methods of hypothermic myocardial protection for myocardial revascularization procedures are comparable regarding the extent of myocardial injury produced, as assessed by clinical, electrocardiographic, and enzymatic criteria.

While cardioplegic techniques provide a flaccid, quiet heart, which facilitates the technical aspects of coronary bypass grafting, hypothermic cardioplegia was not shown in this study to provide any greater protection of the myocardium than hypothermic ischemic arrest.

References

1. Rivera, R., Cantalapiedra, J.L., Trascasa, C.: Aortic crossclamping with local hypothermia versus local occlusion during aorta-coronary bypass grafting, a randomized study. Unpublished data.
2. Griepp, R.B., Stinson, E.B., Oyer, P.E., Copeland, J.G., Shumway, N.E.: The superiority of aortic cross-clamping with profound local hypothermia for myocardial protection during aorta-coronary bypass grafting. J. Thorac. Cardiovasc. Surg. *70*, 995 (1975)
3. Schachner, A., Schimert, G., Lajor, T.Z., Lee, A.H., Montes, M., Chaudry, A., Schaefer, P., Vladutin, A., Siegel, J.H.: Selective intracavitary and coronary hypothermic cardioplegia for myocardial preservation: Clinical physiologic and ultrastructural evaluation. Arch. Surg. *111*, 1197, 1209 (1976)
4. Gay, W.A. (Jr.): Potassium-induced cardioplegia. Ann. Thorac. Surg. *20*, 95, 100 (1975)
5. Nelson, R.L., Goldstein, S.M., McConnell, D.H., Maloney, J.V. (Jr.), Buckberg, G.D.: Improved myocardial performance after aortic cross-clamping by combining pharmacologic arrest with topical hypothermia. Circulation *54* [Suppl. 3], 11 (1976)
6. Kouchoukos, M.T.: Myocardial preservation: hypothermia and anoxic arrest. The first decade of bypass graft surgery for coronary artery disease. International Symposium, The First Decade of Bypass Graft Surgery for Coronary Artery Disease, Cleveland Clinic Anat. *45*, 66 (1978)

Anesthesia for Coronary Artery Surgery

S. Tarhan and J. H. Tinker

Ischemic heart disease is the most common cause of death in most developed countries. More than 675,000 people die from ischemic heart disease each year in the United States and approximately 1,300,000 suffer from myocardial infarction [1]. Surgical revascularization of potentially ischemic myocardium has provided some hope for this dilemma and the number of operations performed each year is increasing. Yet perioperative myocardial infarction surrounding coronary artery bypass is reported to occur at rates ranging from 4.1% - 30%, with a high mortality rate [2]. This creates a major challenge to surgeon and anesthesiologist alike.

More complete understanding of the pathophysiology of the potentially ischemic myocardium, enabling constant intraoperative monitoring of the delicate balance between myocardial O_2 supply and demand, would be likely to reduce the incidence and severity of perioperative MI. Anesthetic management of patients with ischemic heart disease during and after surgery should concentrate on these determinants of myocardial O_2 balance. Myocardial O_2 demand is increased when mean arterial pressure increases due for example, to increased peripheral vascular resistance (an index of afterload). If preload is increased, as monitored by increases in left ventricular filling pressure, oxygen demand will increase also if the heart is capable of increasing its work output. Heart rate may be the single most important clinical determinant of oxygen demand by compromised myocardium. Myocardial oxygen supply is dependent upon coronary blood flow, which in turn is dependent in large part on diastolic arterial blood pressure, especially in areas of compromised coronary vasculature. Obviously O_2 supply also is impaired by arterial hypoxemia from any cause, as well as decreased blood O_2 carrying capacity.

Today, some control of the above is possible with drugs. This task is probably better accomplished primarily by reduction of myocardial oxygen demand ($M\dot{V}_{O_2}$) rather than increasing the coronary artery blood flow. Drugs such as propranolol decrease the heart rate and myocardial contractility leading to reduced $M\dot{V}_{O_2}$. The vasodilators such as nitroglycerin (TNG) (reducing preload mostly) or nitroprusside (SNP) (reducing afterload) reduce cardiac work and decrease cardiac O_2 consumption.

On the other hand, circulatory effects of anesthetics in terms of their effects upon the determinants of myocardial O_2 supply and demand, particularly when coronary blood flow is limited, are relatively unknown. Anesthetics such as halothane do reduce $M\dot{V}_{O_2}$ by reductions in preload, afterload, and inotropic state, in the normal dog heart [3]. Studies have shown that in the absence of ventricular failure, halothane influences the relationship between myocardial O_2 supply and demand in a favorable direction when coronary artery blood flow is limited [4]. However, the situation may be different in the failing heart. Halothane anesthesia may have an adverse effect and cause further elevation of LVEDP, with increased wall tension and $M\dot{V}_{O_2}$, leading to impaired subendocardial blood flow [4].

Anesthetics such as ketamine have been suggested as suitable during cardiovascular surgery because of supposed cardiovascular stability during induction. However, studies have shown that this drug is a potent pulmonary vasoconstrictor even in relatively low dosage. It also increases $M\dot{V}_{O_2}$, making it appear to us to be less than ideal for a patient with limited coronary blood flow [5]. Similar studies with the other anesthetic agents, combined effects of anesthetics and other drugs administered during surgery such as muscle relaxants, adrenergic agonists, and antagonists in terms of myocardial O_2 balance are scarce. It is possible that the combination of the effects of anesthetics and drugs available to us today may be used eventually to protect the myocardium during and after surgery, especially in patients with potentially ischemic myocardium. Therefore, choice of anesthetics and their proper administration to patients with coronary heart disease is probably important for the outcome of surgery in terms of preventing perioperative myocardial infarction and death.

Preoperative Evaluation of the Patient

Poor clinical cardiopulmonary status before operation, such as intractable heart failure, recurrent pulmonary edema, are predictors of the need for intensive therapy postoperatively, such as endotracheal intubation, prolonged mechanical ventilation, and inotropic support.

Drugs that the patient takes before operation may influence the management during and after the procedure. The use of digitalis, diuretics, corticosteroids, beta adrenergic blocking agents, or monoamine-oxidase inhibitors are particularly important to note. Patients who have received cardiac glycosides and diuretics may have reduced total body potassium with or without a low serum K^+ concentration [6]. Potassium depletion increases digitalis sensitivity. Occurrence of arrhythmias is increased with potassium depletion in the presence of therapeutic concentrations of digitalis during and after operations [7]. It is also known that myocardial sensitivity to toxic effects of digitalis may be increased during the first 24 h after cardiopulmonary bypass even if the serum potassium level is normal [8,9]. In our practice we prefer to terminate digoxin 36-48 h and digotoxin 3 days before surgery. Patients seem to tolerate the temporary withdrawal of digitalis well because they are generally at bed rest prior to surgery.

Propranolol hydrochloride is the other drug that causes concern to the anesthesiologists. This beta adrenergic blocking agent is useful in managing angina pectoris, hypertension, and certain cardiac arrhythmias. By blocking cardiac beta receptors, propranolol slows the heart rate and decreases myocardial contractility, thereby reducing cardiac output [10].

During the past 3 years, some reports have described ventricular arrhythmias, severe angina, and even myocardial infarction after the abrupt cessation of propranolol therapy in patients with angina pectoris. The withdrawal phenomenon now has been recognized and may be avoidable [11]. Recent studies also revealed that perioperative infarction ratios were increased significantly among the patients who had abrupt propranolol withdrawal 24 h before surgery [2]. Therefore danger of MI after withdrawal must be weighed against its potential depressant effect on the myocardium during emergence from cardiopulmonary bypass. More recently, anesthesiologists have been less concerned about this potential depression, and the trend today is in the direction of not stopping propranolol prior to surgery.

Hemostasis during and after cardiac operations may be influenced by inherited bleeding disorders, previous intake of salicylates, and vitamin K deficiency.

Electrolyte concentrations may have a significant effect on myocardial function during and after surgery. Potassium is the most important in this regard. Clinically evident hypokalemia usually does not occur until serum potassium concentration is less than 2.5 mEq/liter. Clinical signs include muscle weakness, bradycardia, and arrhythmias. Prolongation of the ST interval and sagging of the ST segment on the electrocardiogram are typical. Occasionally a low amplitude "u" wave can be seen.

Hypokalemia should be corrected before operation. The oral administration of potassium is preferable because abrupt alterations in serum K^+ levels by IV administration can lead to severely decreased cardiac output and even cardiac arrest in diastole. If time is limited, an intravenous route can be employed with caution. We would suggest a maximum replacement rate of 20 mEq KCl/h in an adult.

Preoperative evaluation also includes the data obtained from cardiac catheterization. This may be predictive of the outcome of surgery. Patients undergoing CABG surgery, with marked depression of left ventricular performance (defined as having an ejection fraction equal to or less than 33%, an end-diastolic volume equal to or greater than 103 ml/m^2 or an LVEDP equal to or greater than 18 mmHg have a significantly higher risk of postoperative mortality [12].

Patients undergoing CABG surgery who do not have impaired ventricular function usually require relatively heavy premedication. Different combinations of sedatives, tranquilizers, and opiates can be used successfully. We rely on pentobarbital and morphine for premedication. Pentobarbital is given orally 2 mg/kg maximally to 100 mg 2 h before operation, thus providing adequate sedation.

We do not use belladonna derivatives and related drugs as part of premedication. They may cause increased heart rate [13] and an increased incidence of arrhythmias [14]. If a vagolytic drug is needed during anesthesia, atropine can be given intravenously in small controlled increments until the desired effect is achieved. It is common practice in the United States to premedicate with scopolamine, in an effort to prevent recall of intraoperative events should anesthesia need to be very light due to hemodynamic difficulties. We have not done this, and rely instead on sedation with barbiturates or diazepam.

One of the recent additions to premedication for these patients which we believe is quite useful is the application of Nitrol ointment (Nitroglycerin ointment 2%) to the chest.

Anesthesia

Choice of anesthetics is ideally based on a thorough understanding of the pathophysiology of ischemic myocardium. Effects of anesthetics on the balance of myocardial O_2 supply and demand are of the utmost importance in patients undergoing CABG surgery.

Induction

Induction of patients with coronary artery disease is increasingly recognized as a critical period of anesthetic management. As soon as the patient is placed on the operating table, the ECG electrodes are attached, including the V_5 lead. (This lead is important for patients with disease of the left coronary artery) (Fig. 1).

After the ECG leads are placed, a plastic needle is inserted into a vein of each arm (usually 14 or 16 gauge Teflon). Each needle is attached to an intravenous infusion set containing 250 ml of 5% glucose in water. The patient then breathes 100% O_2 by face mask. Induction starts with small increments of thiopental (50-75 mg) as tolerated and as needed. We then add 0.10-0.12 mg/kg pancuronium intravenously, and rapidly follow with continued thiopental induction so that 3-4 min can elapse to allow adequate relaxation before intubation. Circulatory stability and longer duration of action makes pancuronium reasonably suitable for CABG surgery although tachyarrhythmias do occasionally occur. Before intubation, the trachea is sprayed with topical lidocaine 4% in an effort to prevent arrhythmias in addition to providing additional local tracheal block. This prevention of arrhythmias (if indeed it does occur) is likely more a result of absorption of lidocaine quickly through the tracheal mucosa than it is due to obtundation of tracheal reflexes, especially when a suitable time is allowed to elapse before inserting the endotracheal tube (~30 s - 1 min). We prefer to remove the laryngoscope after the lidocaine spray, and while waiting, observe the effect of that maneuver on arterial pressure and ST segment.

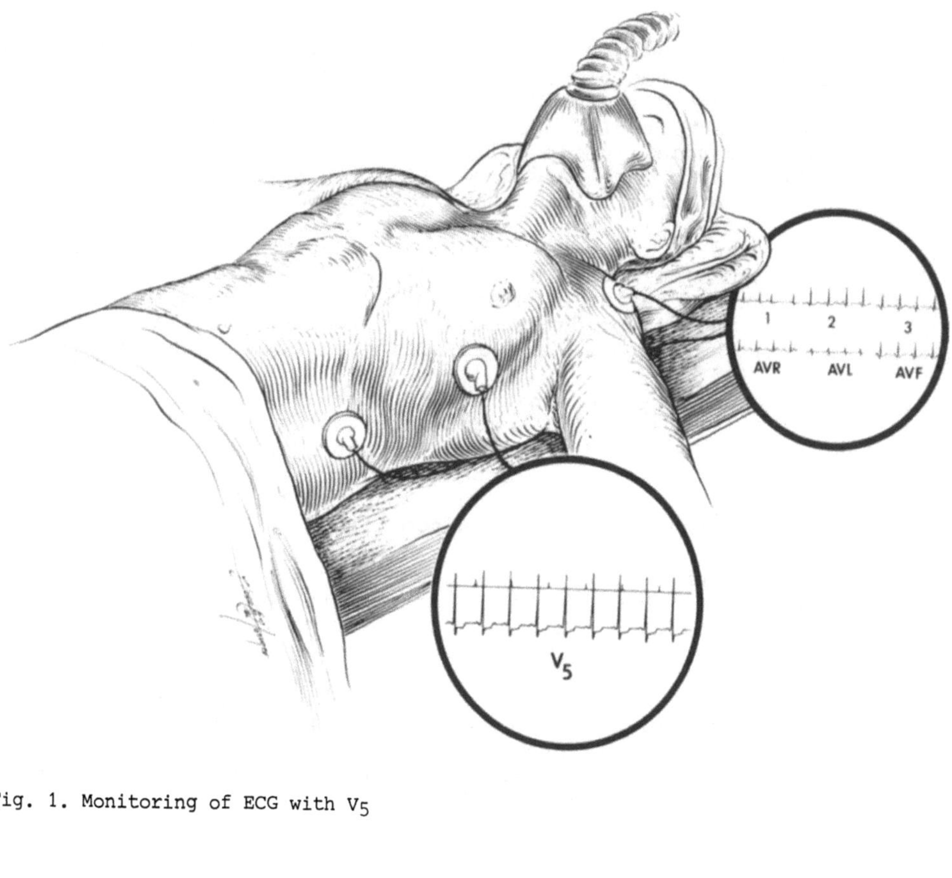

Fig. 1. Monitoring of ECG with V_5

Maintenance

We usually give nitrous oxide (50%-60%) with oxygen and supplement with other drugs such as a narcotic analgesic (meperidine, fentanyl), or a volatile agent (either halothane or enflurane). If meperidine is chosen, we give 20 mg increments intravenously up to a total dose of 200-300 mg.

Morphine has achieved wide popularity for cardiac anesthesia because of its relatively benign effects on the cardiovascular system. Morphine can, however, cause release of endogenous norepinephrine or epinephrine in man [15]. Recent studies comparing morphine N_2O-O_2, versus halothane N_2O-O_2 did not indicate clear superiority for either, but nothing indicated that myocardial depression with halothane was in fact detrimental to the patient. Indeed, myocardial O_2 supply/demand ratio may be somewhat better preserved with halothane anesthesia [16] in patients undergoing CABG surgery.

We find halothane to be of value for use in patients who do not have severely compromised left ventricular function, or who do not have hepatic disease. We try to avoid using halothane in patients to whom it has been given during the previous 12 months. The inspired concentration of halothane is seldom higher than 1.0% with 50% N_2O. If the systolic pressure becomes less than 90 mmHg in a previously normotensive patient, the halothane concentration should be decreased or discontinued, and the anesthetic supplemented with a narcotic such as meperidine (in increments of 10-20 mg). If intense stimulation makes halothane less well tolerated at another, we will administer "balanced" anesthesia at that time.

It has also been amply demonstrated that halothane "sensitizes" the heart to both exogenous and endogenous catecholamines often resulting in arrhythmias. Elevated blood pressure, rapid heart rate, increased serum potassium, and diminished baroreceptor response have all been demonstrated as factors predisposing to these arrhythmias. It is evident that myocardial muscle cells are directly sensitized to epinephrine with halothane anesthesia [17]. This fact should be considered during the usage of halothane for anesthesia.

Enflurane is a recent addition to anesthetic practice. We use 0.5%-2.0% with 50% N_2O-O_2 mixture. No reliable evidence exists yet to implicate enflurane as having a hepatotoxic effect, and it is our clinical impression that it produces less myocardial sensitization to catecholamines, therefore perhaps resulting in fewer arrhythmias.

Patients are heparinized before inserting the arterial and venous cannulas. The initial dose is 90 mg/m^2 body surface. After 1 h of perfusion, one-half of that dose is given and after each subsequent hour one quarter of the initial dose is given. Protamine sulfate (1.3 times the total dose of heparin) is administered to neutralize the heparin after the perfusion is discontinued.

During the perfusion we inflate the lungs with O_2, using a pressure of approximately 5 mm H_2O. We do not attempt to ventilate them. There is little if any evidence that keeping the lungs inflated with this low positive pressure during perfusion minimizes pulmonary damage and postoperative atelectasis, but is seems a logical maneuver. Actually ventilating them might well be preferable, but this delicate surgery requires as still an operating field as possible. Perhaps atelectasis would be better prevented if air were used to inflate the lungs, rather than O_2. No definitive studies have yet answered the question of pulmonary management during bypass.

Monitoring

We routinely monitor arterial and jugular or right atrial pressures, the electrocardiogram, heart sounds, and temperature. Indirect arterial pressure monitoring is unreliable if there is hypotension, thus making direct arterial pressure methods essential in cardiac operations. The percutaneous insertion of an 18 gauge Teflon catheter into the radial artery is effective and seems to be easier to care for postoperatively than a 20 gauge catheter. If ulnar arterial pulsations cannot be palpated and adequate collateral circulation cannot be demonstrated (Allen's test), we use the femoral or dorsalis pedis arteries. If the patient has recently undergone cardiac catheterization or angiography, we prefer not to insert a catheter into the arteries of the arm that was used.

Percutaneous cannulation of the femoral artery can also be easily and safely performed. An 18 gauge, 10 or 15 cm Teflon catheter is used for this purpose. The other method that is commonly used in our institution is a modified Seldinger technique, using a percutaneous puncture and a guide wire, enabling an 18 gauge Teflon catheter to

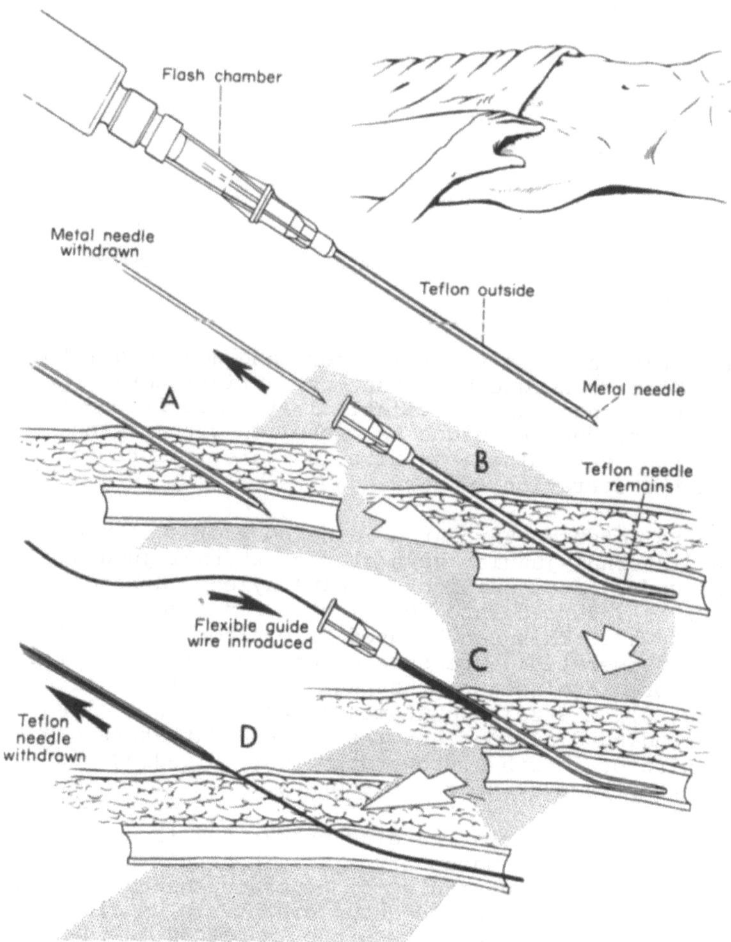

Fig. 2a. Seldinger technique of placing Teflon catheter to the thoracic aorta through the femoral artery

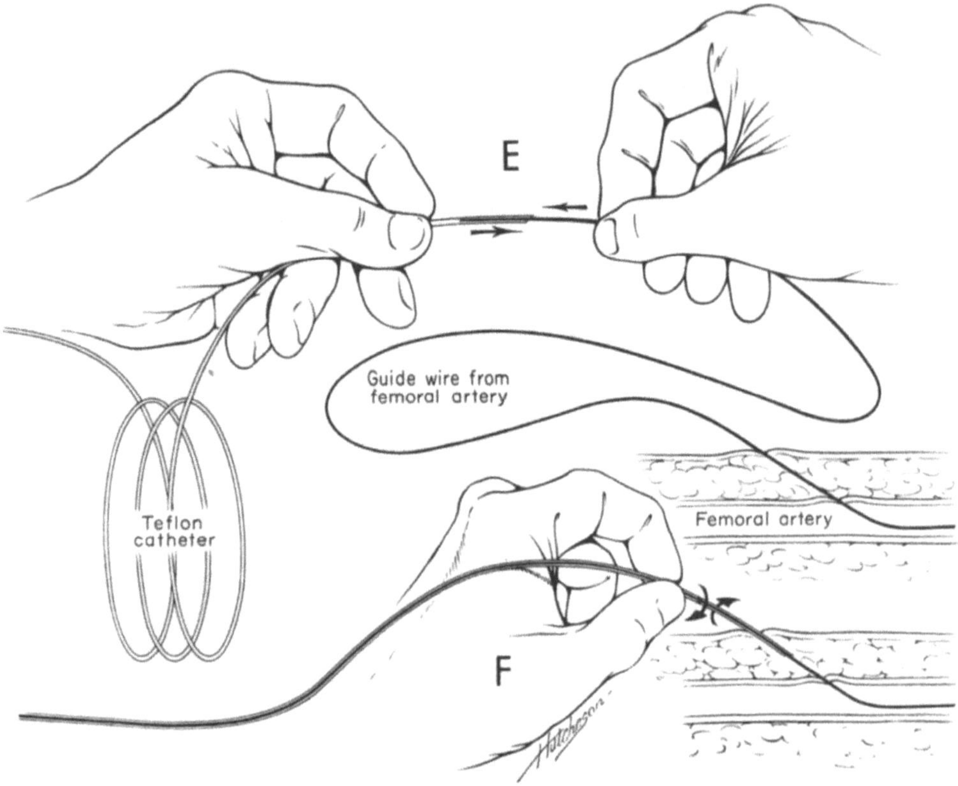

Fig. 2b. Seldinger technique of placing Teflon catheter to the thoracic aorta through the femoral artery

be placed percutaneously into the femoral artery and advanced into the thoracic aorta. This technique has been most satisfactory; the catheter remains patent longer and is relatively trouble free during the postoperative period. The technique is useful in withdrawing blood for cardiac output determinations with indicator-dilution curves during and after operation (Fig. 2).

The venous pressure is measured through a large bore plastic needle placed in the right internal jugular vein or the external jugular vein. After bypass, under direct vision, a polyethylene catheter (1 mm ID, 1.5 mm OD) is inserted into the right atrium and brought out through the chest wall. This can be used to monitor atrial pressure for 24-48 h after operation. Pressure monitoring with a similar catheter inserted before termination of bypass into the left atrium is most helpful (Fig. 3). A strain-gauge manometer, pressure-flush bottle, and direct-reading dial complete the system. Catheters can be removed on the third or fourth postoperative day. Bleeding has not been a problem after removal of the catheters.

The monitoring of temperature during cardiac operations is essential. A probe thermistor placed in the nasopharynx or oropharynx provides a more reliable guide to the temperature of the brain than do rectal and esophageal thermometers. Aortic blood temperature is usually reflected in the reading if the temperature probe is placed in the esophagus. Since the recent reintroduction of hypothermic cardioplegic solutions, we utilize needle thermistor probes to monitor direct myocardial temperature. The heart sounds are monitored by use

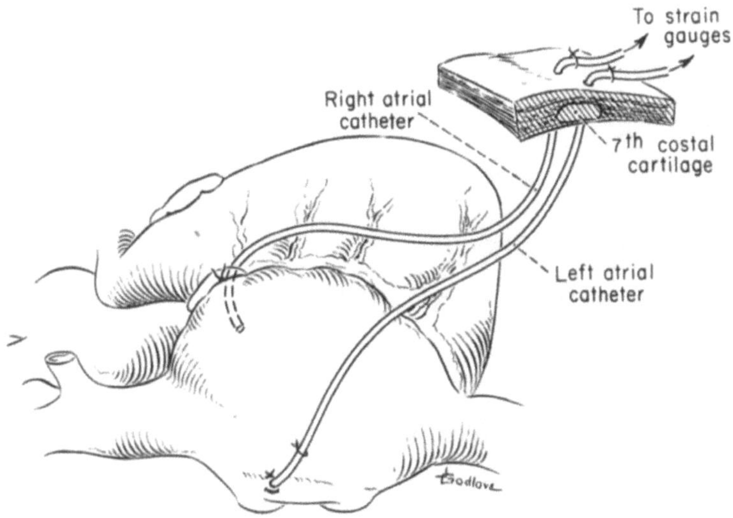

Fig. 3. Catheters placed into atrium before closure of chest and pressures monitored after bypass and during postop period. [27]

of an esophageal stethoscope. Blood oxygen tension, acid-base balance and serum electrolyte concentrations also should be measured at appropriate intervals throughout the procedure.

Cardiopulmonary Bypass

Disposable bubble oxygenators have now become widely accepted because of their economy and practicality. We use the Bentley disposable oxygenator mounted on a Sarns chassis or on a modified Mayo-Gibbon chassis.

The basic components of the Bentley-Temptrol unit are the presterilized oxygenator, a heat exchanger, and a cardiotomy return reservoir. We have incorporated a separate reusable Brown-Harrison heat exchanger into this basic unit to facilitate warming and cooling of the patient. A Bentley blood filter for the cardiotomy reservoir and a bubble trap and/or a filter on the arterial line also have been added to the system. Three sizes of oxygenators are available, and the adult unit can deliver total bypass flows greater than 2.8 liter/min/m^2.

Oxygenator

The shell of the oxygenator is made of polycarbonate, with inlets for blood and an oxygen diffusion assembly at the bottom (Fig. 4). Venous blood enters at the bottom and flows over a funneled base, half of which contains small perforations for gas flow. A tunnel system allows the bubbled blood to flow through. The tunnels are filled with a coarse polypropylene mesh that is coated with silicone antifoam. As the blood passes through the oxygenator for the heat exchanger, it passes through the mesh and is defoamed. A mixture of 98% oxygen and 2% carbon dioxide is fed into the oxygenator at a flow rate of 2-4 liters of gas per liter of blood flow. This rate and mix-

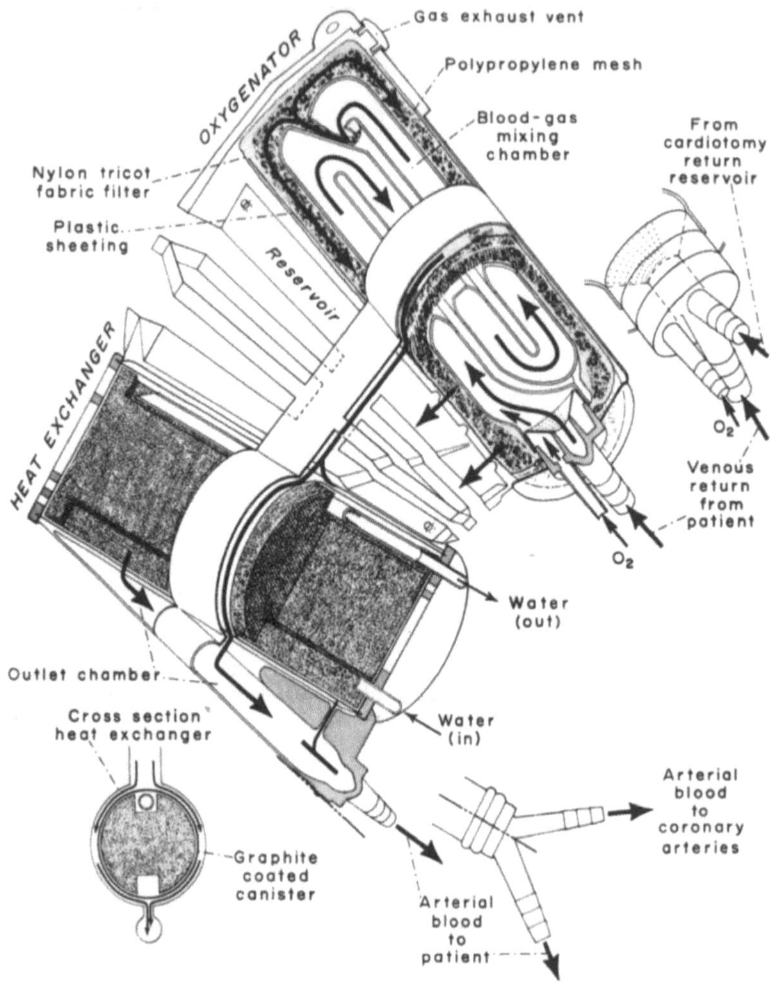

Fig. 4. Bentley-Temptrol oxygenator and heat exchanger. (Courtesy of RA Devloo, M.D.)

ture allow satisfactory arterial oxygen and carbon dioxide tensions. If halothane or enflurane is used for anesthesia, a concentration of 0.5%-1% can be added to the gas mixture through a halothane or enflurane vaporizer incorporated into the system. Arterial line oxygen tension can be monitored by the incorporation of a disposable Clark-type electrode into the arterial line. With this, arterial PO_2 can be adjusted on a minute-to-minute basis.

Priming solutions for adult size oxygenators are given in Tables 1 and 2. Blood constituents are traumatized in the oxygenators; of the bubble oxygenators, the Bentley-Temptrol unit reportedly has a relatively low rate of hemolysis and platelet loss [18]. The membrane oxygenator is still in a developmental stage, but will likely replace the bubble oxygenator in the near future because of its ability to effectively prevent blood trauma.

Table 1. Priming protocol for adult Q-100 oxygenator

Adult Q-100 Short perfusions

Total flow >3.0 liter/min
at 2.0 liter/min/m^2 for patients >1.50 m^2 (≈ 50.0 kg)
at 2.4 liter/min/m^2 for patients >1.25 m^2 (≈ 37.5 kg)

Normosol-R ph 7.4	1,500.0 ml
Heparin sodium 1000 USP units/ml	4.5 ml
Priming volume	1,504.5 ml

Add to this initial priming volume, 30 ml of Normosol per kilogram body weight for each kilogram above 50.0 kg.

Addition

1) Normosol-R ph 7.4	500.0 ml
Heparin sodium 1000 USP units/ml	1.5 ml
	501.5 ml
2) CPD Blood (1 unit)	500.0 ml
Heparin sodium 1000 USP units/ml	3.0 ml
Sodium bicarbonate 8.4%	10.0 ml[a]
Calcium chloride 10%	5.0 ml
	518.0 ml

If patient is less than 1.70 m^2, add addition 1 first then if necessary, addition 2; repeat in order. If patient is larger than 1.70 m^2, add addition 1 first, repeat addition 1 if necessary; if a third addition becomes necessary, add blood as outlined in addition 2.

[a] Use only 5.0 ml Sodium bicarbonate *8.4%) if CPD blood is less than 4 days old.

Table 2. Priming protocol for adult Q-100 oxygenator

Adult Q-100 For coronary perfusion or aortocoronary vein bypass graft

Total flow 3.0-4.8 liter/min
At 2.0 liter/min/m^2 for patients between 1.50 m^2-2.4 m^2 (≈50.0 kg - 106.0 kg)
at 2.4 liter/min/m^2 for patients between 1.25 m^2-2.0 m^2 (≈37.5 kg - 81.0 kg)

CPD blood (2 units)	1,000.0 ml
Heparin sodium 1000 USP units/ml	9.0 ml
Sodium bicarbonate 8.4%	20.0 ml[a]
Normosol-R pH 7.4	1,000.0 ml
Mannitol 15%	100.0 ml
Calcium chloride 10%	10.0 ml
Priming volume	2,139.0 ml

Addition

1. CPD blood (1 unit)	500.0 ml
Heparin sodium 1000 USP units/ml	3.0 ml
Sodium bicarbonate 8.4%	10.0 ml[b]
Calcium chloride 10%	5.0 ml
	518.0 ml
2. Normosol-R pH 7.4	500.0 ml
Heparin sodium 100 USP units/ml	1.5 ml
	501.5 ml

Sequence of addition
For patients between 1.25 m^2 and 1.50 m^2 use addition 1 first, then addition 2. For patients larger than 1.50 m^2 use addition 2 first, then addition 1. Repeat in sequence as needed

[a] Use only 10.0 ml of Sodium bicarbonate (8.4%) if CPD blood is less than 4 days old.
[b] Use only 5.0 ml of Sodium bicarbonate (8.4%) if CPD blood is less than 4 days old.

Cardiotomy Reservoir

The reservoir has a shell also made of rigid polycarbonate, and is placed between the coronary suction line and the oxygenator. The negative surface charge on the outer shell helps to repel hemoglobin and thus perhaps to reduce hemolysis, but it is likely that considerable blood trauma occurs in this part of the bypass setup. The inside of the reservoir is filled with silicone treated polypropylene mesh, which can defoam and filter as much as 3 liters of cardiac suction return per minute [18]. When the technician hears air being suctioned via the cardiotomy suction, he should decrease the vacuum, in a constant effort to minimize blood trauma.

Arterial Line Filter

A filter made of three separate elements of polyester urethane foam with progressively smaller pores (diameter, 150 to 27 μ) is placed between the coronary suction line and the cardiotomy reservoir [18]. The filter allows the removal of both large and small particles without impeding blood flow, although a provision for immediate bypassing of this filter is necessary to have in place should it become clogged.

Hypothermia and Operative Considerations

The patient's temperature during perfusion is dictated by the type of procedure. We decrease body temperature to between 28° and 30° in most patients. Hypothermia also permits the flow rate to be lowered if necessary - for example, if temporary distension of the ventricles occurs, or if an equipment malfunction should take place.

Coronary bypass grafts are done at various degrees of cooling in our institution. Some surgeons prefer cooling the perfusate to 15°-16°C for 6-8 min before crossclamping. After crossclamping, the perfusate is warmed to 30°C. With this technique the heart is cooler than the body, and this may add extra protection to the heart during ischemia. In addition, the heart is almost motionless. Other surgeons accept 30°C as suitable for coronary grafting. Some prefer to perfuse the grafts with blood after distal anastomosis is completed assuming that it would add some protection to the myocardium.

Cardioplegia

Historically, cardiac arrest (cardioplegia) was first induced by the injection of high concentrations of potassium citrate into the coronary circulation. Since then, various cardioplegic methods have been reported. Currently ischemic arrest and hypothermic arrest either singly or in combination are widespread clinical use. Ischemic arrest during cardiopulmonary bypass and open heart surgery can result in severe tissue damage. The concept that this damage might be reduced by the use of specially formulated solutions has attracted considerable attention. These solutions are infused into coronary vessels immediately after aortic crossclamping. Compositions of these solutions vary widely although the basic ideas are twofold: (1) potassium in the solution induces diastolic arrest; (2) "protective" agents in the solution might preserve myocardium from deleterious effects of ischemia [19]. Apparently coronary perfusion with hypothermic solutions or solutions containing high concentrations of potassium chloride which induce arrest without excessively depleting myocardial adenosine triphosphate or creatine phosphate do cause better responses of the myocardium from ischemic cardiac arrest [20]. However, little is at present understood about the mechanism(s) involved in both protection and damage.

In our institution we use two different solutions (Tables 3 and 4) which are stored at 4°C until their use. In CABG surgery cardioplegia is said to be indicated when multiple bypass grafts are required. After initiation of bypass, sites of distal graft anastomosis are found and marked by dissecting epicardial fat from that segment of the vessel, because presence of clear cardioplegia solution in the coronary artery makes their recognition difficult. Once the anastomosis sites are located, the aorta is crossclamped and infusion of cardioplegic solution is begun through a 14 or 18 gauge needle vent inserted proximal to the aortic crossclamp. In order to obtain rapid cessation of electromechanical activity of the heart, preferably without a phase of ventricular fibrillation, the solution should be administered under moderate pressure. We use one of the coronary artery perfusion pumps on the bypass machine for this purpose. Blanching of the myocardium is then observed which is followed by arrest of the heart in diastole. If all distal graft anastomoses are done before the proximal ones, infusion of additional cardioplegic solution is repeated after each distal anastomosis. The volume of the solutions is estimated at 150 ml/m^2/min for about 2 min or 10 ml/kg body weight total.

At the completion of infusion, the temperature of the myocardium should be near 20°C. During the period of myocardial ischemia, measures such as cold saline placed in the pericardial sac, and reducing the perfusate temperature to the range of 22°-25°C can help to reduce the temperature gradient between the body and myocardium, thus help-

Table 3. Cardioplegic solution

Ringers injection	700 ml
Salt poor albumin	12.5 g
Sodium bicarbonate	35 mEq
Potassium chloride	30 mEq
50% dextrose in water	12 ml
Sterile water for injection qs to	1000 ml
Approximate pH = 7.7	
Store at 4°C	

Table 4. Cardioplegic solution

Sodium chloride	5.26 g
Sodium gluconate	5.02 g
Sodium acetate 3 H_2O	3.68 g
Potassium chloride	370 mg
Magnesium chloride	300 mg
Potassium acetate	1.96 g
Calcium chloride 2 H_2O	100 mg
Sodium bicarbonate	1.134 g
Heparin sodium USP 1000 U/ml	2.5 ml
H_2O for injection to make ≈	1,000 ml

ing to maintain the desired degree of hypothermia (Devloo, personal communication).

Circulation During and After Perfusion

As soon as the circulation is taken over by the pump oxygenator, systemic blood pressure declines precipitously. This severe hypotension is due partly to drainage of blood from the patient to the oxygenator, but mostly to vasodilation. A third factor in some patients may be related to the fact that prebypass cardiac output may be somewhat higher than that produced by the pump. Gradually, peripheral vasoconstriction ensues and increases the blood pressure [21]. If morphine is the main anesthetic, arterial pressure may now rise even higher, probably due to release of catecholamines [22]. Such hypertension may be especially hazardous in these heparinized patients, and may contribute to neurologic difficulties.

Perfusion pressures less than 50 mmHg measured in the radial or femoral artery have been blamed for postoperative neurologic complications [23]. Perfusion flow is maintained at 2.0-2.4 liter/min/m^2. Flow alone, without reasonable peripheral blood pressure, does not ensure brain perfusion. Therefore, it is important to monitor blood pressure during bypass.

The period of withdrawal from bypass is a critical time. The patient is rewarmed. The left atrial or ventricular vent is removed. Transfusions from the oxygenator to the patient increase ventricular filling pressure, which in turn hopefully increases stroke volume and blood pressure. The amount of blood transfused depends on the left and right atrial pressures, both of which should be directly monitored during this step (Fig. 5). We do not consider it adequate to estimate left atrial pressure by palpation or inspection at this time, whether or not a left atrial catheter is to be left in place.

Transfusion until a mean left atrial pressure of 10-15 mmHg is reached is usually satisfactory. If increasing the filling pressure up to 20 mmHg does not produce adequate arterial pressure, perfusion should be restarted. Circulatory inadequacy at this point may be caused by coronary air embolism, and this is usually transient. Acute ST segment changes, along with impaired hemodynamics, may be helpful in recognition of this problem.

Allowing time for air bubbles in the coronary arteries to be absorbed or to pass into the venous circulation or administering drugs to improve contractility often leads to a more successful outcome when perfusion is again discontinued. Needless to say, nitrous oxide administration is contraindicated during emergence from bypass and probably for at least 15 min thereafter, because of the possibility of expansion of any air which might have remained in any vessel.

Transfusions of additional small amounts of blood through the arterial cannula are given until the largest blood volume that is compatible with a reasonable left atrial pressure is reached (i.e., LAP $\approx$ 20).

With normal atrial pressure some patients tend to have high arterial pressures when anesthetics are withdrawn at the end of the operation. We generally control this tendency to high arterial pressure with vasodilators (e.g., nitroprusside) which should be gradually added as the anesthetic is tapered at the end of the case. This avoids the necessity of deliberately keeping the patient hypovolemic.

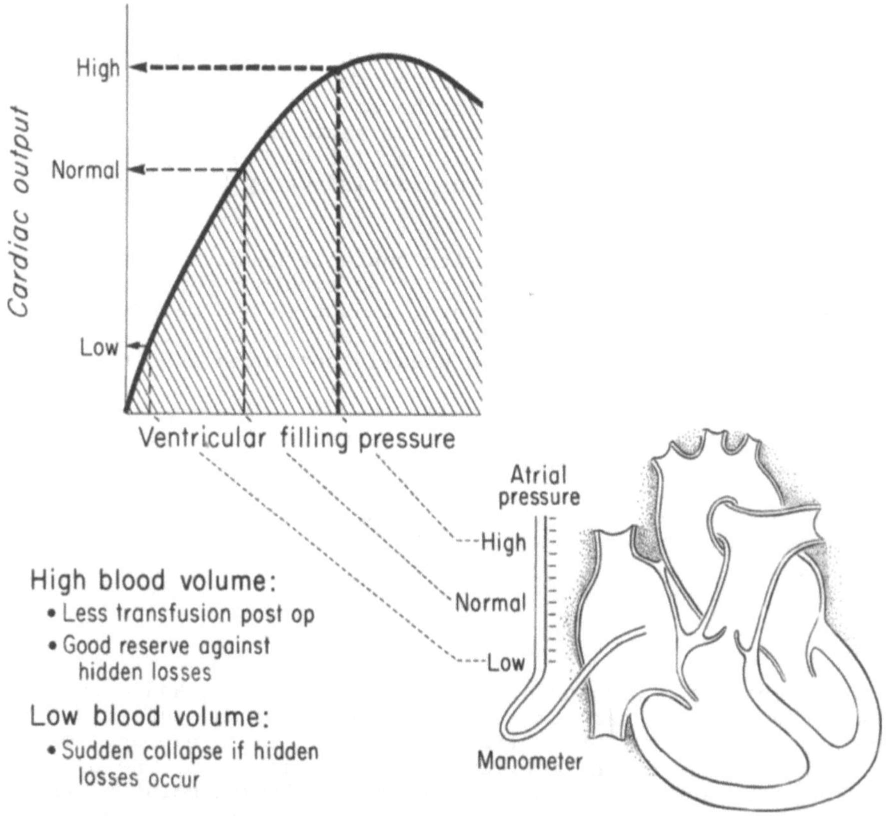

Fig. 5. Management of blood volume after cardiopulmonary bypass. Monitoring blood volume on higher level without overloading patient may provide improved ventricular function and reserve against blood losses. [27]

Intraaortic Balloon Assist (IABA)

Sometimes bypass cannot be terminated because of inadequate myocardial performance and impaired coronary blood flow. If other methods to support hemodynamics fail, an IABA technique can be used for circulatory support. Its use during the operative and immediate postoperative periods to support the failing circulation is sometimes lifesaving. The usual pharmacologic agents employed in treating intraoperative and postoperative cardiogenic shock are vasopressors and inotropic drugs. These drugs increase either afterload or inotropic state, increasing myocardial oxygen requirements during a time when total oxygen availability and delivery may be decreased. IABA lowers myocardial oxygen requirements [24] by decreasing systolic blood pressure, resulting in reduced left ventricular work. Diastolic blood pressure is increased, which increases coronary blood flow, leading at the same time to greater oxygen availability [24].

The insertion of the balloon is a simple procedure during extracorporeal circulation. A Dacron or Teflon graft is sutured to the common femoral artery. The balloon is inserted into the thoracic aorta distal to the origin of the left subclavian artery. When counterpulsation is begun, extracorporeal circulation is discontinued gradually. Since placement of an intraaortic balloon does not require systemic anticoagulation, heparin given for extracorporeal circulation can be neutralized with protamine. Circulatory assistance is maintained for 24-72 h after the operation and then is gradually decreased in such a way that the ratio of balloon inflations to heartbeats is reduced from 1:1 to 1:2 to 1:4 and, finally, to 1:8. When the patient can maintain a satisfactory blood pressure for 12 h, the balloon is removed.

We now also apply IABA to patients with unstable hemodynamics before emergency coronary arteriography or left ventriculography [25], often proceeding then with CABG surgery. Induction and maintenance of anesthesia in these patients has been relatively well tolerated. After completion of surgery, IABA is usually continued into the postoperative period.

An alternative method for management of anesthesia for a patient with unstable hemodynamics is to establish extracorporeal circulation before induction of anesthesia (Fig. 6). The femoral artery and veins can be cannulated under local anesthesia and connected to the oxygenator. Bypass can then be started if the circulation fails [26].

Air Embolism

Air embolism must be a constant concern to both surgeon and anesthesiologist (Fig. 7). The seriousness of air entering the systemic circulation and then the cerebral circulation requires no explanation. The heart itself also can be afflicted with air embolism. The ostium of the right coronary artery is located at the highest point of the aortic root when the patient is supine, thus increasing the chance of air embolism of the right coronary artery. It is manifested as poor right ventricular contractility, arrhythmias, ST segment elevation on the electrocardiogram, and especially higher pressures in the right atrium than in the left.

Air entrapment in the left atrium and ventricle creates the danger of arterial air embolism. A useful instrument to prevent air embolism is a needle vent connected to a suction line (Fig. 8). The needle vent has a slit along the needle shaft. With the needle vent in the ascending aorta, accumulated bubbles and foam can be continuously suctioned [27].

Embolism into the coronary arteries can be prevented if the aortic clamp is released slowly while the proximal right coronary artery is gently occluded. This allows blood to fill the proximal aorta and forces any entrapped air in the aortic root out via the needle vent.

Before perfusion is terminated, every effort must be made to eliminate air from the left heart. The surgeon should elevate the ventricle, after invaginating and massaging the left atrial appendage to expel trapped air. If the lungs are hyperinflated at the same time, blood from the pulmonary veins will be pushed to the left atrium and ventricle, carrying air that can then be removed through the left ventricular vent. This is also the proper time to try to overcome any pulmonary atelectasis which may have occurred during bypass.

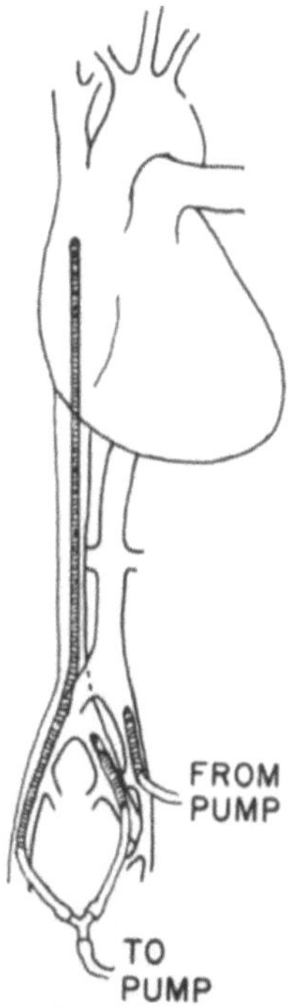

Fig. 6. Cannulation of femoral veins and artery using local anesthesia. Note position of cannulas in femoral veins. In some patients cannulation of one femoral vein may provide sufficient venous return to oxygenator to keep flow at 2 liters/min/m^2. [26]

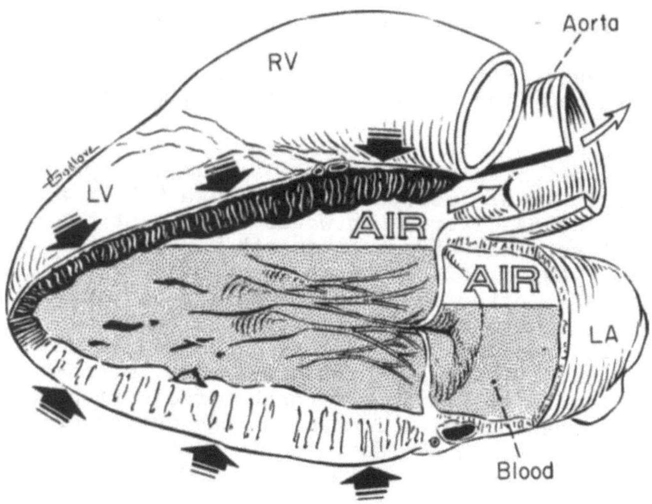

Fig. 7. Mechanism of air embolism. Contraction left ventricle would eject blood and air to unclamped aorta if mitral valve is competent and air would enter the systemic circulation. [27]

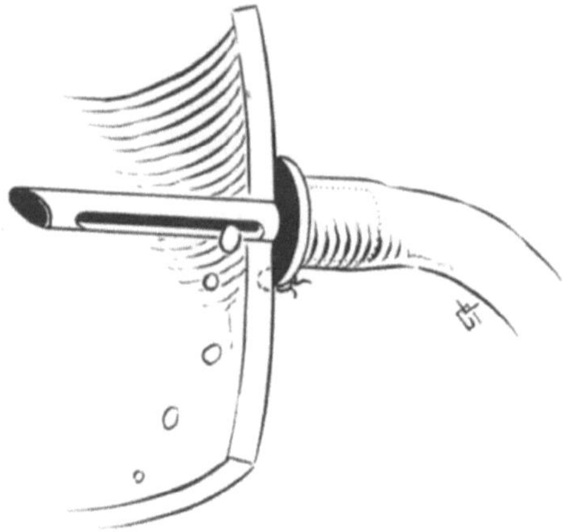

Fig. 8. Air bubbles in aorta can be evacuated continually with a thumbtack needle vent placed in the ascending aorta and connected to the suction line.[27]

Circulatory Care

Proper intraoperative anesthetic management of a patient with ischemic myocardium dictates careful regulation of hemodynamics. A light anesthetized patient, especially a patient receiving morphine as an anesthetic can have greatly increased blood pressure (increased afterload) or heart rate, there an increase of $M\dot{V}O_2$ which may exceed O_2 supply. Pharmacologically induced vasodilation has gained popularity recently for the therapy of inadequate hemodynamic function. Vasodilator drugs have been used in the treatment of refractory heart failure and myocardial ischemia. Rationale of this therapy is as follows: Arterial vasodilation reduces afterload, decreases the tension generated in the left ventricle and reduces O_2 consumption.

Also venous vasodilation causes pooling of blood which in turn decreases venous return (preload) and LVEDP, thus reducing myocardial O_2 consumption.

The drugs most commonly used for this purpose are sodium nitroprusside (SNP) and nitroglycerin (TNG) intravenously. We use SNP in a concentration of 50 mg/250 cc 5% dextrose in water. The agent has rapid action and rapidly reversible effect on smooth muscle. One drawback is its potential cyanide toxicity with overdosage. Nitroglycerin (TNG) is a remarkably effective drug for angina pectoris. It reduces $M\dot{V}O_2$ by dilating venous capacitance vessels, reducing venous return (preload). It has long been used as a sublingual medication, but its intravenous (IV) usage is relatively new. Nitroglycerin has also been shown to result in a favorable redistribution of coronary blood flow to subendocardial ischemic areas during experimental myocardial infarctions in the dog. The IV route has advantages such as easy reversal, control of the dose, and the drug has no cyanide toxicity. The solution must be prepared under sterile conditions. Eight mg TNG is dissolved in 250 ml dextrose in water resulting in a concentration of 32 µg/cc [28]. A reasonable starting dosage is 1.0 µg/kg/min.

Although TNG and SNP exhibit grossly similar hemodynamic effects, TNG may reduce electrocardiographic ischemic injury partly by increasing perfusion of the ischemic areas. On the other hand, SNP may worsen electrocardiographic ischemic injury, at least in part by reducing regional perfusion. Therefore TNG seems preferable to SNP for reducing preload and afterload in patients during the early phase of acute MI. [29] This experimental evidence seems immediately applicable to the OR.

Metabolic acidosis develops secondary to low flow states and may create a vicious cycle. If the acidosis is severe enough, cardiac contractility is depressed, antagonizing the action of the sympathomimetic drugs. Pulmonary vascular resistance is increased also, with concomitant decreases in blood oxygen-carrying capacity. [7] We use sodium bicarbonate to correct acidosis. The required dose is calculated in milliequivalents (base deficit x 0.3 of total body weight in kilograms).

The heart with impaired function (pump failure) may require pharmacologic inotropic support. All known positive inotropes increase $M\dot{V}_{O_2}$ by increasing preload, afterload, or both, as well as by increasing contractility and heart rate. Epinephrine (0.02-0.04 µg/kg/min) is sometimes helpful. Dopamine, a norepinephrine precursor, increases cardiac output by augmenting stroke volume with somewhat less effect on heart rate than epinephrine. This agent also decreases renal vascular resistance, increasing renal blood flow and sodium excretion [30]. We use 200-400 mg dopamine in 250 ml of 5% glucose in water and infuse it intravenously 5-20 µg/kg/min.

A relatively new inotropic agent is dobutamine, a derivative of dopamine. It has been reported to have less arrhythmogenicity and less chronotropic effect than isoproterenol, yet it has a strong inotropic effect. A dose of 10 µg/kg/min increased cardiac output by 27% with little increase in heart rate during actual emergence from bypass. [31] Few arrhythmias were noted in this study [31].

In the absence of specific contraindications, cardiac glycosides also can be given to patients with postoperative low cardiac output. Digoxin is our choice because of its rapid effect and relatively short biological half-life. The digitalizing dose is estimated as 0.9 mg/m^2 of body surface area. Initially, one-half of the estimated dose is administered intravenously, followed by one-fourth or one-eighth of the total calculated dose given every 1-2 h during careful electrocardiographic monitoring, until the desired effect is obtained or adverse effects appear. A maintenance dose of approximately one-eighth the digitalizing dose is given daily, beginning on the day after digitalization has been achieved. Patients usually, however, have been previously digitalized. In this situation, redigitalization must be monitored with digitalis blood levels.

Intravenously administered calcium chloride is commonly used as an inotropic agent in critically ill patients, yet reports on its effectiveness have been controversial. [32] Clinically, an increase of blood pressure after intravenous injection of calcium chloride is often observed. In a comparative study of three calcium salts, we noted only after the administration of the chloride preparation, a consistent, reproducible, and predictable relationship between total and ionic plasma calcium concentrations. In addition, plasma ionic calcium was higher after calcium chloride administration than after administration of either the gluconate or the gluceptate salt [33]. Undoubtedly, length of cardiopulmonary bypass and induced myocardial ischemia are related to the possibility of maintaining a good cardiac output after operation. Studies have shown that cardiopulmonary bypass longer than 1 h increased the ratio of perioperative infarcts significantly. [2] Recent reports indicate that postoperative acute cardiac deaths can be predicted reliably from the combination of cardiac index and mixed venous oxygen levels ($P\bar{V}_{O_2}$) [34]. Therapy in these acutely ill patients should be directed toward keeping the cardiac index greater than 2.0 $l/min/m^2$ and the $P\bar{V}_{O_2}$ greater than 30 mmHg.

Arrhythmias

Arrhythmias may be deleterious to myocardial performance, and they may be warning signals of the development of life-threatening arrhythmias. For example, an episode of ventricular extrasystoles or bigeminy may presage ventricular tachycardia and fibrillation.

The mechanism of myocardial excitation is complex, but factors that cause ectopic activity during and after operation are understood relatively well. These include myocardial ischemia, hypoxemia, alterations in serum potassium concentrations, postbypass myocardial failure, and high blood concentrations of certain drugs such as digitalis.

Before anti-arrhythmia therapy is undertaken, the type of arrhythmia should be identified by the electrocardiogram. Then the cause should be treated, such as correcting acid-base imbalance or low total-body potassium by the intravenous infusion of potassium chloride. Deficient release and activity of insulin during and after extracorporeal circulation may contribute to the failure of potassium and glucose uptake by all cells. The administration of insulin, potassium, and glucose may improve tissue perfusion and correct the arrhythmia. Insulin probably enhances the entry of glucose and potassium into the myocardial cell [35].

Another specific method of treating arrhythmias is cardiac pacing [36] with temporary epicardial electrodes placed during the operation. The heart should be paced at a rate sufficient to suppress ectopic beats and to correct bradycardia. For atrial fibrillation or heart block, wires are carried externally, inferior to the sternum [37], and are attached to an external temporary pacemaker. Electrocautery must be used with care, because current may be induced in the wires which may induce ventricular fibrillation.

If supraventricular tachycardia develops before the chest has been closed, the surgeon may massage or compress the right atrial junction of the inferior vena cava. This is often sufficient to return the heart rate to normal.

Ventricular extopic beats can be suppressed by one of several drugs such as lidocaine (Xylocaine), dipheylhydantoin (Dilantin), quinidine, and procainamide hydrochloride (Pronestyl). With the possible exception of lidocaine, these drugs depress contractility and vascular tone to the same extent that they depress ectopic beats [38].

During the past decade, lidocaine has become the most widely used agent for the treatment and prevention of cardiac arrhythmias. The drug is presently administered for the treatment of ventricular tachycardia and of frequent or multifocal premature ventricular beats and after electric reversion of ventricular fibrillation. Its prophylactic use is indicated if the number of unifocal premature ventricular beats exceeds 5/min, in the presence of multifocal premature ventricular beats, and R-on-T wave premature ventricular beats. The drug is not effective for atrial arrhythmias.

For intravenous administration, a bolus injection of 100 mg of lidocaine is generally acceptable treatment. The half-life of effective blood levels to ensure therapeutic action after a single injection is 12-15 min [39]. Infusion of lidocaine, usually approximately 2 mg/min, should most often be started simultaneously. This will sustain blood levels within the therapeutic range [39].

Diphenylhydantoin sodium is valuable in treating digitalis-induced arrhythmias, even those of supraventricular origin [37,40]. Our dose is 100 mg administered intravenously at 3-5 min intervals, and it is repeated every 5 min until therapeutic or toxic effects are produced. A total dose of up to 1,000 mg has been advocated [38].

Digitalis overdosage can produce almost any type of cardiac arrhythmia. Premature ventricular beats in heart failure are often an indication for more, not less, digitalis [41]. If there is doubt, serum digoxin blood levels should be determined at least 6 h after the last dose of the drug. Levels above 2.0 ng/ml indicate a need for caution, and definite toxicity is indicated by a digoxin level above 3.0 ng/ml.

When digitalis overdosage occurs, medication is withheld. If ventricular arrhythmias are present, 50-100 mEq of potassium should be given in an intravenous solution at a rate of 0.5 mEq/min [41]. If the arrhythmia persists, lidocaine or diphenylhydantoin can be given as previously described.

The beta adrenergic blocking agent propranolol (Inderal) slows or terminates tachyarrhythmias caused by excess circulating catecholamines or increased sympathetic tone. The drug lengthens the refractory period of the atrioventricular node and prolongs atrioventricular conduction time. It slows the ventricular rate in patients with atrial fibrillation or flutter even when such arrhythmias do not respond to digitalis. Propranolol is also effective in treating digitalis-induced tachyarrhythmias of supraventricular or ventricular origin. It is given in 0.25 mg increments as needed to a total dose of 2.0-3.0 mg. The drug is very potent intravenously and should be used with caution because it can cause bradycardia and myocardial depression. Isoproterenol can be used to counteract excessive beta adrenergic blockade, and a large dose usually is needed to overcome myocardial depresssion or bradycardia (or both). Atropine may be helpful for the bradycardia caused by propranolol [10].

Atrioventricular block, bradycardia, pulmonary hypertension, and advanced cardiac failure are relative contraindications to the use of propranolol.

Ventricular tachycardia requires immediate action, because it usually progresses to ventricular fibrillation. Direct current electroshock is applied as soon as possible along with intravenous administration of lidocaine. Lidocaine should be given as previously described in order to suppress ventricular ectopic activity.

Postoperative Respiratory Care

Patients who have undergone saphenous vein grafting for coronary artery disease often remain intubated overnight. Recent publications have emphasized the value of controlled earlier extubation after uncomplicated CABG surgery [42]. Tracheal intubation may be occasionally extended to between 48 and 72 h.

The endotracheal tube generally is well tolerated, although sedation may be necessary. A drug such as diazepam 2.5-5 mg intravenously is usually sufficient.

If the patient had narcotic analgesics during operation, emergence from anesthesia may be slow and respiration depressed. It may be difficult to determine if the unresponsiveness is due to the narcotic, air embolism of the central nervous system, or inadequate cerebral perfusion during extracorporeal circulation. Naloxone (Narcan), a narcotic antagonist, is useful in determining the case of the unresponsiveness. If the unresponsiveness is narcotic related, the patient usually will be aroused by intravenous administration of 0.5-1.0 mg (0.2-0.4 mg) of naloxone.

If an endotracheal tube is in place and inspired gas is not artificially warmed and humidified, the inspired mixture bypasses the natural humidifier provided by the nose and pharynx and can be humidified and warmed only by the remaining moisture and heat from the bronchi and lower airways. As a result, the blanket of mucus that lines the airways dries, ciliary activity decreases, and accumulated secretions become dry and obstruct the airway [43].

Controlled ventilation should be discontinued when the cardiovascular system has stabilized and the arterial oxygen tension (Pa_{O_2}) is satisfactory. The ratio of dead space to tidal volume (V_D/V_T) is also an indication of whether or not the patient can maintain an adequate alveolar ventilation. Patients with a V_D/V_T of more than 0.6 are unlikely to be successfully weaned from mechanical ventilation [43]. If cardiac index is low, weaning from mechanical ventilation may again be difficult. Obviously, patients actively bleeding or requiring inotropic support are unlikely candidates for weaning.

Before extubation, a T-piece adapter should be connected to the endotracheal tube and the patient allowed to breathe oxygen spontaneously. Vital signs and cardiac rhythm are monitored closely, and arterial blood gases are determined after weaning has started. If arrhythmia, tachycardia, cyanosis, or agitation develops, arterial blood gases should be redetermined and the patient connected to the ventilator immediately. A patient with a low blood pH, hypercapnia, and a low Pa_{O_2} ($<$ 70 mmHg) requires further mechanical ventilation.

If the patient's condition is stable, with good vital signs for another half hour, the endotracheal tube may be removed. After extubation, most patients can maintain a satisfactory Pa_{O_2} when breathing oxygen in a concentration of 30%-40% through a face tent or nasal tube.

References

1. Hillis, L.D., Braunwald, E.: Myocardial ischemia (Part I). N. Engl. J. Med. *296*, 971-982 (1977)
2. Langou, R.A., Wiles, J.C., Peduzzi, P.N., Hammond, G.L., Cohen, L.S.: Incidence and mortality of perioperative myocardial infarction in patients undergoing coronary artery bypass grafting. Circulation *56* [Suppl. 2], II-54 - II-58, (1977)
3. Theye, R.A.: Myocardial and total oxygen consumption with halothane. Anesthesiology *28*, 1042-1047 (1967)
4. Bland, J.H.L., Lowenstein, E.: Halothane-induced decrease in experimental myocardial ischemia in the non-failing canine heart. Anesthesiology *45*, 287-293 (1976)

5. De Master, R.J., Fogdall, R.P.: The effects of ketamine on the pulmonary and systemic circulations in patients with coronary artery disease. Annual Meeting of the American Society of Anesthesiologists *1977*, 721-722 (Abs.)
6. Lown, B., Black, H., Moore, F.D.: Digitalis, electrolytes and the surgical patient. Am. J. Cardiol. *6*, 309 (1960)
7. Gilston, A.: Anaesthesia for cardiac surgery. Br. J. Anaesth. *43*, 217 (1971)
8. Morrison, J., Killip, T.: Serum digitalis and arrhythmia in patients undergoing cardiopulmonary bypass. Circulation *47*, 341 (1973)
9. Rose, M.R., Glassman, E., Spencer, F.C.: Arrhythmias following cardiac surgery: relation to serum digoxin levels. Am. Heart J. *89*, 288 (1975)
10. Department of Drugs, American Medical Association: Current status of propranolol hydrochloride (Inderal). JAMA *225*, 1380 (1973)
11. Shand, D.G.: Propranolol withdrawal (editorial). N. Engl. J. Med. *293*, 449 (1975)
12. Hammermeister, K.E., Kennedy, J.W.: Predictors of surgical mortality in patients undergoing direct myocardial revascularization. Circulation *50* [Suppl. 2], 112 (1974)
13. Moffitt, E.A.: Anesthesia and supportive care during operation. In: Surgery for acquired mitral valve disease. Ellis, F.H. (Jr.) (ed.), p. 145. Philadelphia: Saunders 1967
14. Eger, E.I. II: Atropine, scopolamine, and related compounds. Anesthesiology *23*, 365 (1962)
15. Hasbrouck, J.D.: Morphine anesthesia for open-heart surgery. Ann. Thorac. Surg. *10*, 364 (1970)
16. Kistner, J.R., Miller, E.D. (Jr.), Lake, C.L., et al: Indices of myocardial oxygenation during coronary revascularization with morphine versus halothane anesthesia in man. Annual Meeting of the American Society of Anesthesiologists *1977*, 509 (Abs.)
17. Khan, A.A., Miletich, D.J., Albrecht, R.F.: "Direct" sensitization of myocardial muscle cells to epinephrine by halothane. Annual Meeting of the American Society of Anesthesiologists *1977*, 93 (Abs.)
18. Barnhorst, D.A., Moffitt, E.A., McGoon, D.C.: Clinical use of the Bentley-Temptrol oxygenating system. In: Current techniques in extracorporeal circulation. Ionescu, M.I., Wooler, G.H. (eds.), p. 91. London: Butterworth 1976
19. Jynge, P., Hearse, D.J., Braimbridge, M.V., et al: Myocardial protection during ischemic cardiac arrest, a possible hazard with calcium-free cardioplegic infusate. J. Thorac. Cardiovasc. Surg. *73*, 848 (1977)
20. Hearse, D.J., Stewart, D.A., Braimbridge, M.V.: Hypothermic arrest and potassium arrest, metabolic and myocardial protection during elective cardiac arrest. Circulation Res. *36*, 481 (1975)
21. Gordon, R.J., Ravin, M., Rawitscher, R.E., et al: Changes in arterial pressure, viscosity, and resistance during cardiopulmonary bypass. J. Thorac. Cardiovasc. Surg. *69*, 552 (1975)
22. Hasbrouck, J.D.: Morphine anesthesia for open-heart surgery. Ann. Thorac. Surg. *10*, 364 (1970)
23. Stockard, J.J., Bickford, R.G., Chir, B., et al: Pressure-dependent cerebral ischemia during cardiopulmonary bypass. Neurology (Minneap) *23*, 521 (1973)
24. Housman, L.B., Bernstein, E.F., Braunwald, N.S., et al: Counterpulsation for intraoperative cardiogenic shock: successful use of intra-aortic balloon. JAMA *224*, 1131 (1973)
25. Curtis, J.J., Barnhorst, D.A., Pluth, J.R., et al: Intra-aortic balloon assist, initial Mayo Clinic experience and current concepts. Mayo Clin. Proc. *52*, 723-730 (1977)
26. Danielson, G.K., Hasbrouck, J.D., Bryant, L.R.: Cannulation under local or regional anesthasia for the "salvage" cardiac patient. J. Thorac. Cardiovasc. Surg. *55*, 864 (1968)
27. McGoon, D.C.: Technics of open-heart surgery for congenital heart disease. In: Current Problems in Surgery. Ravitch, M. (ed.), p. 3. Chicago: Yearbook Medical Publishers 1968
28. Kaplan, J.A.: The pharmacological treatment of the cardiovascular system. Annual Meeting of the American Society of Anesthesiologists *1976*, 212 (Abs.)

29. Chiariello, M., Gold, H.K., Leinbach, R.C., et al: Comparison between the effects of nitroprusside and nitroglycerin on ischemic injury during acute myocardial infarction. Circulation *54*, 766 (1976)
30. Rosenblum, R., Frieden, J.: Intravenous dopamine in the treatment of myocardial dysfunction after open-heart surgery. Am. Heart J. *83*, 743 (1972)
31. Tinker, J.H., Tarhan, S., White, R.D., et al: Dobutamine for inotropic support during emergence from cardiopulmonary bypass. Anesthesiology *44*, 281 (1976)
32. Denlinger, J.K., Kaplan, J.A., Lecky, J.H., et al: Cardiovascular responses to calcium administered intravenously to man during halothane anesthesia. Anesthesiology *42*, 390 (1975)
33. White, R.D., Goldsmith, R.S., Rodriguez, E., et al: Plasma ionic calcium levels following injection of chloride, gluconate, and gluceptate salts of calcium. J. Thorac. Cardiovasc. Surg. *71*, 609 (1976)
34. Parr, G.V.S., Blackstone, E.H., Kirklin, J.W.: Cardiac performance and mortality early after intracardiac surgery in infants and young children. Circulation *51*, 867 (1975)
35. Moffitt, E.A., Rosevear, J.W., Molnar, G.D., et al: Effects of giving glucose-insulin-potassium solution on metabolism after cardiac surgery. Circulation *39*, [Suppl. 3], 149 (1969) (Abs.)
36. Danielson, G.K., Ellis, F.H. (Jr.): Low cardiac output and cardiac arrhythmias after open-heart surgery. In: Critical surgical illness. Hardy, J.D. (ed.), p. 587. Philadelphia: Saunders 1971
37. McGoon, D.C., Pluth, J.R.: Postoperative care of the open-heart patient: general considerations. In: Cardiovascular surgery, current practice. Burford, T.H., Ferguson, T.B. (eds.), Vol. 1, p. 33. St. Louis: Mosby 1969
38. Harrison, D.C., Kerber, R.E., Alderman, E.L.: Pharmacodynamics and clinical use of cardiovascular drugs after cardiac surgery. Am. J. Cardiol. *26*, 385 (1970)
39. Harrison, D.C.: Practical guidelines for the use of lidocaine: prevention and treatment of cardiac arrhythmias. JAMA *233*, 1202 (1975)
40. Karliner, J.S.: Intravenous diphenylhydantoin sodium (Dilantin) in cardiac arrhythmias. Dis. Chest. *51*, 256 (1967)
41. Walker, W.J.: Treatment of heart failure. JAMA *228*, 1276 (1974)
42. Klineberg, P.L., Geer, R.T., Hirsh, R.A., et al: Early extubation after coronary artery bypass graft surgery. Crit. Care Med. *5*, 272 (1977)
43. Feeley, T.W., Hedley-Whyte, J.: Weaning from controlled ventilation and supplemental oxygen. N. Engl. J. Med. *292*, 903 (1975)

Myocardial Protection by a Calcium Antagonist

R. E. Clark, Ph. D. Henry, I. Y. Christlieb,
J. R. Williamson, and B. E. Sobel

Calcium plays an essential role in the regulation of energy metabolism in cardiac muscle. It controls activation of the contractile apparatus and is a major determinant of myocardial energy expenditure. Calcium is essential in oxidative phosphorylation and modulates the effects of catecholamines.

Ischemic injury results in abnormal ion exchanges between the interstitial fluid and intracellular compartments. These ionic shifts occur along prevailing electrochemical concentration gradients and result in a loss of intracellular potassium, magnesium, and phosphate and a gain in calcium, sodium, chloride, and water. The free calcium ion concentration is approximately 1,000 to 10,000 times greater outside than inside the cell. When the active processes that maintain the ionic ratio within cells are impaired by ischemia, calcium accumulates within the cell and is consistently found in large concentrations in irreversibly injured myocardial cells.

The increase in intracellular calcium concentration as a result of ischemic injury results in inappropriate activation of the myocardium and impairment of synthesis of ATP. This process accelerates the depletion of high energy phosphate stores. Muscle relaxation also requires ATP so that when ATP stores are severely depleted, myocardial relaxation is impaired and ischemic contracture ensues. In its most extreme form, this lesion is manifest as myocardial rigor or "stone heart".

The rationale of our experiments was that by prevention of the accumulation of intracellular calcium and subsequent depletion of high energy phosphate stores, the consequent stiffness and decrease in contractility associated with ischemic injury and reperfusion could be ameliorated. The drug chosen for blockade of transmembrane calcium flux was nifedipine, Fig. 1. It appears to have specific membrane effects for blockade of calcium and is an extraordinarily potent vasodilator. Its mechanisms of action have not been fully delineated. It is known that it exerts a strong negative inotropic effect on myocardium but it is not a beta adrenergic blocker. The drug has been widely used in Europe, Asia, and Central and South America for the treatment of angina and appears to work in concert and synergistically with propranolol. It has a rapid onset of action of 5-20 min when given in sublingual form and, in contrast to nitroglycerin, its effects last 4-6 h.

The intravenous form of the drug is not widely available nor has it been used therapeutically in humans. This form is rapidly degraded when exposed to light, a property that may make nifedipine attractive for use in myocardial protection in the setting of cardiopulmonary bypass since any escape of drug into the extracorporeal circuit will result in its rapid deactivation. Experiments detailed here were designed to demonstrate amelioration of the biochemical and pathologic alterations caused by ischemia by selective blockade of the calcium transmembrane flux.

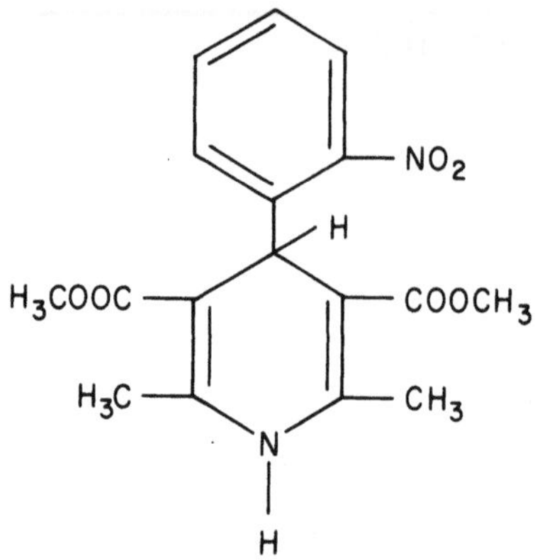

NIFEDIPINE
BAY A 1040

Fig. 1

Methods

Four preparations have been used: (1) isolated perfused rabbit hearts, (2) closed chest conscious dogs given myocardial infarction, (3) open chested dogs with occlusion of the left anterior descending coronary artery for various time periods, and (4) global myocardial ischemia using cardiopulmonary bypass at 28° or 37°C.

Isolated Perfused Rabbit Hearts

Albino rabbits weighing between 2.0 and 2.5 kg were used. Hearts were isolated and perfused retrograde at 37°C through the aorta. The perfusate contained (mM) NaCl, 118; KCl, 2.8; KH_2PO_4, 1.2; $CaCl_2$, 2.5; $MgSO_4$, 1.2; $NaHCO_3$, 25; and glucose, 5. After equilibration at 37°C with a 5% CO_2-95% O_2 gas mixture, the pH of the perfusate was 7.38. The rate of the perfusion was maintained at 22 ml/min with a roller pump. A latex balloon mounted around a micromanometer was inserted into the left ventricular cavity for measurement of left ventricular pressure and LVDP/dt. The balloon was filled slowly with deaerated saline with the use of a micrometer syringe until end diastolic pressure stabilized between 5 and 8 mmHg. A bipolar electrode was attached to the right ventricular wall and the heart was paced at a frequency of 180 beats per minute. Thus, the major determinants of cardiac performance; ventricular preload; afterload, heart rate, coronary flow, and temperature were controlled.

All hearts were equilibrated for 30 min at a flow rate of 22 ml/min. Then a slow perfusion was started at the rate of 0.2 ml/min with the perfusate containing nifedipine or its vehicle and maintained for 60 min. Nifedipine or its vehicle was infused with a syringe pump into the perfusion system at a rate not exceeding 1% of the total flow.

The calcium content of the myocardial mitochondral fraction was determined using copper as a mitochondral marker.

Protection of Ischemic Myocardium by Nifedipine in Conscious Dogs
Mongrel dogs were anesthetized with pentabarbitol sodium (25 mg/kg), intubated and placed on a volume ventilator and had a left thoracotomy through the 5th left intercostal space. The left anterior descending coronary artery was dissected and a balloon occluder passed around it. Catheters were inserted into the left atrium, jugular vein, and central aorta and an electromagnetic flow probe placed around the aorta. The free ends of the transducer cables, snare, and catheters were exteriorized dorsally at the base of the neck. The chest was closed and each animal was allowed to recover 11-17 days. The hemodynamic measurements were made in conscious, loosely restrained dogs while they were lying quietly on the right side. Regional coronary blood flow was estimated by the microsphere method with carbonized microspheres, a 15 ± µ 3 uM labelled with ^{85}Sr, ^{141}Ce, ^{51}Cr. After control data was obtained, the left anterior descending coronary artery was occluded. Twenty-nine minutes after occlusion an initial injection of microspheres was given and the administration of nifedipine or its vehicle was begun. Drug treated animals received a loading dose of nifedipine of 5 µg/kg followed by a continuous intravenous infusion of the drug. A second injection of microspheres was given 3 min after the onset of the infusion of the drug or its vehicle and hemodynamic monitoring was continued for three hours. In four control and four treated animals an injection was administered at the end of the three hour interval. Finally, an injection of microspheres was given 24 h after the occlusion and the animal sacrificed. Creatine kinase activity as well as radioactivity in core samples was determined for three zones of the myocardium: The nonischemic zone, the peripheral ischemic zone and the central ischemic zone.

Regional Ischemia in Open Chested Dogs
Mongrel dogs were anesthetized, intubated, and ventilated and had a left thoracotomy. Catheters were placed through the groin vessels to the level of the right atrium and the ascending aorta. Two catheters were inserted into the left atrium, one of which was passed through the mitral valve into the left ventricle. Catheters were applied to strain gauge transducers and the phasic and mean pressures were recorded. An electromagnetic flow probe was applied to the ascending aorta for determination of phasic and mean flows. The left ventricular pressure was differentiated and recorded directly as LVDP/dt. Occlusion of the left anterior descending coronary artery was accomplished with fine silicone rubber tubing. Animals were treated with nifedipine during the ischemic period of one or two hours duration, during the two-hour reperfusion period which was constant for all animals or during both periods. Each animal had an infusion of either saline or saline plus nifedipine at a rate of 40 ml/h through an aortic root needle controlled by a Harvard infusion pump. The solutions were at room temperature and the dosage of nifedipine was 5 µg/kg/h at an average concentration of 3.0 ± 0.3 mg/ml. Infusions were begun simultaneously with an LAD occlusion or LAD release. After 120 min of reperfusion, 100/mg/kg of colloidal carbon was injected through the left atrial catheter. After 5 min the heart was flushed and fixed in situ. The heart was cut in approximately 5 mm slices perpendicular to the apical aortic root axis with a calibrated slicer. After complete fixation each slice was photographed and the volume of the ischemic reperfusion injury determined morphometrically and the results expressed as a percent of total volume.

Global Ischemia Using Cardiopulmonary Bypass
Two groups of experiments have been performed: one under conditions mimicking clinical practice employed for myocardial preservation and the second under normothermic conditions.

Mongrel dogs were placed on total cardiopulmonary bypass with systemic hypothermia of 28°C and topical cardiac hypothermia was produced with 4°C Ringer's lactate. Each animal received substrate priming with insulin, glucose, and potassium and osmolality was briefly raised with an infusion of 12.5 g of mannitol prior to clamping of the ascending aorta. Two hours of global ischemia were induced following which each animal was reperfused for 30-60 min while in normal sinus rhythm with an empty beating nonworking heart. The experimental group received five µg/kg/h of nifedipine through an aortic root catheter during ischemia. The control animals received the vehicle in an identical volume of 50 ml/h.

A second group of mongrel dogs were placed on total cardiopulmonary bypass and had 60 min of global ischemia at 37°C. Each animal received an infusion of either saline or saline plus nifedipine at a rate of 240 ml/h. The concentration of the drug was 0.167 µg/ml. Each animal received an infusion of 2.5 g of calcium chloride in 100 ml of Ringer's lactate solution. The infusion of this solution was begun during the last 15 min of ischemia and was continued during the reperfusion period until the animal was stable off cardiopulmonary bypass. All data was statistically analyzed and stroke work, cardiac index, and total peripheral vascular resistance were calculated.

Results

Isolated Perfused Rabbit Hearts

The effects of low flow of 0.2 ml/min resulted in a marked decline of developed left ventricular pressure and dP/dt in all animals initially. Upon reperfusion of the nondrug treated hearts, peak pressure recovered to a level of 78% of preischemic values and recovered only 38% of preischemic values for peak dP/dt. These controls showed a marked elevation of the end diastolic pressure to 40 mmHg. Those rabbit hearts perfused with the same protocol except for the infusion of nifedipine 10^{-7} M during the low flow period showed a marked return of mechanical activity with an 87 and 85% recovery of peak pressure and peak dP/dt, respectively. Importantly, the enddiastolic pressure increased only 2 mmHg in contrast to 40 mmHg for the control hearts.

The calcium determinations demonstrated that control values for calcium in units of nanograms-Atom/mg protein for hearts perfused for 60 min with high flow was 7.6 ± 0.4. Hearts perfused under low flow conditions for 60 min without the presence of nifedipine in the perfusate resulted in a calcium index of 28.2 ± 1.9 while those treated with nifedipine yielded a normal value of 8.0 ± 0.5. The latter value was statistically not different than the control values while the hearts not receiving nifedipine had a value that was statistically significant at the 0.001 level.

Protection of Ischemic Myocardium by Nifedipine in Conscious Dogs

Treatment with nifedipine induced modest and transient decreases in aortic and left atrial pressures and significant increases in the heart rate 33 min and 3.5 h after coronary occlusion. Cardiac output was significantly increased at all times in dogs given nifedipine in comparison to animals that did not receive this drug. Cardiac output was increased by 39% 33 min after coronary occlusion and by 22% 3.5 h and 24 h after occlusion. Blood flow to all zones of the myocardium was markedly increased by the use of nifedipine. Blood flow to the nonischemic area in placebo treated animals was 83 ± 10 ml/100 g/min versus 162 ± 18 for animals treated with nifedipine. In the peripheral ischemic zone the control values were 34 ± 4 versus 72 ± 7 ml/100 g/min for the nifedipine treated dogs. Finally, in the central ischemic zone, blood flow was 12 ± 2 for the controls versus 39 ± 5 ml/100 g/min for the nifedipine treated animals.

Myocardial CK activity in IU/g wet weight 24 h after creation of myocardial infarction was similar in the nonischemic zone for both the placebo and nifedipine treated dogs, 2450 ± 126 versus 2460 ± 117 respectively. For the peripheral ischemic zone, CK activity was 342 ± 58 versus 2080 ± 118 for the nifedipine treated dogs. For the central ischemic zone the control value was 208 ± 31 versus 789 ± 63 for drug treated dogs.

Regional Ischemia in Open Chested Dogs

There was a marked difference between animals which received nifedipine and those that did not with respect to hemodynamics and injury volume. Hearts that received nifedipine during both periods had a stroke work index of 19 g-M/M^2 versus 9.6 g-M/M^2 for animals that did not receive nifedipine. Similarly, the dP/dt was 3125 and 2294 mmHg/s for nifedipine dogs and control dogs, respectively. Use of nifedipine resulted in an injury volume of 2.6% in animals treated with drug versus 4.8% for those not so treated. Similar results were found for the 2 h ischemic period where controls and treated animals had 8.9% and 3.1% injury volumes, respectively. When drug was given during ischemia only, there was good preservation of contractility but injury volume was 4.1 at 1 h of ischemia and 8.0 for 2 h of ischemia. If the drug was given during the reperfusion period only the injury volume was 4.4 for 1 h of ischemia and 4.9 for 2 h of ischemia. Clearly, the most efficacious mode was the infusion of nifedipine at the onset of ischemia and its continuation during the reperfusion period.

Global Ischemia With Cardiopulmonary Bypass

A. Hypothermia
None of the seven control animals could be weaned from cardiopulmonary bypass after 2 h of ischemia at 28°C with a saline infusion at room temperature during the ischemic period. All had a marked loss of stroke work. LVDP/dt, a marked reduction of 70% of cardiac output, and no response to volume loading. There was an 85% depression of stroke work and 53% decrease in LVDP/dt. In marked contrast, the animals receiving nifedipine during the 2 h of global ischemia had a 27% reduction of cardiac output, a 17% reduction in stroke work, and a 19% reduction in LVDP/dt. All animals were weaned from cardiopulmonary bypass and all had a normal response to volume loading. Histologic studies revealed marked subendothelial injury in the control animals whereas two-thirds of the drug treated hearts were determined to be normal.

B. Normothermic Animals
There was a striking difference between animals treated with nifedipine and those that were not. The saline treated controls had a 53% reduction in stroke work index, a 27% reduction in LVDP/dt, and 29% reduction in cardiac index. In contrast, the nifedipine treated animals had a 10% increase in stroke work index, a 6% decrease in LVDP/dt, and 1% increase in cardiac index. The values for the latter group are not statistically significant in comparison to the preischemic values.

Discussion

It is clear from all experiments to date that nifedipine, a specific blocker of transmembrane calcium flux provides a highly significant protective effect to ischemic myocardium. The isolated rabbit heart experiments clearly demonstrated that use of this drug prevented the characteristic increase in wall stiffness associated with ischemia with nearly normal preservation of peak developed pressure and LVDP/dt.

The conscious dogs that received myocardial infarction and drug demonstrated a nearly fourfold increase in myocardial creatine kinase activity (CK) in the central ischemic zone of biopsies taken 24 h post infarction. Similarly, there was a nearly fourfold increase of CK in the ischemic peripheral zone with no difference in the non-ischemic areas. These data correlated well with the blood flow data demonstrating that there was a threefold increase of blood flow to the central ischemic zone and a twofold increase in the peripheral ischemic zone in drug treated animals versus controls.

The marked preservation of ventricular mechanics and the impressive reduction of the ischemic reperfused injury volume again demonstrates the efficacy of nifedipine when used in the setting of acute myocardial infarction.

The animals placed on cardiopulmonary bypass under both normothermic and hypothermic conditions demonstrate yet another potential use for this drug. It appears to have a marked protective effect as demonstrated by both groups of experiments regardless of temperature. Inasmuch as myocardial ischemia is required in cardiac surgery for prolonged periods of time to accomplish multiple revascularization procedures, this drug has great potential for extending methods currently in use. The prospect of 2-3 h of complete global ischemia with normal recovery is perhaps within grasp.

Summary

Four groups of experiments utilizing the isolated perfused rabbit heart, myocardial infarction in conscious dogs, regional ischemia in the open-chested dog, and global ischemia under normothermic and hypothermic conditions have demonstrated the marked efficacy of nifedipine in the setting of myocardial ischemia and reperfusion. The potential for this drug to have an impact on myocardial infarction in man and markedly improved myocardial protection during cardiac surgery is discussed.

Myocardial Protection and Postoperative Care with Vasodilator Therapy (Nitrates)

S. Piepenbrock and G. Hempelmann

Patients undergoing aortocoronary bypass surgery may present problems because of relative imbalance between cardiac oxygen supply and demand.

During anesthesia in these patients it is therefore essential to influence the oxygen supply-to-demand ratio in such a way, that a positive net effect results in adequate supply of cardiac O_2 needs.

Neuroleptanalgesia has been proven to be the anesthesia of choice for this purpose. Different variations with morphine, piritramid, or sulfentanil may also be employed.

If there is any tendency toward hypertension during surgical procedures we try to "deepen" anesthesia using additional drugs, such as diazepam or flunitrazepam.

Apart from their sedative effects, flunitrazepam (Rohypnol) as well as diazepam (Valium), have vasodilating properties which may lead to a reduction in arterial blood pressure and a distinct decrease in left ventricular enddiastolic pressure (Fig. 1).

A further possibility in protecting the myocardium from inadequate oxygen demand-supply ratio caused by an extensive increase in pressure-work is the use of nitroglycerin or sodium nitroprusside. In recent years these two substances have gained a considerable amount of interest in connection with inducing controlled hypotension, treatment of congestive heart failure, and treatment of acute myocardial infarction.

Nitroglycerin

The mechanism of cardiovascular action of nitroglycerin in coronary artery disease is related to a predominant reduction in peripheral venous resistance as compared to arteriolar resistance. The diagram from Dobbs and Povalski [1] illustrates this mechanism (Fig. 2). Nitroglycerin appears to have a rather selective action on the venous capacitance vessels, although it also has some influence in reducing pressure on the arterial side. This combined effects results in a reduction in both preload (filling pressures) and afterload (arterial impedance), which contribute mainly in reducing myocardial wall stress [2-4].

Reduction in venous resistance and return will also lead to a decrease in enddiastolic pressure and volume, which in turn results in a reduction in ventricular size and, therefore, wall tension. The net effect is a decrease in oxygen requirements [1,5].

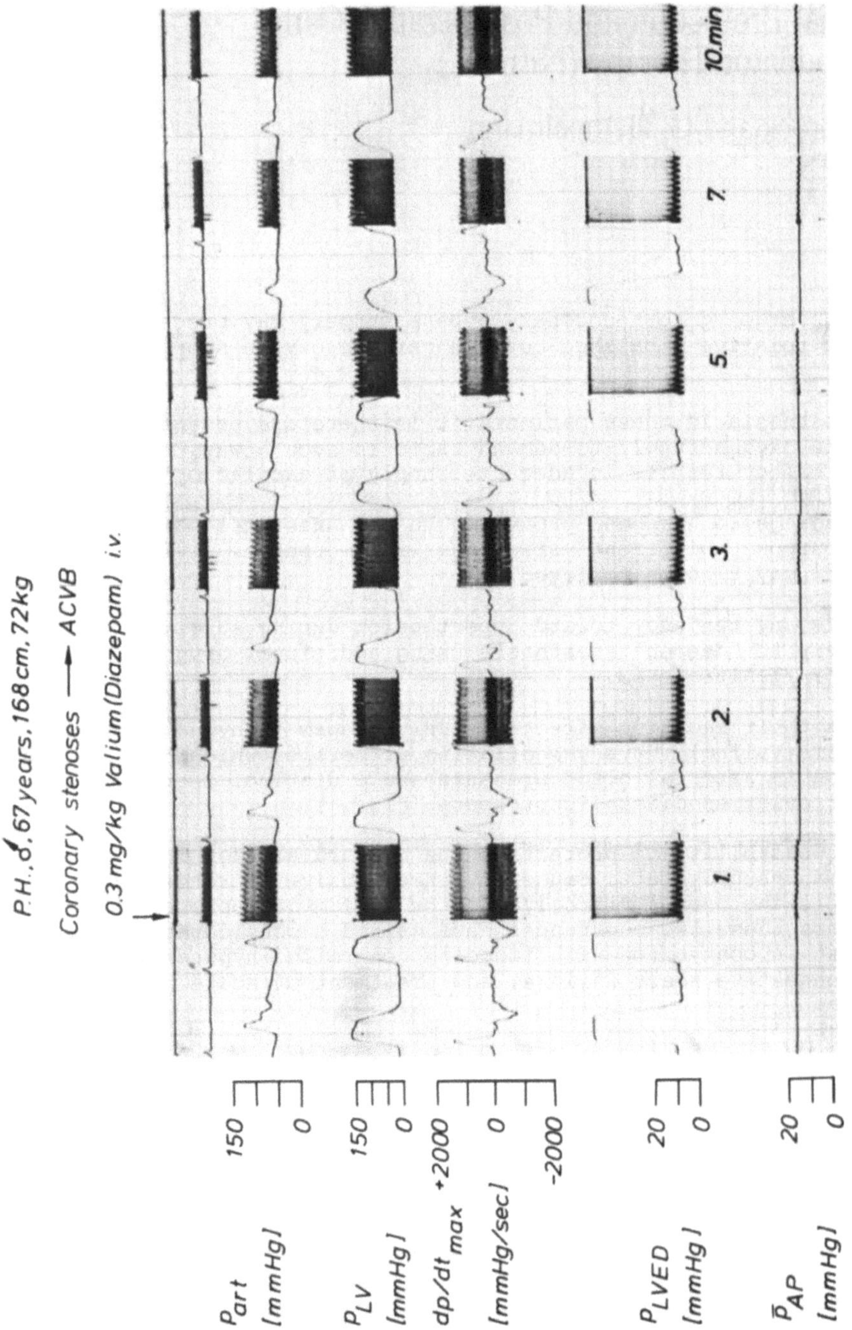

Fig. 1. Changes in hemodynamic parameters following administration of 0.3 mg/kg diazepam in a patient with coronary heart disease during cardiac surgery (neuroleptanalgesia was used). p_{art} arterial pressure; p_{LV} left ventricular pressure; dp/dt first time derivative of left ventricular pressure; p_{LVED} left ventricular enddiastolic pressure; $\bar{p}_{AP}$ mean pulmonary artery pressure

In coronary artery disease nitroglycerin may not increase total coronary blood flow.

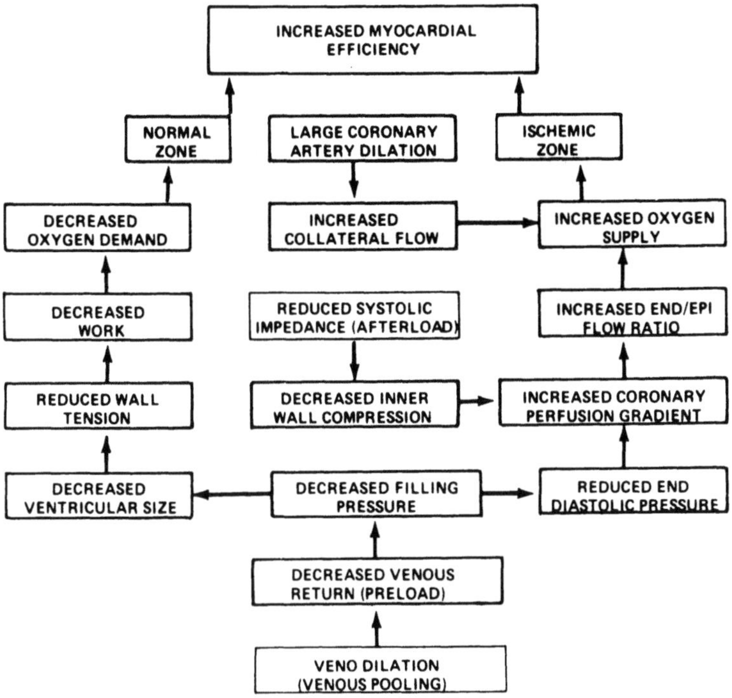

Fig. 2. Therapeutic hemodynamic changes caused by vasodilators (nitrates) according to W. Dobbs and H.J. Povaski [1]

Coronary arteries may be completely or almost completely dilated already in response to the underlying obstruction, therefore, additional dilation by drugs may not be obtainable and arterial pressure fall can reduce coronary perfusion pressure. But there is evidence that the drug may cause a beneficial redistribution of flow, increasing preferentially endocardial blood flow [6,7].

Finally, experiments in dogs with acute coronary insufficiency have demonstrated that nitroglycerin also has a beneficial effect in raising ventricular fibrillation threshold [8]. Apart from these beneficial aspects of nitroglycerin there are some potential limitations of this drug [1]:

1) Excessive drug-induced hypotension can cause reflex tachycardia and increased contractility leading to an augmentation in oxygen demand.
2) Inappropriate decrease in blood pressure can reduce coronary perfusion pressure.
3) Reflex tachycardia can reduce diastolic coronary perfusion interval.

In our anesthesiologic routine work we often use single injections of nitroglycerin to reduce, for example, an increase in blood pressure after sternotomy or to facilitate an easier cannulation of the aorta.

After injection of 0.2 mg nitroglycerin, mean values of eight patients with coronary artery disease showed a reduction in left ventricular enddiastolic pressure of 43%, arterial pressure of 20% and

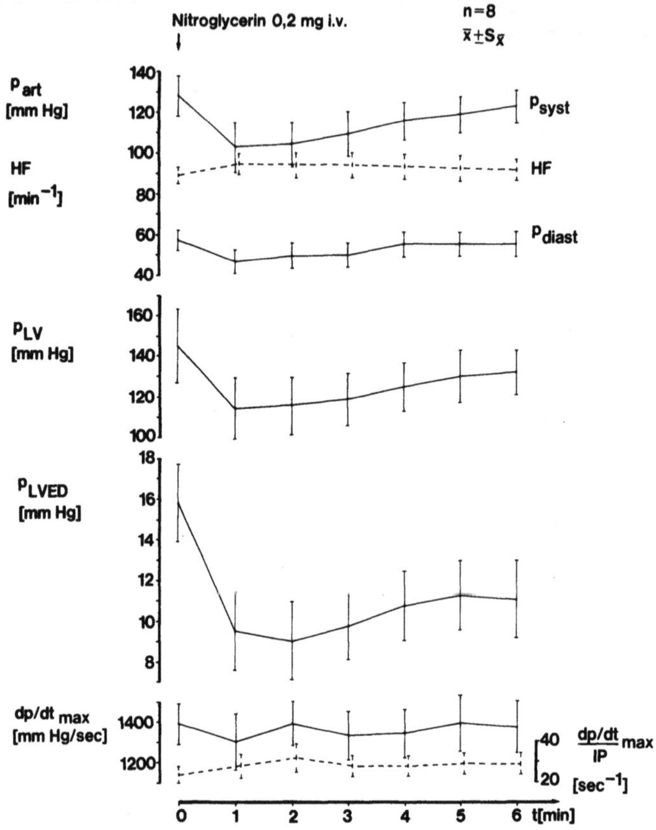

Fig. 3. Mean changes in arterial pressure (p_{art}), heart rate (*HF*), left ventricular pressure (p_{LV}); left ventricular enddiastolic pressure (p_{LVED}); peak *dp/dt* (dp/dt_{max}), and dp/dt_{max}: IP in 8 patients during heart operations after injection of 0.2 mg nitroglycerin. Neuroleptanalgesia was used for anesthesia [9]

dp/dt_{max} of 7% (N.S.), whereas heart rate increased only by 6% (Fig. 3). Calculated myocardial oxygen-consumption decreased from 7.5 ml O_2/min·100 g to 6.1 ml O_2/min·100 g (19%) and the cardiac effort index (p_{LV} x HR) decreased by 18.5% [9].

In contrast to bolus injections, a continuous infusion of nitroglycerin 2 mg/h caused a more gradual change in hemodynamics. Again a marked decrease in p_{LVED} can be demonstrated (Fig. 4). In ten patients myocardial oxygen consumption decreased by 16% (8.1 → 6.8 ml O_2/min·100 g) and the cardiac effort index (the product of p_{LV} x HR) by 14% [9].

The period of extracorporeal circulation during open heart surgery with induced myocardial fibrillation allows examination of vascular reactions of any agent without cardiac interference. Figure 5 demonstrates that an infusion of 4 mg/h nitroglycerin reduces arterial perfusion pressure ($\bar{p}_{art}$) and blood volume (ΔV) in the reservoir of the oxygenator. These effects prove that there is both a venous and arterial vasodilation. After stopping the nitroglycerin infusion both parameters rise again [10].

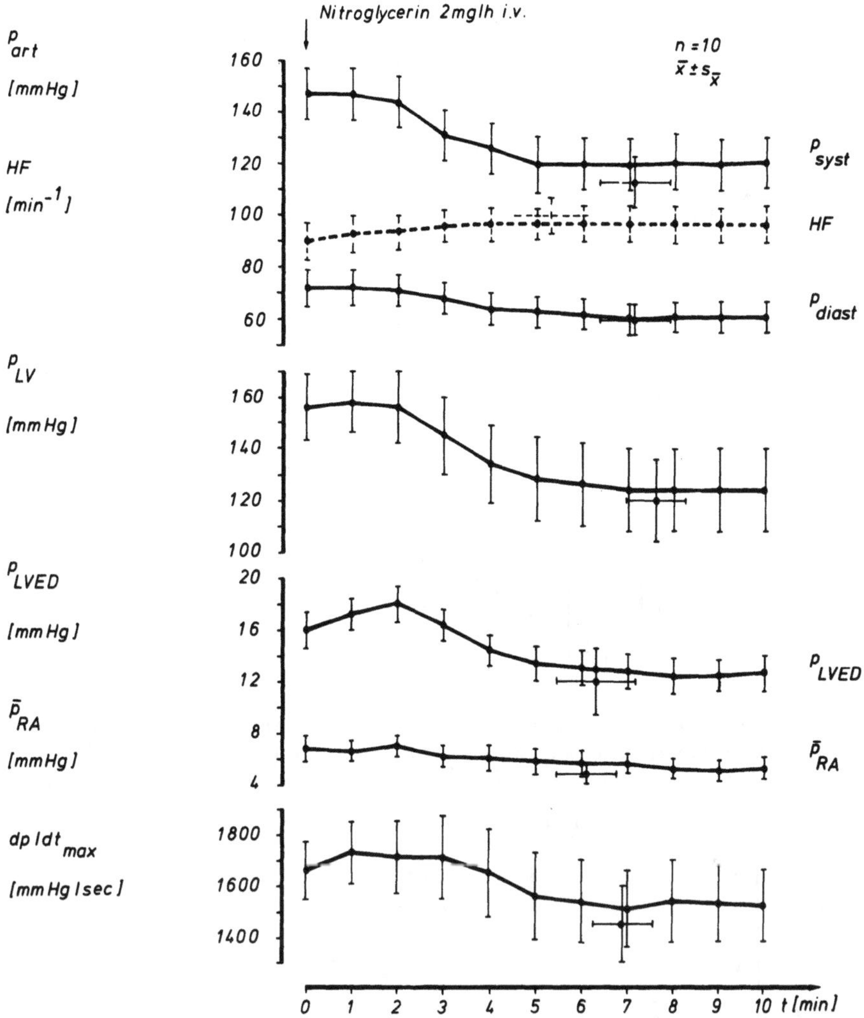

Fig. 4. Influence of an infusion of 2 mg/h nitroglycerin on arterial pressure (p_{art}), heart rate (*HF*), left ventricular pressure (p_{LV}); left ventricular end-diastolic pressure (p_{LVED}); right atrial pressure ($\bar{p}_{RA}$) and peak dp/dt (dp/dt_{max}) in 10 patients during cardiac surgical procedure performed with the use of neuroleptanalgesia [9]

Sodium Nitroprusside

Sodium nitroprusside seems to be the most potent short-acting vasodilator [11]. It also relaxes vascular smooth muscle in both the arterial and venous vessels. But in comparison to nitroglycerin, sodium nitroprusside causes a more severe decrease in arterial blood pressure at comparable left ventricular filling pressures, which can be shown in Fig. 6: After infusion of sodium nitroprusside the decrease in arterial perfusion pressure in relation to the reduction of oxygenator-blood-volume is more pronounced than with nitroglycerin [10].

Sodium nitroprusside is the substance of choice in the treatment of hypertensive crisis [2]. It has also been widely employed in the acute management of cardiac failure from a variety of causes [13,14]. Side effects other than hypotension from overdosage are surprisingly

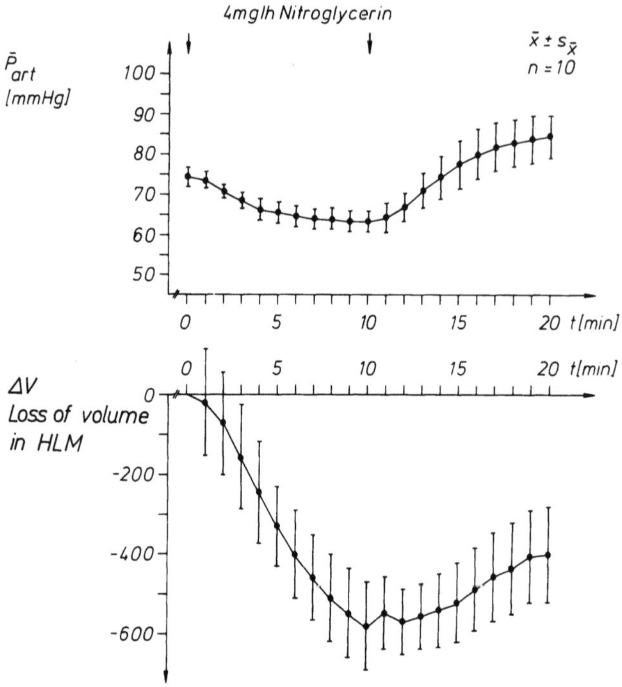

Fig. 5. Mean changes of arterial perfusion pressure ($\bar{p}_{art}$) and of oxygenator blood volume (ΔV) during extracorporeal circulation following an infusion of 4 mg/h nitroglycerin and after stopping the infusion [10]

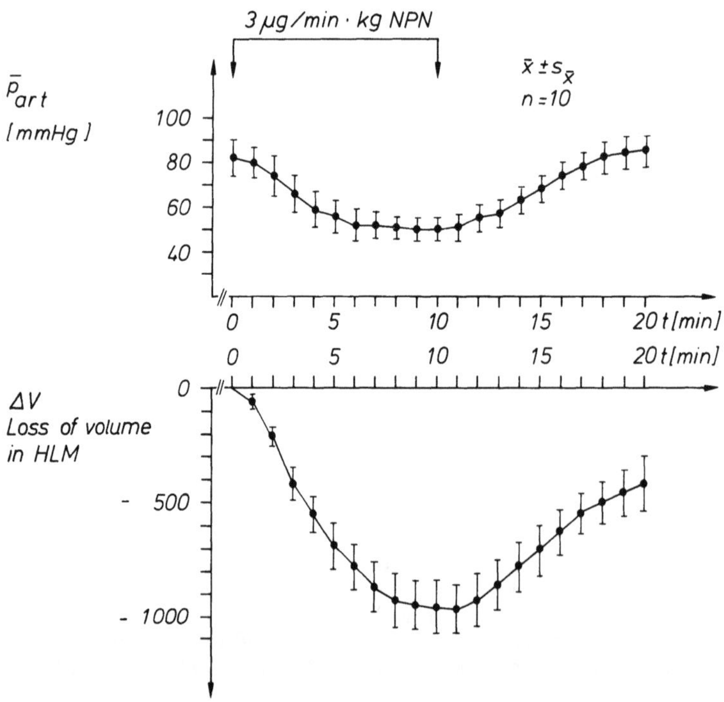

Fig. 6. Effects of an infusion of 3 µg/min·kg sodium nitroprusside on arterial perfusion pressure ($\bar{p}_{art}$) and oxygenator blood volume (ΔV) during extracorporeal circulation [10]

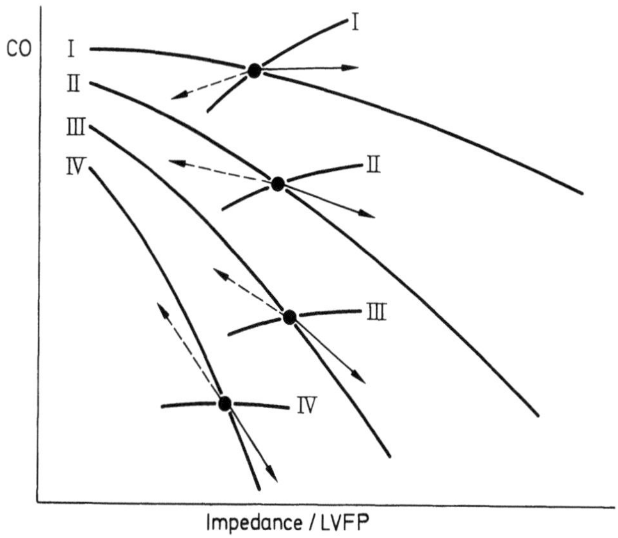

Fig. 7. Interrelations between preload (ventricular filling, LVFP) and outflow resistance (impedance) in the control of left ventricular output (CO). Small segments of preload curves are superimposed on outflow resistance curves. Sodium nitroprusside, which dilates both arteries and veins, may improve cardiac output (*dotted lines*) in patients with severe myocardial disease (*curves III and IV*), because in these cases impedance effect predominates over preload effect [15].

uncommon. But prolonged administration may result in an accumulation of thiocyanate in the blood and cerebral signs of thiocyanate toxicity may occur. The danger of this complication can be prevented by measurement of blood thyocyanate levels [15-17].

Since sodium nitroprusside dilates both venous capacitance and arterial resistance vessels, its hemodynamic response represents a combination of venous pooling and reduced arterial impedance [15]. The expected hemodynamic changes depend on the pre-existing cardiovascular state. This can be illustrated by a diagram (Fig. 7) taken from Cohn and Franciosa [15]. Small segments of preload curves (LVEP) are superimposed on outflow resistance curves (impedance). Curves I and II represent normal or slightly impaired cardiac function. Under these circumstances preload reduction has a greater effect than impedance reduction. The net effect is a fall in cardiac output, which is symbolized by the dotted line. Curves III and IV characterize severe myocardial disease. The heart is operating on a flat Frank-Starling curve and a markedly depressed impedance curve. Thus the impedance effect of sodium nitroprusside predominates over the preload effect and cardiac output rises.

Figures 8 and 9 demonstrate hemodynamic effects of a sodium nitroprusside infusion in cardiosurgical patients with slightly impaired left ventricular function [18]. In these patients either an aortic valve replacement or an aortocoronary bypass operation has been performed. Postoperatively, mean arterial pressure was decreased to a 60% level from the initial value using individual dosages of sodium nitroprusside. These dosages ranged from a mean initial dose of 125 µg/min sodium nitroprusside up to 290 µg/min. Left atrial pressure was reduced from 15 to 7 mmHg (53.4%); after stopping the infusion an

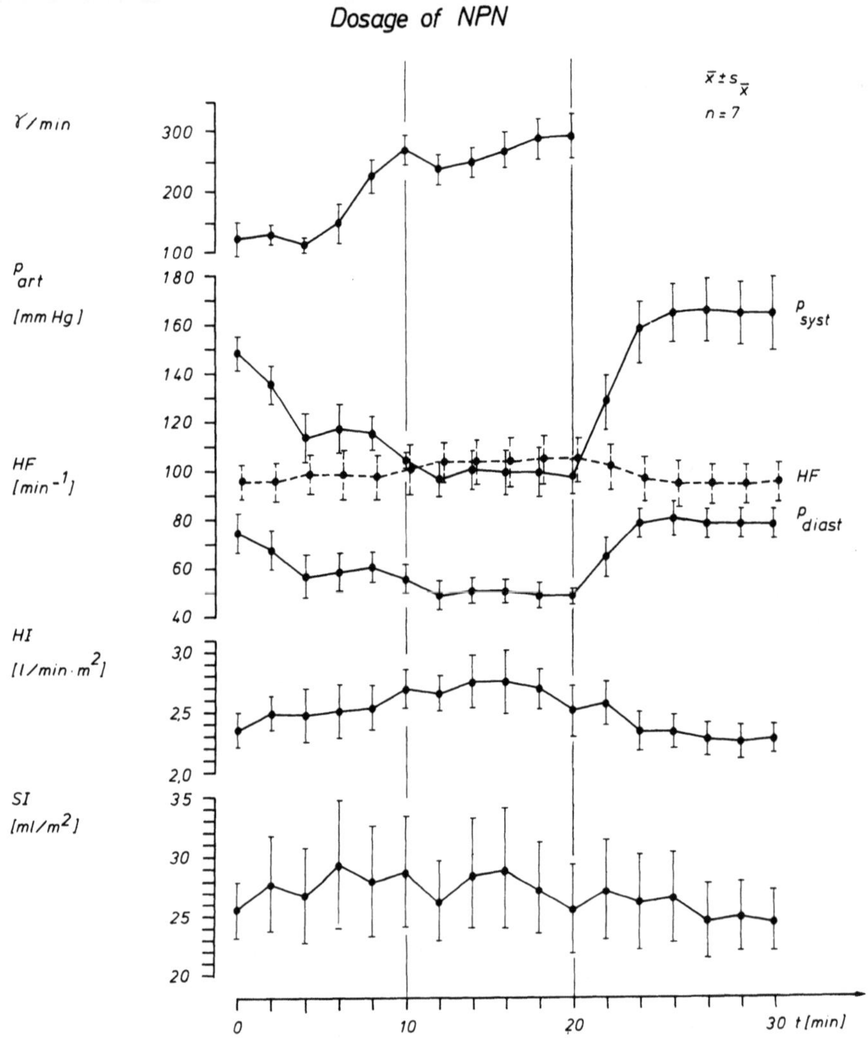

Fig. 8. Changes of hemodynamic parameters by an infusion of sodium nitroprusside in 7 patients immediately after open heart surgery. Mean arterial pressure was decreased to a 60% level from the initial value using individual dosages of sodium nitroprusside. Mean dosage of sodium nitroprusside (NPN) in γ/min; p_{art} arterial pressure; *HF* heart rate; *HI* cardiac index; *SI* stroke index [18]

increase to mean values of 18 mmHg was reached within a few minutes. Right atrial pressure (10.5 mmHg) was decreased by 33.4%, mean pulmonary artery pressure (23.6 mmHg) by 36.4%, and total peripheral resistance (1,846 dyn·s·cm^{-5}) by 40.4%. The increase in cardiac index (2.4 → 2.7 l/min·m^2) was more pronounced than the increase in stroke index due to a change in heart rate from 96 min^{-1} to 105 min^{-1}. The diminuation in myocardial oxygen consumption can be estimated by the product HR x p_{syst}, which was reduced by 27%.

Heart rate generally increases moderately when sodium nitroprusside reduces arterial pressure in normal subjects or patients with minor myocardial impairment. In heart failure, however, infusion of sodium nitroprusside usually does not alter heart rate but may even reduce it, according to Guiha, Cohn, Franciosa, and co-workers [13-15].

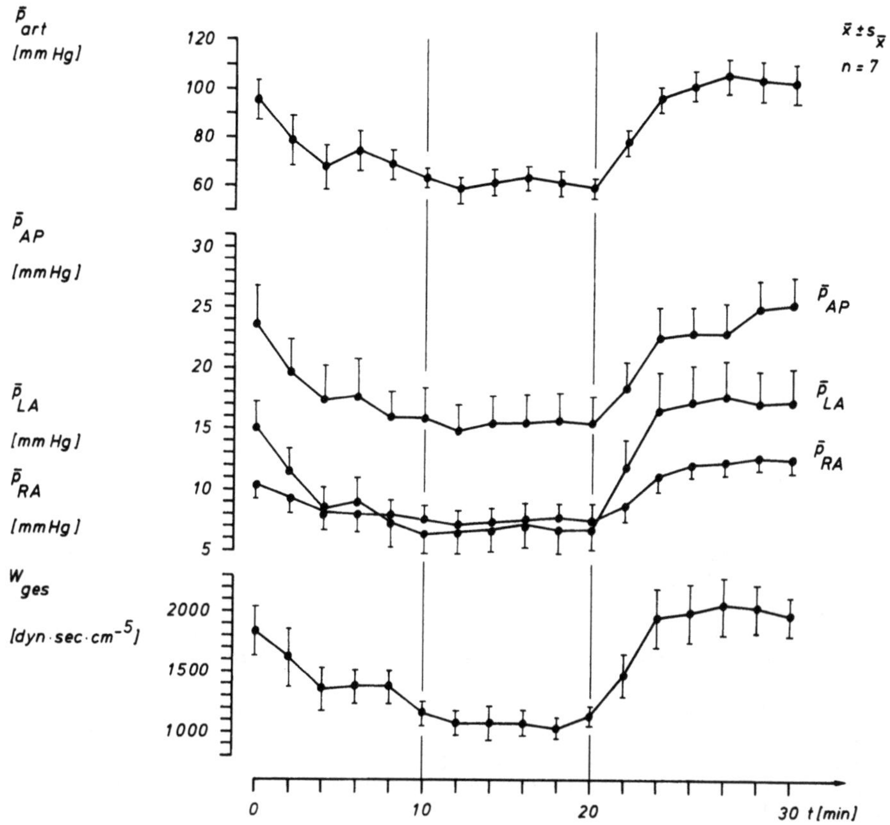

Fig. 9. Continuation of Fig. 8; $\bar{p}_{art}$ mean arterial pressure; $\bar{p}_{AP}$ mean pulmonary artery pressure; $\bar{p}_{LA}$ mean left atrial pressure; $\bar{p}_{RA}$ mean right atrial pressure; W_{ges} total systemic resistance [18]

Myocardial protection from extreme oxygen demand caused by an increase in pressure-work or improvement in pump performance in acute heart failure during or after coronary heart surgery may be achieved by vasodilator administration. Because of their potency, rapid onset and short duration of effect, nitroglycerin and sodium nitroprusside are of major interest in this respect. In comparing nitroglycerin with sodium nitroprusside, the predominant preload-reducing action of nitroglycerin over its effect of reducing impedance must be considered.

Caution must be observed, since the fall in arterial pressure might compromise coronary perfusion. While instituting vasodilator therapy, therefore, careful hemodynamic monitoring is mandatory. Otherwise, a potential, beneficial, therapeutical approach may turn out to be a hazardous one, particularly in patients with ischemic heart disease.

References

1. Dobbs, W., Povalski, H.J.: Coronary circulation, angina pectoris and anti-anginal agents. In: Cardiovascular pharmacology. Antonaccio, M.J., pp. 461-521. New York: Raven 1977
2. Chiong, M.A., West, R.D., Parker, J.O.: Influence of nitroglycerin on myocardial metabolism and hemodynamics during angina induced by atrial pacing. Circulation *45*, 1044 (1972)
3. Raff, W.K., Lochner, W.: Wirkungsmechanismus von Nitroglycerin. Med. Klin. *69*, 1100 (1974)
4. Shell, W.E., Sobel, B.E.: Protection of jeopardized ischemic myocardium by reduction of ventricular afterload. N. Engl. J. Med. *291*, 481 (1974)
5. Sonnenblick, E., Ross, J., Braunwald, E.: Oxygen consumption of the heart. Am. J. Cardiol. *22*, 328 (1968)
6. Horwitz, L.D., Gorlin, R., Taylor, W.J., Kemp, H.G.: Effects of nitroglycerin on regional myocardial blood flow in coronary artery disease. J. Clin. Invest. *50*, 1578 (1971)
7. Winburg, M.M., Howe, B.B., Weiss, H.R.: Effect of nitroglycerin and dipyridamole on epicardial and endocardial oxygen tension - further evidence for redistribution of myocardial flow. J. Pharmacol. Exp. Ther. *176*, 184 (1971)
8. Kent, K.M., Smith, E.R., Redwood, D.R., Epstein, S.E.: Beneficial electrophysiologic effects of nitroglycerin during acute myocardial infarction. Am. J. Cardiol. *33*, 513 &1973)
9. Hempelmann, G., Piepenbrock, S., Seitz, W., Karliczek, G.: Changes in hemodynamic parameters, inotropic state, and myocardial oxygen consumption owing to intravenous application of nitroglycerin. J. Thorac. Cardiovasc. Surg. *73*, 836 (1977)
10. Piepenbrock, S., Hempelmann, G.: Möglichkeiten medikamentöser Vasodilatation bei kardiochirurgischen Eingriffen. In: Anästhesie bei kardiochirurgischen Eingriffen. Götz, E., Lawin, P., (eds.), 8 pp. 82-99. Stuttgart: Thieme 1978
11. Kreye, V.A.W.: Zum zellulären Wirkungsmechanismus von Natrium-Nitroprussid. Herz *2*, 125 (1976)
12. Rahn, K.H.: Die Behandlung hypertensiver Notfälle. Herz *1*, 180 (1976)
13. Franciosa, J.A., Guiha, N.H., Limas, C.J.: Improved left ventricular function during nitroprusside infusion in acute myocardial infarction. Lancet *1972/I* 650
14. Guiha, N.H., Cohn, J.N., Mikulic, E.: Treatment of refractory heart failure with infusion of nitroprusside. N. Engl. J. Med. *291*, 587 (1974)
15. Cohn, J.N., Franciosa, J.A.: Vasodilator therapy of cardiac failure. N. Engl. J. Med. *297* (1977)
16. Höbel, M., Kreye, V.A., Raithelhuber, A.: Natrium-Nitroprussid: Toxizität, Stoffwechsel und Organverteilung. Herz *1*, 130 (1976)
17. Palmer, R.F., Lasseter, K.C.: Drug therapy: sodium nitro-prusside. N. Engl. J. Med. *292*, 294 (1975)
18. Karliczek, G., Hempelmann, G., Piepenbrock, S., Dragojevic, D.: Blutdrucksenkung durch Nitroprussid-Natrium. Hämodynamische Untersuchungen bei herzchirurgischen Patienten. Thoraxchirurgie [Special Issue 1], 27 (1976)

Can Postoperative Care be Facilitated by Preoperative Preparation?

P. Suter and A. Bloch

Summary

The experience in postoperative intensive care has shown that the patient who is prepared physically and psychologically has a greater facility to adapt to the situation immediately after coronary artery surgery and will collaborate actively to achieve complete recovery.

Among the most important factors to assure a rapid recovery and to avoid postoperative complications are the nutritional status, the pulmonary function, fluid and electrolyte balance. A precise assessment of the fluid and electrolyte status before surgery will allow a pre- and peroperative correction of important disturbances. In particular, the estimation of total body sodium and potassium can direct the postoperative treatment and help to avoid cardiac dysfunction due to inadequate intravascular volume or arrythmias secondary to a potassium deficit. Preoperative drug therapy must be adapted to the individual patient's needs.

Obesity or malnutrition and hypoproteinemia are associated with an increased postoperative morbidity secondary to problems related to weakness and lack of coordination of respiratory muscles, edema formation, and a decrease in the defense mechanisms against secondary infection. Chronic obstructive pulmonary disease and bronchitis must be treated aggressively to avoid postoperative pulmonary infection and to spare the respiratory forces of the patient at a time when his cardiovascular system may not be able to adapt to increased respiratory work.

Preoperative Examination

A precise preoperative examination of the clinical and biochemical status facilitates pre- and postoperative therapy as well as anesthetic management. Early recognition of electrolyte imbalances, renal, or hepatic dysfunction allows a rational treatment of these problems and helps to avoid postoperative complications. Preoperative assessment should include graded exercise testing in patients who have had no recent infarction and who do not have unstable angina, to provide a basis of comparison for postoperative studies [1,2]. The systolic pressure heart rate product at which angina or electrocardiographic changes occur provides a useful guide for the anesthesiologist and for postoperative care. If this product is not exceeded, intra- or postoperative infarction is less likely to occur [1,3].

In this paper, we will focus on some aspects of preoperative preparation, namely drug treatment, fluid and electrolyte status, nutrition, respiratory, and psychological factors.

Preoperative Considerations for Patients on Continuous Drug Therapy

Digitalis may be indicated in some patients to improve myocardial function or to control the ventricular rate when atrial fibrillation exists preoperatively or develops in the postoperative phase [4]. However, it is not recommended to use this drug routinely in all cardiac surgery patients, because it increases postoperative ventricular irritability [5]. Unless the effects of digitalis are imperative for the patient, this drug should be withheld for 1 to several days before surgery.

A great number of patients undergoing coronary artery surgery receive beta blocking agents such as propranolol to decrease the myocardial oxygen demand and to decrease angina and arrythmias. Some surgeons wish to discontinue this type of drug 1 to several weeks before cardiac surgery because of its potential side effects such as negative inotropy, negative chronotropy, bronchoconstriction, and an inhibition of the glycogenolytic action of catecholamines [1,6,7].

However, we have convincing evidence that the activity of propranolol disappears within 24-48 h and this allows a safe intervention [8-10]. Hug, Kaplan, and Rigel have shown that the plasma levels of propranolol decrease dramatically before, during, and after cardiopulmonary bypass, depending on the dose administered, when the drug is discontinued 9-15 h before induction of anesthesia [11]. Accordingly, the cardiac responses to isoproterenol increased in these patients. In a randomized, prospective study by Slogoff, Keats, and Ott in patients receiving continuous propranolol therapy before coronary artery surgery, there was an increase in preoperative angina, intraoperative ventricular arrythmias, and ischemic ST changes in the group where propranolol was discontinuend 24-72 h before surgery [12], when compared to the group where the drug was continued within 12 h of operation.

Reserpine and ganglion blocking agents should be omitted several days before surgery to allow norepinephrine repletion and adequate autoregulation of peripheral vascular tone. L-dopa, utilized for the treatment of Parkinson's disease, reduces renin release and norepinephrine production and this results in a lower arterial blood pressure [13]. Orthostatic hypotension is common with L-dopa treatment, and hypotension is a potential threat during and after anesthesia [14]. In addition, drugs utilized frequently in the postoperative period such as chlorpromazine and droperidol can precipitate a parkinson-like syndrome by blocking the action of L-dopa [15]. Monoamine oxidase (MAO) inhibitors should be discontinued for at least 2 weeks before anesthesia, because administration of sympathicomimetic amines will release stored catecholamines and may precipitate severe hypertensive states in patients on this therapy. Hypertensive crises or other adverse reactions may also occur when potent analgesics are administered [16]. Tricyclic antidepressants reduce the amount and the effect of catecholamines in myocardial tissue. They may induce hypotension and congestive heart failure [17]. These drugs should be discontinued before coronary artery surgery to eliminate their potential cardiotoxic effect.

Pre- and Postoperative Correction of Heart Failure, Fluid, and Electrolyte Disorders

Patients presenting with congestive heart failure preoperatively must be treated with rest, salt and fluid restriction, diuretics, and digitalis until they reach their normal dry weight. This medical therapy may produce blood volume depletion and electrolyte imbalances, and these patients tolerate anesthesia poorly. The most frequently observed abnormalities are a hyponatremia and hypokalemia. During cardiopulmonary bypass, an additional loss of potassium is observed. The decrease of total body potassium and hypokalemia can cause cardiac arrythmias, increased susceptibility to glycosides, salt and water retention and hypotension. This potassium deficiency must be corrected rapidly. One must remember that the serum potassium level gives only an incomplete picture of the total potassium content of the body and dangerous arrythmias can occur in the postoperative period in the presence of a normal serum potassium [18].

After an acute myocardial infarction, a minimum of 6 weeks is generally allowed for healing before operation. The mortality by elective coronary bypass surgery decreases progressively during the first 2 months following acute infarction, from a level more than six times the usual rate during the first week to control levels after 1 month [19]. However, refractary cardiogenic shock following myocardial infarction can in selected cases be regarded as an indication for emergency operation for coronary artery revascularization or correction of a mechanical defect of the myocardium [1]. Pre- and postoperative circulatory support with an intra-aortic balloon pump is helpful in these patients [20,21].

Nutritional Status

In addition to the correction of fluid retention, the patient presenting with malnutrition or obesity has to be treated with an appropriate diet in order to improve muscle strength and to avoid respiratory failure in the postoperative period. Muscle weakness can lead to inappropriate ventilatory reserves, uncoordinated respiratory movement, decreased capability to cough effectively, and a delayed mobilization after surgery. Hypoproteinemia is associated with an increased postoperative morbidity secondary to problems related to edema formation, a deficiency in the defense mechanisms, and retarded wound healing.

Diabetes mellitus has been identified as a risk factor in coronary heart disease, and the left ventricular performance is impaired in diabetic patients even without clinical evidence of cardiac involvement or myocardial ischemia [22].

All patients must stop smoking several weeks before cardiac surgery to improve small airway function and to avoid pulmonary complications postoperatively.

Respiratory Problems

Derangements of pulmonary function are common in patients with cardiac disease. A minimum of pulmonary function tests in necessary to assess the respiratory status. The forced expiratory volume in 1 second (FEV_1) and the maximum minute ventilation (MMV) are two simple and useful examinations to estimate the ventilatory reserves. The pulmonary gas exchange can be assessed by measuring arterial blood gases and these measurements additionally provide a useful baseline value for the postoperative evaluation. Bronchitis or bronchiectasis associated with significant obstruction, sputum production, and infection must be treated aggressively before surgery, because these patients are very likely to develop respiratory insufficiency after operation. This is a dangerous complication appearing at a time when the cardiovascular system may not be able to adapt to increased respiratory work.

Chester et al. examined the effect of physical training on cardiopulmonary performance in patients with chronic obstructive pulmonary disease [23]. After 4 weeks of physical exercise there were no significant changes in cardiovascular function and gas exchange except for a small increase in pulmonary capillary wedge pressure. However, an improvement in the capacity for exercise with a decrease in minute ventilation and oxygen consumption was observed after the training period.

Psychological Orientation

To obtain a maximal cooperation in the postoperative period and to aid in the prevention of postoperative psychosis [24], the motivation of the patient is important. He should receive adequate information concerning the intensive care unit or recovery room, monitoring equipment, ventilators, nursing routines, and function of tubes and catheters that will be used. The possibility and purpose of prolonged endotracheal intubation and mechanical ventilation should be discussed [1]. When the patient is staying in the postoperative intensive care unit, he should be frequently reinformed on his clinical status and progress, the environment, and the duration of his stay in the ICU. In the majority of the coronary surgery patients psychological support from the staff and the visiting family makes the recovery easier and avoids postoperative discouragement and depression.

Conclusions

An optimal preoperative preparation for coronary artery surgery includes an adaptation of drug therapy, the achievement of a good nutritional status, the treatment of chronic airway disease, and psychological orientation.

These measures decrease the risk of adverse drug reactions, the overall potential cardiotoxic effects, and allow a good adaptation during the postoperative period. Weaning from ventilatory support, recovery, and the return to an active life are enhanced by individual assessment and treatment of these factors, and severe complications are less likely to occur.

References

1. Behrendt, D.M., Austen, W.G.: Patient care in cardiac surgery, 2nd ed. Boston: Little, Brown 1976

2. Lapin, E.S., Murray, J.A., Bruce, R.A., Winterscheid, L.: Changes in maximal exercise performance in the evaluation of saphenous vein bypass surgery. Circulation *47*, 1164 (1973)
3. Nelson, R.R., Gobel, F.L., Jorgensen, C.R., Wang, K., Wang, Y., Taylor, H.L.: Hemodynamic predictors of myocardial oxygen consumption during static and dynamic exercise. Circulation *50*, 1179 (1974)
4. Selzer, A., Walter, R.M.: Adequacy of preoperative digitalis therapy in controlling ventricular rate in postoperative atrial fibrillation. Circulation *34*, 119 (1966)
5. Selzer, A., Kelly, J.J., (Jr.), Gerbode, F., Keith, W.J., Osborn, J.J., Popper, R.W.: Case against routine use of digitalis in patients undergoing cardiac surgery. JAMA, *195*, 141 (1966)
6. Shand, D.G.: Propranolol. N. Engl. J. Med. *293*, 280 (1975)
7. Viljoen, J.F., Estafanous, F.G., Kellner, G.A.: Propranolol and cardiac surgery. J. Thorac, Cardiovasc. Surg. *64*, 826 (1972)
8. Faulkner, S.L., Hopkins, J.T., Boerth, R.C., et al.: Time required for complete recovery from chronic propranolol therapy. N. Engl. J. Med. *289*, 607 (1973)
9. Leaman, D.M., Levenson, L.W., Shiroff, R.A., Babb, J.D., De Joseph, R.L., Hayes, A.H., Zelis, R.: Persistence of biologic activity after disappearance of propranolol from the serum. J. Thorac. Cardiovasc. Surg. *72*, 67 (1976)
10. Moran, J.M., Mulet, J., Caralps, J.M., Piffarré, R.: Coronary revascularization in patients receiving propranolol. Circulation *49-50* [Suppl. 2], 116 (1974)
11. Hug, C.C., Kaplan, J.A., Rigel, E.P.: The effect of cardio-pulmonary bypass on plasma propranolol concentrations and the response to isoproterenol. Annual Meeting of the American Society of Anesthesiologists *1977*, 501 (Abs.)
12. Slogoff, S., Keats, A.S., Ott, E.: Propranolol and coronary surgery: a prospective study. Annual Meeting of the American Society of Anesthesiologists *1977*, 499 (Abs.)
13. Barbeau, A., Gillo-Joffroy, L., Boucher, R., et al.: Renin-aldosterone system in Parkinson's disease. Science *165*, 291 (1969)
14. Schwartz, A.J., Wollmann, H.: Anesthetic considerations for patients on chronic drug therapy. ASA Refresher courses in anesthesiology *4*, 99 (1976)
15. Wiklund, R.A., Ngai, S.H.: Rigidity and pulmonary edema after Innovar in a patient on levodopa therapy: report of a case. Anesthesiology *35*, 545 (1971)
16. Perks, E.R.: Monoamine oxidase inhibitors. Anaesthesia *19*, 376 (1964)
17. Williams, R.B., Sherter, C.: Cardiac complications of tricyclic antidepressant therapy. Ann. Intern. Med. *74*, 395 (1971)
18. Badka, R., Piffarré, R.: Potassium replacement during cardiopulmonary bypass. J. Thorac. Cardiovasc. Surg. *73*, 212 (1977)
19. Dawson, J.T., Hall, R.J., Hallmann, G.L., Cooley, D.A.: Mortality in patients undergoing coronary artery bypass surgery after myocardial infarction. Am. J. Cardiol. *33*, 483 (1974)
20. Buckley, M.J., Craver, J.M., Gold, H.K., Mundth, E.D., Daggett, W.M., Austen, W.G.: Intra-aortic balloon pump assist for cardiogenic shock after cardiopulmonary bypass. Circulation *47-48* [Suppl. III], 90 (1973)
21. Buckley, M.J., Mundth, E.D., Daggett, W.M., De Sanctis, R.W., Sanders, C.A., Austen, W.G.: Surgical therapy for early complications of myocardial infarction. Surgery *70*, 814 (1971)
22. Zoneraich, S., Zoneraich, O., Rhee, J.J.: Left ventricular performance in diabetic patients without clinical heart disease. Chest *72*, 748 (1977)
23. Chester, E.H., Belman, M.J., Bahler, R.C., Baum, G.L., Schey, G., Buch, P.: Miltidisciplinary treatment of chronic pulmonary insufficiency. 3. The effect of physical training on cardiopulmonary performance in patients with chronic obstructive pulmonary disease. Chest *72*, 695 (1977)
24. Weiss, H.J.: Psychological aspects of intensive care. In: Handbook of critical care. Berk, J.J., Sampliner, J.E., Artz, J.S., Vinocur, B., (eds.) pp. 419-430. Boston: Little, Brown 1976

5. Functional Results of Coronary Heart Surgery

Factors Influencing Long-Term Improvement of Angina Pectoris, Exercise Tolerance, and Exercise Electrocardiography in Patients After Vein Bypass Surgery

M. H. Ellestad and R. J. Stuart, Jr.

In the minds of many physicians and some laymen, the stress test is the first of a series of events leading toward coronary angiography and eventually coronary bypass surgery. Because of this we should ask ourselves some critical questions about what the procedure can and cannot accomplish. In preoperaitve testing they are:

1) Can the severity of coronary disease be predicted?
2) Can the postoperative result be predicted?
3) Does pain during testing have predictive value?
4) Does ischemia at low work loads predict surgical result?
5) Does sex help predict the surgical result?

In those with postoperative testing:

1) Does postoperative ST depression predict graft patency or lack of patency?
2) Does the ST depression correlate with the relief of angina?
3) Does exercise tolerance correlate with graft patency?
4) Does comparison of pre- and postoperative testing aid in evaluation?
5) Does serial postoperative testing aid in evaluation?

It can be stated with considerable reliability that stress testing is an aid in the prediction of serious disease, although there are a significant number of errors. Follow-up studies in our laboratory [1] and correlations with angiographic data by Goldschlager [2] and Thompson [3] have established that the onset of deep ST segment depression at low work loads or a drop in blood pressure is usually correlated with high grade three vessel disease or left main disease. In order to answer the questions about the usefulness of stress testing in the prediction of the outcome of vein graft surgery, we conducted a study on 387 operated patients, 196 of whom had completed pre- and postoperative treadmill stress tests. Of this latter group 54 were excluded because of abnormal tracings at rest, i.e., ST depression or elevation, patient taking Digitalis, or a conduction defect. Postoperative angiograms were not done.

We found a 61% improved double product (pulse X pressure product) at the point of ST depression, and a 58% improvement in the peak double product obtained (Fig. 1). In those 73 patients with 2 or more postoperative stress tests, 57% had continuous improvement or improved on later tests (Fig. 2). Twenty-six patients demonstrated chronotropic incompetence (inappropriately slow pulse response to exercise). Of these, 17 (65%) had it appear postoperative, persist or appear later on in subsequent tests, suggesting a deteriorization of left ventricular function. It disappeared in 6 (23%) or became intermittent with successive stress test in 3 (12%).

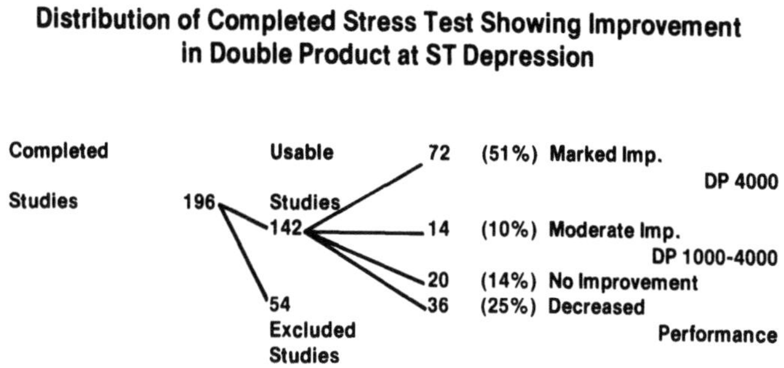

Fig. 1. Sixty-one percent exhibited marked to moderate improvement as estimated by the double product at the time of onset of ST segment depression. Fourteen percent showed no improvement and twenty-five percent actually had a lower double product at onset of ST depression

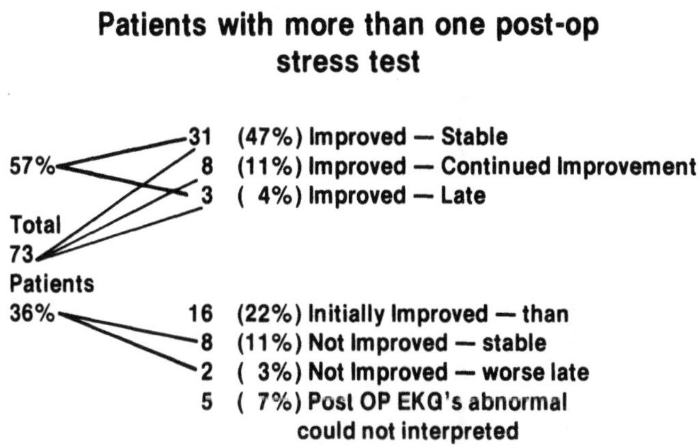

Fig. 2. In those patients having more than one postoperative stress test, forty-seven percent were initially improved and remained improved over the testing interval. Eleven percent actually were found to have a higher double product at onset of ST depression as time passed. Twenty-two percent actually improved initially, and then on subsequent testing showed deterioration

We attempted to identify if any of the information in the preoperative stress test would predict the postoperative results of saphenous vein bypass surgery (Fig. 3). Our findings showed that the patient's sex, angina during stress testing, and the work load associated with ischemia failed to discriminate those who could benefit from surgery (Fig. 4). Our study like others demonstrated the disparity between symptomatic and functional improvement following surgery (Fig. 5).

A number of studies have been published showing the correlation between exercise stress test results and angiographically demonstrated patent grafts (Fig. 6) [4-6]. Recently published studies, however, have cast doubt on whether the postoperative stress test correlates with angiographic complete or incomplete revascularization [7].

McConahay et al. [8] showed a poor correlation between stress testing and the completenes of revascularization. They went on to conclude that an electrocardiographically abnormal treadmill exercise test (TET) was as frequently associated with residual coronary disease

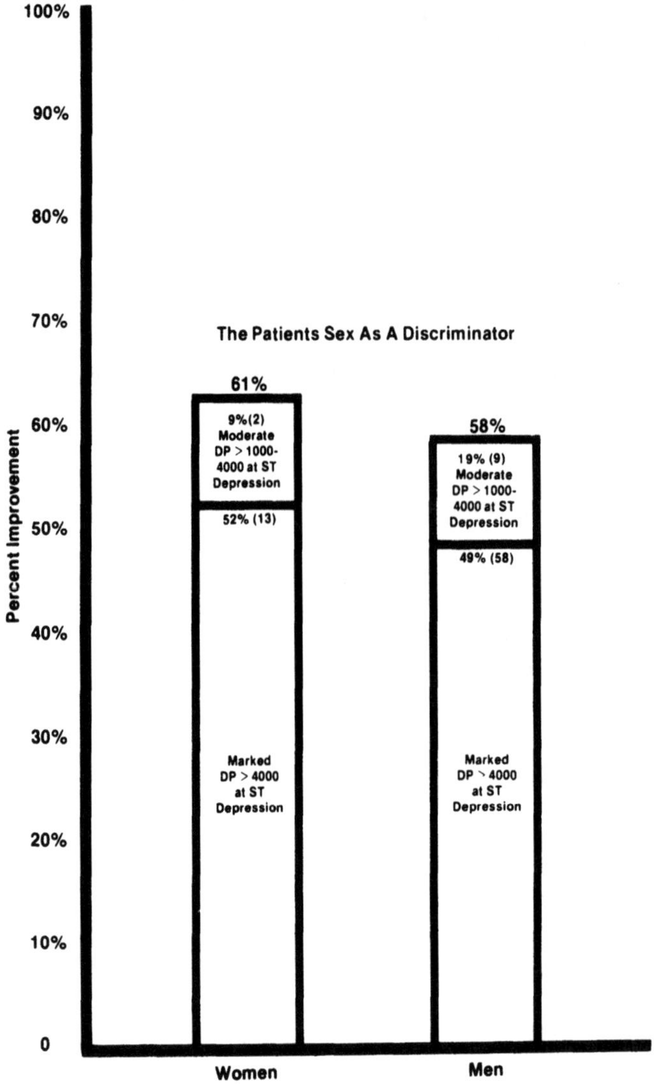

Fig. 3. The percentage of those improvement after surgery was not significantly different in men and women

postoperatively as preoperatively. A normal TET was of limited value. With an abnormal preoperative TET, a normal or improved postoperative TET correlated with at least one patent graft, no residual disease, or single coronary artery disease successfully bypassed. Treadmill exercise test induced angina correlated with residual coronary disease or incomplete revascularization. The absence of angina on a postoperative TET was of no value in estimating completeness of myocardial revascularization or saphenous vein graft patency.

Block, et al. [7] found an improved exercise performance following unseccessful myocardial revascularization. Their study group of 23 patients showed a statistically significant improvement in maximal heart rate and lesser improvement in functional aerobic impairment,

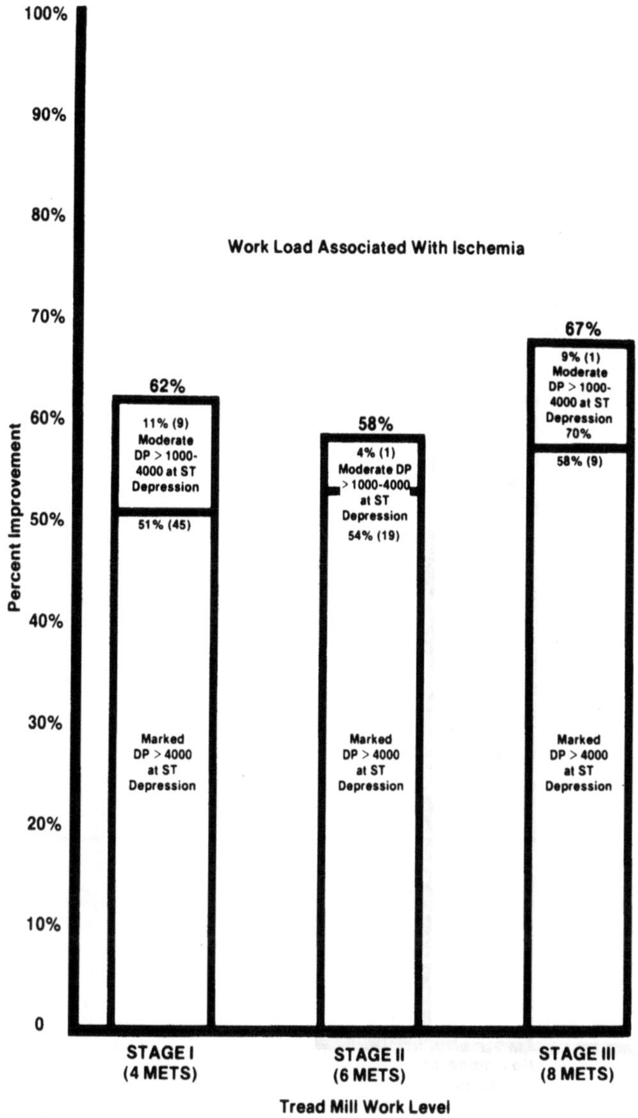

Fig. 4. The work load at which ischemia was first found in the preoperative stress test was not a good predictor of the ventual results. There seemed to be somewhat more of those who had first developed ischemia at high work loads showing marked improvement, but the difference is not statistically significant

absolute duration of exercise, and pressure rate products, while having occlusion of all implanted grafts (Fig. 7). There appeared to be a good correlation between disappearance of treadmill induced angina and improvement in overall exercise capacity as measured by exercise duration or work load achieved, irrespective of mechanism.

A rough correlation existed between improvement in exercise capacity and loss of ischemic ST changes postoperatively. Merrill et al. [9] reports a pressure rate product at maximal exercise of 25,000 or less does not differentiate patent from nonpatent grafts.

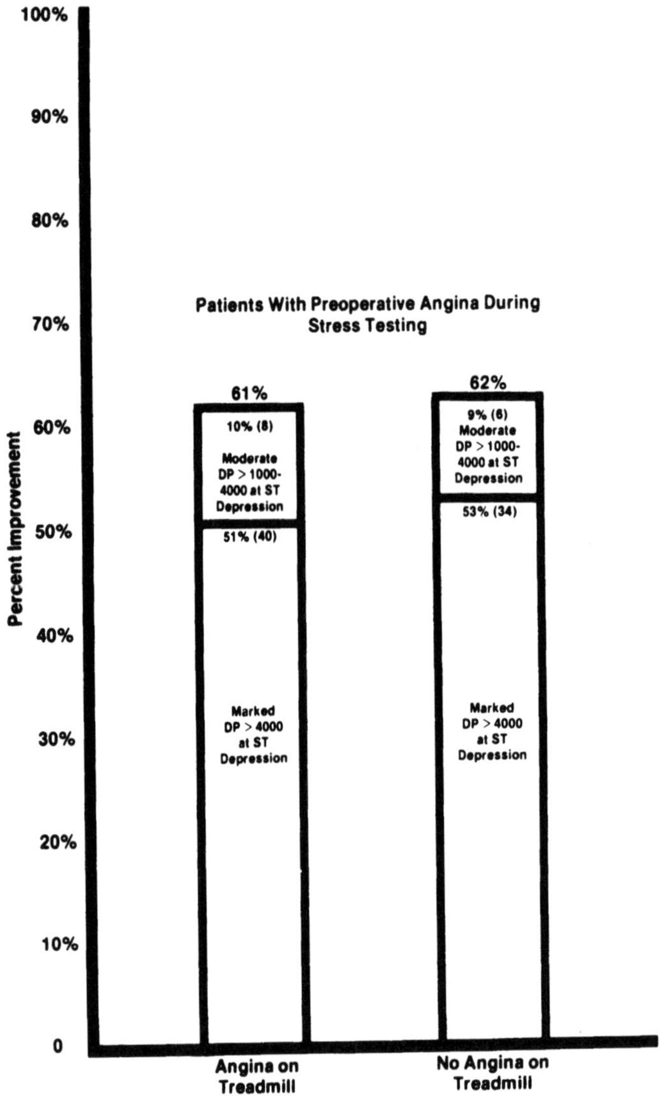

Fig. 5. Those patients showing angina preoperatively did not have a better result than those who failed to show angina on stress testing preoperatively

In summary, interpretation of postoperative exercise tests must be done with great care. Although improvement in ST segments and exercise performance may occur postoperatively, it may not correlate with graft patency. Stress testing is useful in evaluating postoperative patients, but the findings must be considered in light of the above data.

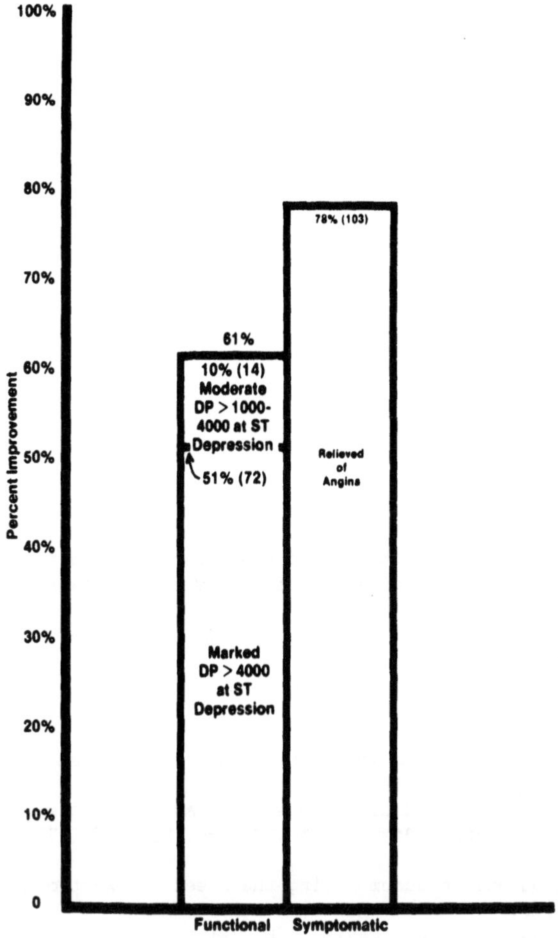

Fig. 6. Although seventy-eight percent were relieved of their angina by history, only sixty-one percent actually demonstrated a definite improvement in the time of onset of ST segment depression, a more functional way of evaluating their results

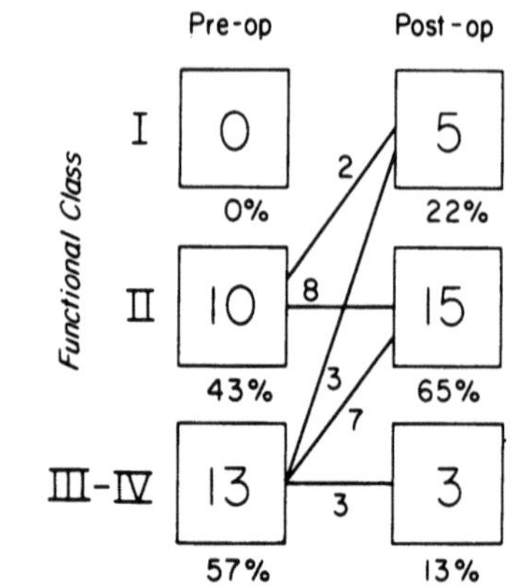

Change in functional class in 23 patients after unsuccessful myocardial revascularization. Post-op = postoperative; pre-op = preoperative.

Fig. 7. In twenty-three patients reported by Brock who had unseccessful myocardial revascularization, an improvement in functional classification was seen in twenty. Reproduced with permission, Ref. [7]

References

1. Ellestad, M.H., Halliday, W.K.: Stress testing in the prognosis and management of ischemic heart disease. Angiology *28*, 149-159 (1977)
2. Goldschlager, H., Selzer, A., Cohn, K.: Treadmill stress tests as indicators of presence and severity of coronary artery disease. Am. Intern. Med. *85*, 277-286 (1977)
3. Thompson, P.D., Kelemen, M.H.: Hypotension accompanying the onset of exertional angina. Circulation *52*, 28-32 (1975)
4. Assad-Morell, J.L., Frye R.L., Connolly, D.C., Davis, G.D., Pluth, J.R., Wallace, R.B., Barnhorst, D.A., Elveback, L.R., Danielson, G.K.: Aorta-coronary artery saphenous vein bypass surgery, clinical and angiographic results. Mayo Clinic Proc. *50*, 379-386 (1975)
5. Busch, U., Garcia, E., Hall, R.J., Mathur, V.S., DeCastro, C.M., Guttin, J., Dear, W.E., Cooley, D.A.: Serial graded exercise testing in follow-up of coronary artery bypass: a preliminary report. Cardiovasc. Dis. Bull. Texas Heart Inst. *4*, 149-16+ (1977)
6. Lawrie, G.M., Morris, G.C., Howell, J.F., Ogura, J.W., Spencer, W.H., Cashion, W.R., Winters, W.L., Beazley, H.L., Chapman, D.W., Peterson, P.K., Lie, J.T.: Results of coronary bypass more than 5 years after operation in 434 patients; clinical, treadmill exercise and angiographic correlations. Am. J. Cardiol. *40*, 665-672 (1977)
7. Block, T.A., Murray, J.A., English, M.T.: Improvement in exercise performance after unseccessful myocardial revascularization. Am. J. Cardiol. *40*, 673-680 (1977)
8. McConahay, D.R., Valdes, M., McCallister, B.D., Crockett, J.E., Conn, R.D., Reed, W.A., Killen, D.A.: Accuracy of treadmill testing in assessment of direct myocardial revascularization. Circulation *56*, 548-552 (1977)
9. Merrill, A.J.: Abstract. Circulation *51*, 144 (1975)

Long-Term Effect of Coronary Bypass Surgery on Exercise Tolerance: A 2-Year Randomized Study

M. H. Frick, P-T. Harjola, and M. Valle

Introduction

The well established relief of symptoms of coronary heart disease by bypass surgery is based on a number of factors among which the completeness of revascularization, patency of grafts, and progression of disease in both grafted and nongrafted arteries are most significant [1]. In principle there are two alternatives in analyzing the relief of symptoms: 1) comparison of patients with patent grafts with patients having graft occlusions, and 2) the use of randomized, medically treated controls. The first alternative elucidates the role of graft patency, while the latter approach gives the overall results of bypass surgery, regardless of the mechanism of action.

We have recently completed a 2-year follow-up of a randomized series. The preliminary data of this comparison form the basis of this report.

Material and Methods

Between 1973 and 1976, we randomly allocated 100 patients with coronary heart disease into two groups of 50 patients each. One group was subjected to coronary bypass surgery and additional medical therapy when indicated, the other group received medical therapy alone. The criteria for inclusion and exclusion are given in Table 1. The primary requirement was that medical management did nod result in a satisfactory control of the symptoms. The success of randomization is given in Table 2. No major differences existed between the groups (χ^2-test, Yates correction). Three patients of the surgical group refused operation and two patients died between randomization and the scheduled operation reducing the number of patients to 45 in the surgical subset. There were no operative deaths.

Table 1. Characteristics of the series

Criteria for Inclusion	Exclusion
Males under 65 years	Uncontrolled hypertension
Significant angina pectoris despite optimal antianginal therapy	Only 1-vessel disease (left main stenosis = 2-vessel disease)
Positive exercise test	Ejection fraction less than 50%
At least 2-vessel disease by angio	Other concomitant cardiac surgery
Suitable coronary anatomy	

Table 2. Results of randomization

	Medical group	Surgical group
Age, years	47 ± 0.9[a]	46 ± 0.9
Duration of angina, months	37 ± 5.0[a]	39 ± 5.2
Patients with past myocardial infarction	14 (28%)	22 (49%)
Patients with 2-vessel disease	10 (20%)	13 (29%)
Patients with 3-vessel disease	40 (80%)	32 (71%)
Left ventricular ejection fraction, %	67 ± 1.4[a]	66 ± 1.6
Total work at entry, kpm	3331 ± 326[a]	3366 ± 314

[a]Mean ± s.e.

The surgical procedures were as earlier described [2]. The left internal mammarian artery was exclusively used to bypass lesions in the left anterior descending coronary artery and/or its diagonal branch. The surgical subset exhibited altogether 121 coronary arteries with ≧ 50% stenosis; 106 bypass grafts were inserted. This resulted in complete revascularization of 29 patients while 16 patients had one lesion each which was not bypassed. Eleven of these were in the right coronary artery, 4 in the left circumflex artery, and 1 in the left anterior descending artery. All these arteries were diffusely damaged; discouraged by our results with gas endarterectomy, [3] they were not bypassed.

Postoperative control angiographies were performed early after operation (mean of 3 weeks) and 1 year after operation. Both the inserted grafts and the native arteries were injected on both occasions [4]. The medical subset was not subjected to repeated angiography.

Using a bicycle ergometer exercise testing was performed at entry and 6 months, 1 year, and 2 years after randomization. The endpoint was angina and/or dyspnea requiring short-acting nitroglycerin or in a number of patients, who were without symptoms after operation, a heart rate exceeding 85% of age-predicted maximum. In the testing at entry beta blocking drugs were discontinued a week before the test, in the subsequent testing these drugs were allowed if indicated. The following parameters were calculated: total work (TW, kpm), representing all the loads accomplished multiplied by the respective times in minutes, maximal tolerated load (MaxL, kpm/min), maximal heart rate (MaxHR, beats/min), rate-pressure product at pain (RPP, mmHg·min 10^{-2}), and maximal ST segment depression ($MaxST_d$, mm).

The statistical significance of the observed differences were assessed by Student's t-test for unpaired data.

Results

The follow-up data of the medical subgroup are given in Table 3. None of the changes during follow-up differed significantly from the data at entry. There was a steady decline in the number of patients tested at various intervals after randomization. This was due to a number of reasons, e.g., six patients had died before testing at 2 years, two patients refused prolonged follow-up, one was operated because of in-

Table 3. Data on repeated exercise testing of the medical subgroup

	At entry	At 6 months	At 1 year	At 2 years
No. of pts	50	47	44	40
Total work, kpm	3331 ± 326[a]	3424 ± 296	3544 ± 334	3589 ± 382
Maximal load, kpm/min	567 ± 31	583 ± 29	603 ± 37	603 ± 37
Maximal heart rate, beats/min	120 ± 2.7	108 ± 2.6	110 ± 3.2	109 ± 3.2
Rate-pressure product, mmHg·min 10^{-2}	214 ± 7.7	176 ± 7.6	177 ± 8.0	178 ± 8.3
Maximal ST depression, mm	3.1 ± 0.3	2.7 ± 0.2	2.8 ± 0.3	2.3 ± 0.3

[a]Mean ± s.e.

Table 4. Data on repeated exercise testing of the surgical subgroup

	At entry	At 6 months	*P*	At 1 year	*P*	At 2 years	*P*
No. of patients	45	39		42		41	
Total work, kpm	3366±314[a]	5265±495	<0.01	5186±396	<0.01	5578±427	<0.01
Maximal load, kpm/min	569±32	718±34	<0.01	718±40	<0.01	768±39	<0.01
Maximal heart rate, beats/min	124±2.8	132±3.5	N.S.	135±3.2	<0.02	134±3.6	<0.05
Rate-pressure product, mmHg·min 10^{-2}	213±7.5	232±10.0	N.S.	235±8.9	N.S.	243±8.6	<0.01
Maximal ST depression, mm	2.8±0.3	1.7±0.2	<0.05	1.5±0.2	<0.001	1.4±0.2	<0.001

[a]Mean ± s.e.; N.S. not significant

tractable angina, and one patient moved abroad. The fraction of patients on beta blockade during the follow-up was as follows: 89% at 6 months, 93% at 1 year, and 92% at 2 years. As stated, all the patients were off beta blockade in testing at entry.

Table 4 gives the data of the surgical subgroup. A considerable improvement was observed at 6 months control without any decline with time up to 2 years. In the last control TW was 66% higher and $MaxST_d$ 50% smaller than at entry. There were no postoperative deaths, but for a number of reasons, e.g., refusal of follow-up, myocardial infarctions at the time of scheduled testing, and severe sciatica, the number of patients at each testing vary. The fraction of patients on beta blockade for residual angina pectoris, hypertension, arrhythmias, or combinations of these were as follows: 43% at 6 months, 52% at 1 year, and 55% at 2 years.

The early postoperative angiography revealed seven occluded grafts (patency rate 93%) and the late angiography added five more yielding a patency rate of 89% at 1 year.

The rate of progression in bypassed arteries and those not bypassed is still under analysis and cannot be incorporated into the present data.

Discussion

The unchanged exercise tolerance of the medical subset (Table 3) despite treatment with beta blocking substances is worth noting. This is evidently due to the selection of the patients to represent a group without satisfactory response to medical therapy (Table 1). In comparing the follow-up data it is further important to recognize that about 50% of the patients in the surgical subset were on beta blockade during the postoperative testing. Thus the comparison elucidates the effect of bypass surgery and beta blockade when indicated over the response to medical management alone.

Treatment with beta blocking substances has been repeatedly demonstrated to evoke a decrease in MaxHR and RPP at pain, [5,6], and is again demonstrated by the data of the medical subset during the follow-up (Table 3). This is also operable in the surgical subset by decreasing the response of both the MaxHR and RPP to surgery (Table 4), but evidently the improved coronary perfusion was responsible for significantly increased values at 2 years. The decreased $MaxST_d$ is additional evidence for improved myocardial perfusion after the bypass procedure.

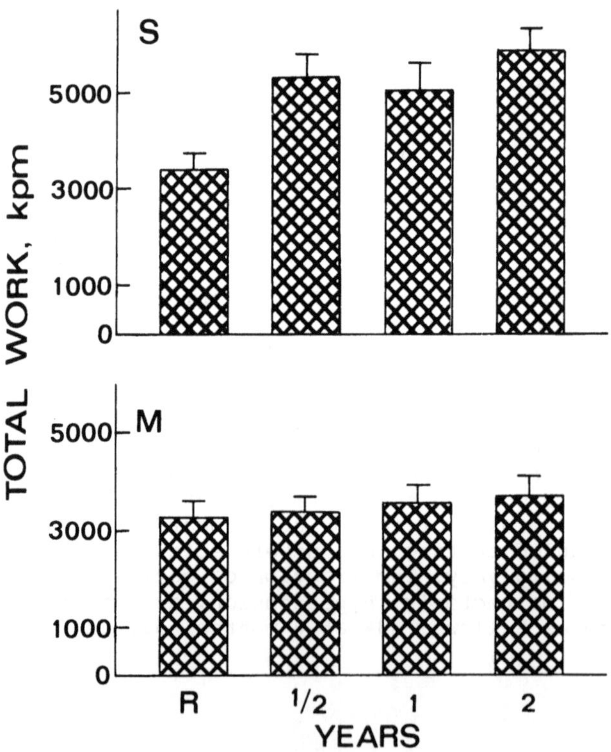

Fig. 1. Persistence of the improved exercise tolerance after bypass surgery. *S* surgical subgroup; *M* medical subgroup; *R* at randomization

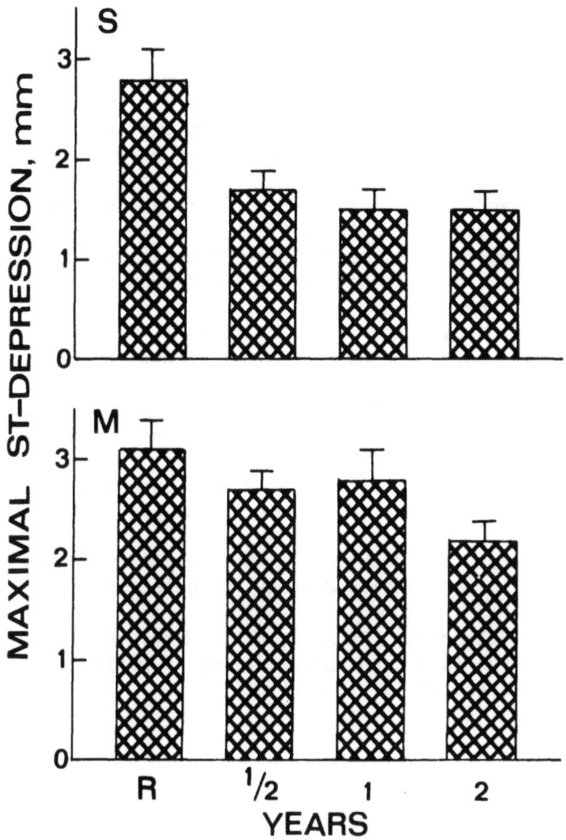

Fig. 2. Persistence of the decrease in maximal ST depression after bypass surgery. *S* surgical subgroup; *M* medical subgroup; *R* at randomization

The present data are in accord with some earlier series of randomized materials, which show that the exercise tolerance of surgically treated patients is superior to that achieved by medical management [7,8]. Schwade et al. [9] observed that this clear difference was evident at 12 months control but not at 18 months follow-up. It has been recently suggested that the initial symptomatic improvement may not be maintained on longer follow-up up to 30 months postoperatively [10]. Our data do not agree with this, but show a consistent improvement up to 24 months postoperatively (Figs. 1 and 2). Different rates of postoperative graft occlusion and progression of the underlying vascular pathology may explain the difference. This will be analyzed by combining graft occlusion to progression of the disease in the native circulation in the present series.

References

1. Frick, M.H.: An appraisal of symptom relief after coronary bypass grafting. Postgrad. Med. J. *52*, 765 (1976)
2. Frick, M.H., Harjola, P-T., Valle, M.: Effect of aorto-coronary grafts and native vessel patency on the occurrence of angina pectoris after coronary bypass surgery. Br. Heart J. *37*, 414 (1975)
3. Harjola, P-T., Valle, M.: Fate of gas endarterectomized coronary artery segments. J. Cardiovasc. Surg. [Special Issue], 95-101 (1973)
4. Valle, M.: Postoperative coronary angiography. Acta Radiol. [Suppl. 333] (1973)
5. Frick, M.H., Katila, M.: Cardio-selective beta-adrenergic inhibition by practolol in angina pectoris. Ann. Clin. Res. *2*, 96 (1970)
6. Frick, M.H., Luurila, O.: Double-blind titrated-dose comparison of metoprolol and propranolol in the treatment of angina pectoris. Ann. Clin. Res. *8*, 385 (1976)
7. Tilkian, A.G., Pfeifer, J.F., Lipton, M.J., Hultgren, H.N.: The effect of coronary bypass surgery on exercise induced ventricular arrhythmias: a randomized study. Circulation *50* [Suppl. 3], 34 (1974)
8. Mathur, V.S., Guinn, G.A., Anastassiades, L.C., Chahine, R.A., Korompai, F.C., Montero, A.C., Luchi, R.J.: Surgical treatment for stable angina pectoris. N. Engl. J. Med. *292*, 709 (1975)
9. Schwade, J.L., Pope, J.R., Mierzwiak, D.S., Shapiro, W.: Work capacity before and after therapy for angina pectoris: a randomized study. Circulation *48* [Suppl. 4], 217 (1973)
10. Tecklenberg, P.L., Alderman, E.L., Miller, C., Shumway, N.E., Harrison, D.C.: Changes in survival and symptom relief in a longitudinal study of patients after bypass surgery. Circulation *51* [Suppl. 1], 98 (1975)

Improvement of Hemodynamics During Exercise

A. Holmgren and P. Carlens

Coronary bypass surgery has been shown to improve the performance capacity of the patient as well as to reduce angina pectoris in the majority of patients currently accepted for bypass surgery [1-3]. We want to report some observations in connection with a 1-year follow-up study in 64 patients after bypass surgery [4]. The patients were accepted for surgery only if they suffered from intractable angina and had a coronary angiogram that made surgery feasible.

The work capacity (W_{max}) was determined sitting and supine on a bicycle ergometer. The loads were increased by 10 W every minute [5]. The end point of the work test was determined by the severity of the angina before surgery and the angina, dyspnea, or fatigue after surgery. The angina was evaluated by psychophysical scaling [6]. Before surgery there was a marked difference between work capacity in the seated and supine positions, the latter being only about 25% of that in the seated position (Fig. 1).

The work capacity in the seated positon 1 year after surgery is illustrated in Fig. 2 in relation to the preoperative value. W_{max} increased on the average 40 W in this group of patients. The scatter is, however, large indicating the presence of both spectacular improvements but also of reductions in work capacity. The effect on W_{max} for supine exercise is illustrated in Fig. 3, which shows a marked increase in "supine" W_{max} expressed as a fraction of "sitting" W_{max}. This fraction might be a better index of improvement in patients with ischemic heart disease than sitting W_{max} alone.

What evidence of true improvement of the heart's pump function can be found in these patients? It is obvious that since the end point of the test is determined by the patient and related to the severity of symptoms, pain and/or dyspnea, the elimination of pain alone or in combination with the knowledge of both patient and the person who conducts the test that the patient has been treated surgically will influence the outcome of the test. It is also obvious that the definition of the breaking point in patients who no longer suffer from angina may play a role.

The question then arises as to whether any significant changes in the dimensions and functional capacities of the cardiovascular system can explain the observed increases in work capacity.

One important determinant of the oxygen transport capacity is blood volume. Preoperatively, marked reductions in blood volume have been reported [7] (Fig. 4). One year after surgery, blood volume remains on the average unchanged, with a large scatter indicating both marked increases but also decreases. A return of blood volume to normal would tend to increase the ability to maintain a large stroke volume in the upright position during exercise and thereby the work capacity, but on the other hand, such an increase in blood volume would tend to increase the volume load on the heart during exercise in the supine position.

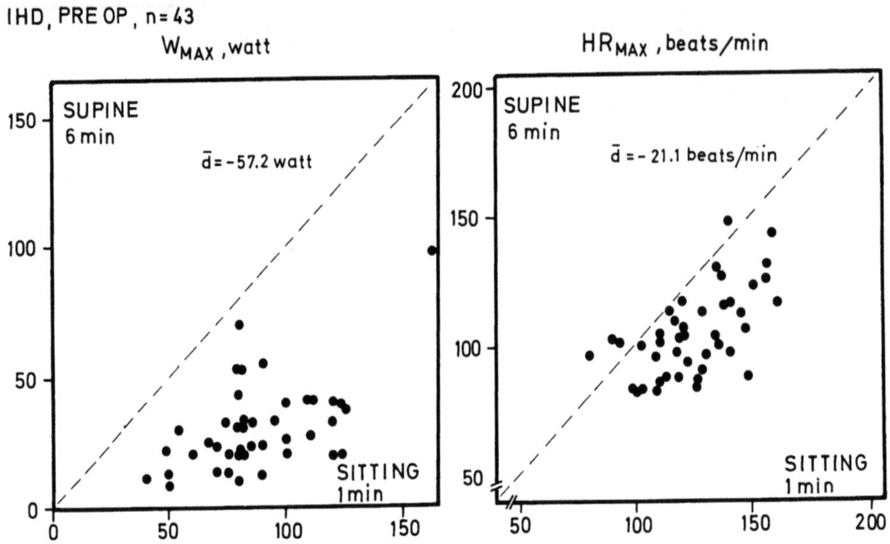

Fig. 1. Symptom of limited work capacity (W_{max}, watts) and maximal heart rate, (HR_{max}, dpm), in 43 patients with ischemic heart disease (*IHD*). Patients compared at breaking point. In seated position, stepwise increases of 10 W every minute were used; in supine position, the patients worked for 6 min at each load

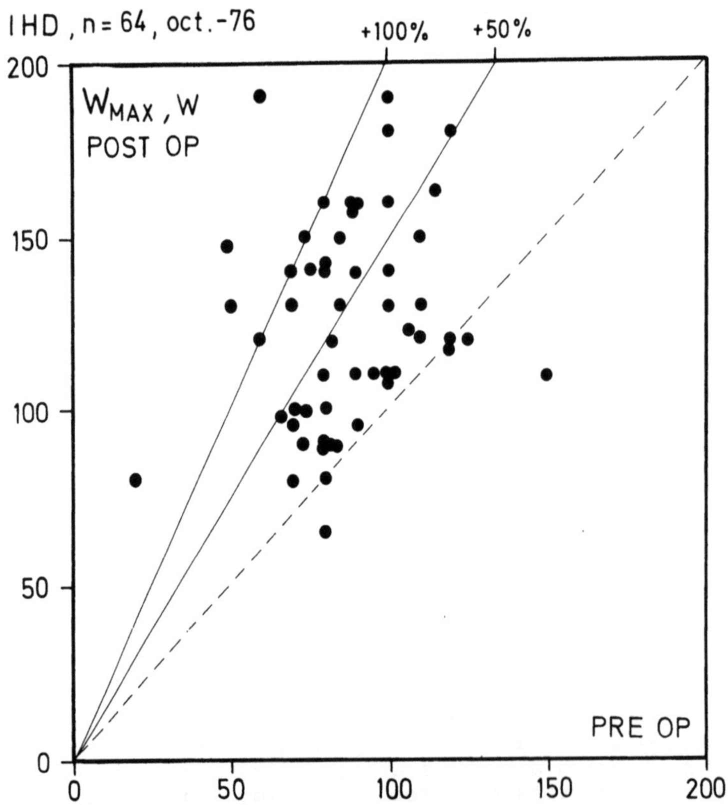

Fig. 2. W_{max}, watts in seated position before and 1 year after bypass surgery in 64 patients with IHD. Breaking point highest tolerable angina. *Closed circles* indicate individual values post-operatively, *solid line* indicates 50% and 100% improvement post-operatively, respectively

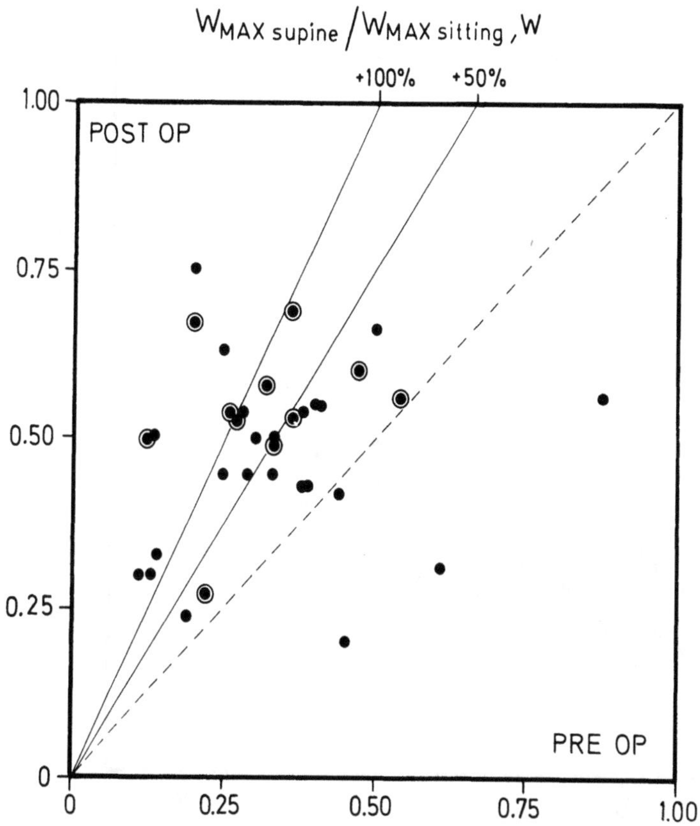

Fig. 3. Supine W_{max} expressed as a fraction of sitting W_{max} in 35 patients with IHD before and 1 year after bypass surgery. *Circles around dots* indicate patients with complete, successful correction. Closed circles indicate not completely successful correction

The submaximal work capacity has been shown to be related to the product of cardiac output and arteriovenous oxygen difference in subjects not limited by symptoms. The preoperative circulation is hypokinetic with a low cardiac output in relation to oxygen uptake both at rest and during exercise (Fig. 5). After surgery, there is on the average a tendency toward a higher arteriovenous oxygen difference in relation to oxygen uptake, i.e., toward an even more hypokinetic circulation. However, as for the other variables studied, the interindividual variation is large. Neither of the parameters, i.e., stroke volume and stroke work index, seem to offer any explanation for the increased work capacity, being on the average unchanged after surgery.

Let us now turn to the filling pressures of the two ventricles. Before surgery, exercise in the supine positon producing angina pectoris is accompanied by marked increases in both right and left end-diastolic pressures (Figs. 6 and 7). When plotted as a function curve, stroke work index versus end-diastolic pressure of the left ventricle, there are only small changes in stroke work, and at the end of work even decreases can be observed (Fig. 8 and 9).

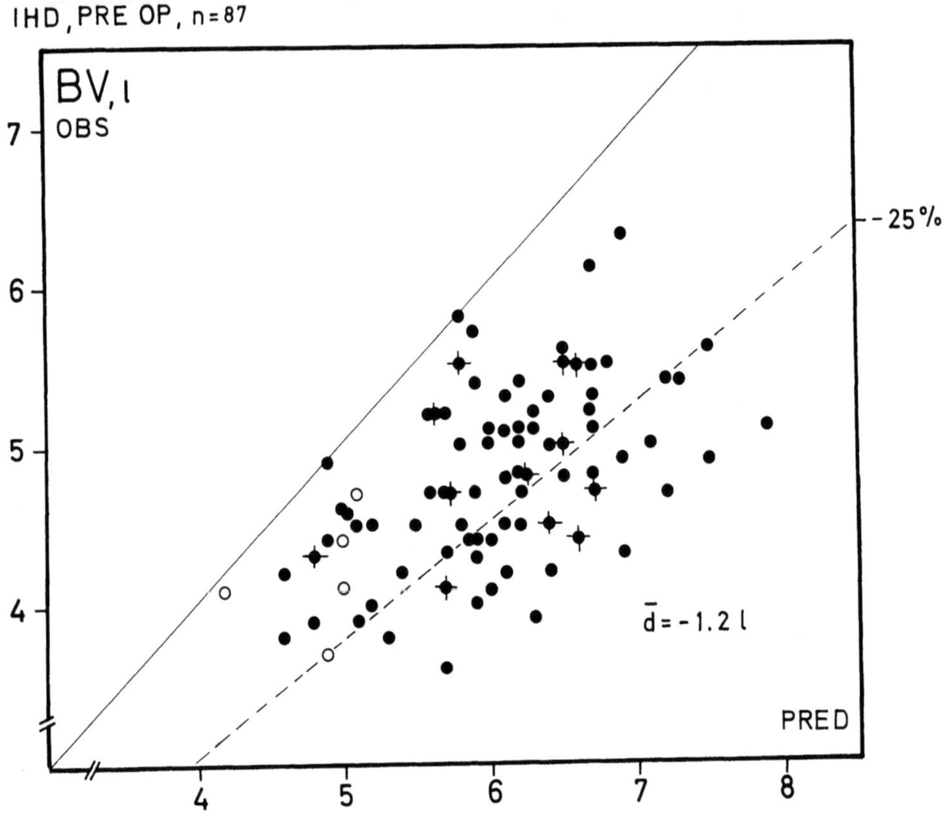

Fig. 4. Blood volume (*BV*, liters) in 87 patients with IHD, accepted for bypass surgery, in relation to normal value predicted from body weight. *Closed circles* male; *open circles* female; *crossed circles* patients with completely successful revascularization

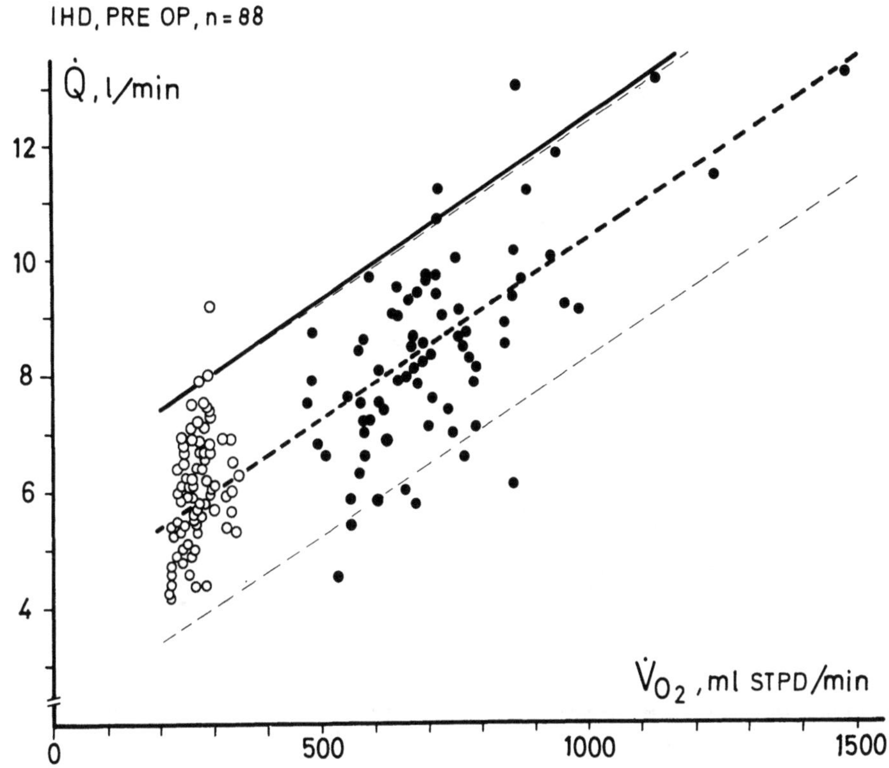

Fig. 5. Cardiac output ($\dot{Q}$, liters) at rest and during supine exercise that causes tolerable angina. *Solid line* indicates normal regression in healthy young subjects [9]. *Thick broken line* indicates regression in healthy old men (>65 years) [10]. *Thin broken line* indicates -2 SD for regression in old men. Open symbols indicate observations at rest, closed symbols observations during exercise

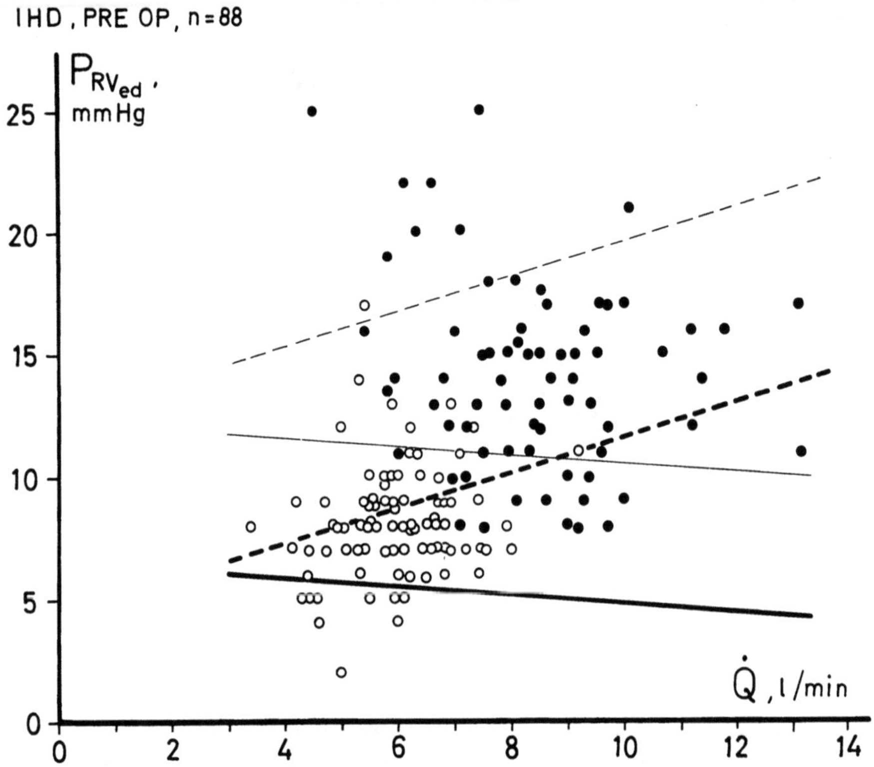

Fig. 6. Right ventricular end-diastolic pressure ($P_{RV\ ed}$, mm Hg), at rest (*open symbols*) and during exercise (*closed symbols*) that produces tolerable angina of an intensity that the patient can continue to exercise long enough that $\dot{Q}$ can be measured with direct Fick technique in 88 patients with IHD. *Solid line* indicates normal regression in healthy young subjects [9] with +2 SD. Broken line indicates observed regression in healthy old subjects [10]

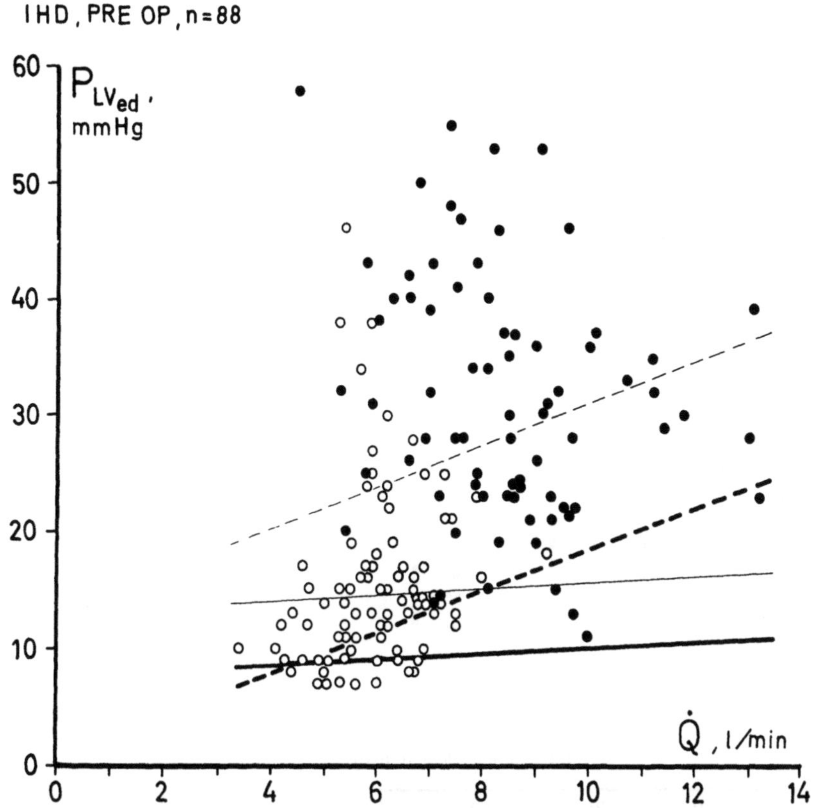

Fig. 7. Left ventricular end-diastolic pressure ($P_{LV\,ed}$, mm Hg) at rest (*open symbols*) and during supine steady-state exercise (*closed symbols*) in the same patients as in Fig. 6. Regression indicates the relatioship in healthy young and old subjects as in Fig. 6

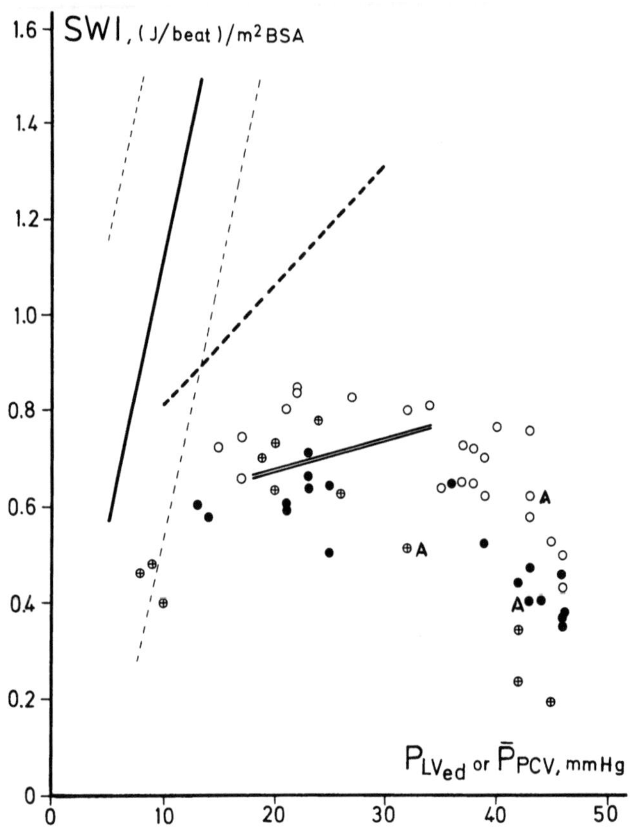

Fig. 8. Stroke work index (*SWI*, J/beat/m^2 BSA) at rest and during supine exercise in three patients with severe effort angina. *A* represents onset of angina. Regression lines as in Fig. 9. Double-contoured line indicates regression for observations in the present preoperative studies. Note the marked decrease in stroke work work index at filling pressures above 40 mm Hg

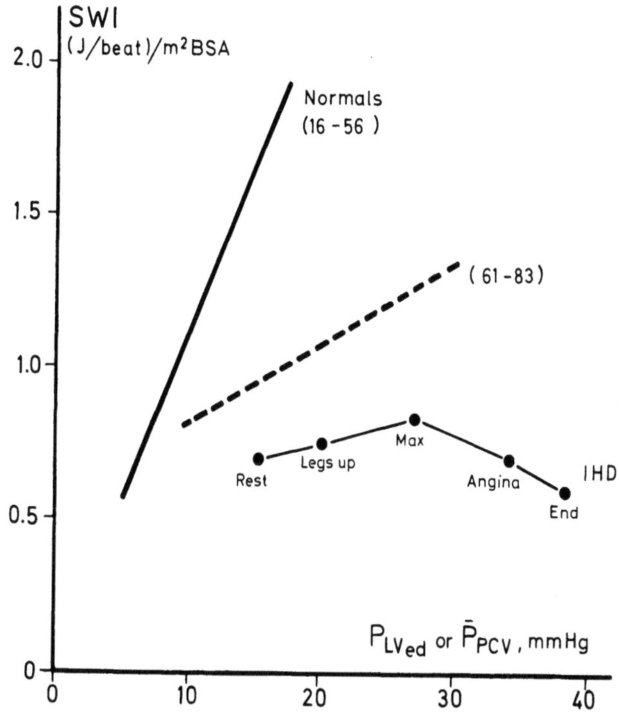

Fig. 9. Stroke work index (*SWI*, J/beat/m^2 BSA) at rest and during supine non-steady-state exercise with stepwise increase work load until the patient stops because of angina, in 20 patients investigated before bypass surgery, in relation to left ventricular end-diastolic pressure (mm Hg). *Solid line* indicates relationship in normal subjects (Ekelund et al., 1967), *broken line* in healthy old men [10]

One year after surgery, marked reductions of both left and right ventricular filling pressure are observed (Figs. 10 and 11), but stroke volume and stroke work seem on the average to remain unchanged; with the other variables studied, the variation is marked indicating the great inhomogeneity of material and surgical results. In a selected group including only patients with sucessful, complete grafting of all stenosed vessels, a significant improvement of the function curve can be observed [8] (Fig. 12).

In conclusion, we find from these preliminary data that the work capacity increases after surgery in most patients. The work capacity in the supine position also increases, both absolutely and as a fraction of the sitting work capacity. This increase is to a large extent due to the relief from pain. There are only minor changes in blood volume and the kinetics of the circulation after surgery but rather marked reductions of the supine filling pressures of both right and left ventricles. In successful cases, the increase in work capacity is also accompanied by marked improvement in pump function as demonstrated by function curves.

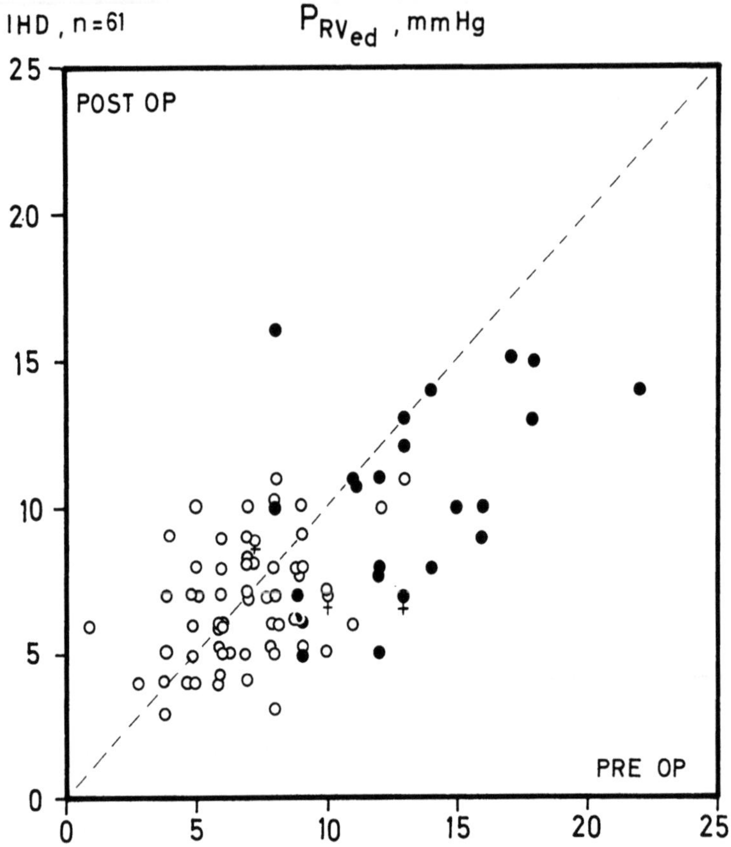

Fig. 10. Right ventricular end-diastolic pressure (mm Hg) before and 1 year after bypass surgery. Symbols and conditions as in Fig. 7

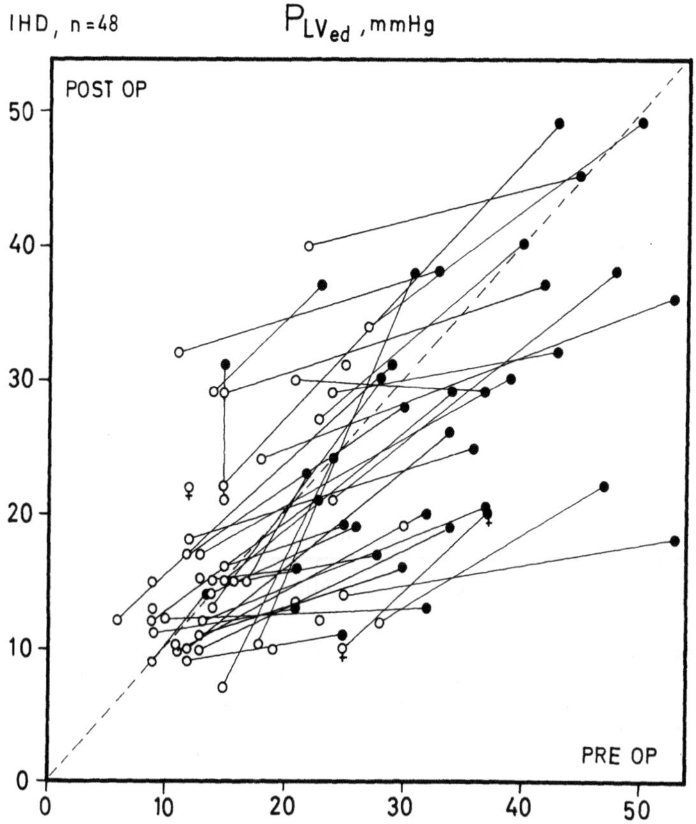

Fig. 11. Left ventricular end-diastolic pressure ($P_{LV\ ed}$, mm Hg) in 48 patients with IHD, at rest and during exercise at identical work loads, before and after bypass surgery. Symbols as in Fig. 4

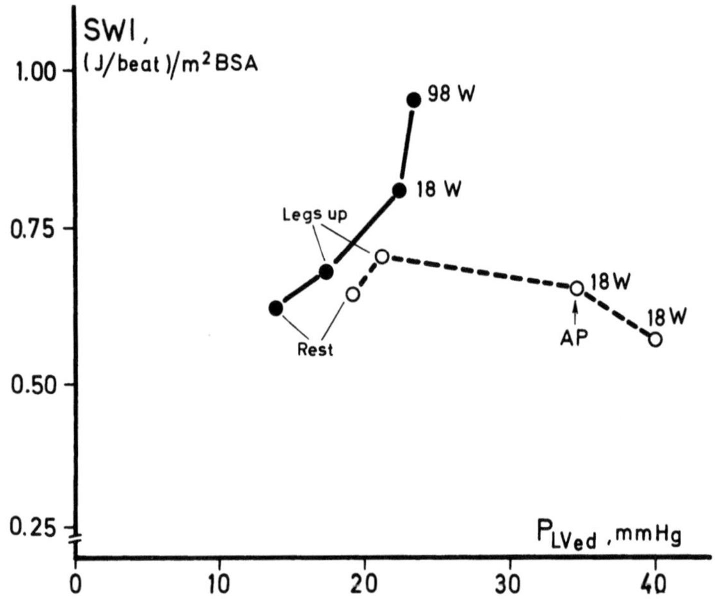

Fig. 12. Stroke work index (*SWI*, J/beat/m^2 BSA) in relation to left ventricular end-diastolic pressure, at rest and during exercise in five patients with IHD before (*open circles, broken line*) and 1 year after bypass surgery (*closed circles*, solid line). *AP* indicates onset of effort angina. Figures indicate mean work load (watts). Note the normalization of the "function curve" after surgery [8]

References

1. Cannom, D.S., Miller, D.C., Shumway, N.E., Fogarty, T.J., Daily, P.O., Hu, M., Brown, B., Jr., Harrison, D.C.: The long-term follow-up of patients undergoing saphenous vein bypass surgery. Circulation *49*, 77-85 (1974)
2. Dunkman, W.B., Perloff, J.K., Kastor, J.A., Shelburne, J.C.: Medical perspectives in coronary artery disease - a caveat. Ann. Intern. Med. *81*, 817-837 (1974)
3. Assad-Morell, J.L., Frye, R.L., Connolly, D.C., Davis, G.D., Pluth, J.R., Wallace, R.B., Barnhorst, D.A., Elvebeck, L.R., Danielson, G.K.: Aorta-coronary artery saphenous vein bypass surgery: clinical and angiographic results. Mayo Clin. Proc. *50*, 379-386 (1975)
4. Björk, V.O., Henze, A., Hindmarsch, T., Holmgren, A., Jonsson, B.: Central hemodynamics of Bypass-Surgery. A 1-year follow-up study. In preparation (1978)
5. Åström, H., Jonsson, B.: Design of exercise test with special reference to heart patients. Br. Heart J. *38* (3), 289-296 (1976)
6. Borg, G.: Relative response and stimulus scale. Rep. Inst. Appl. Psychol., No.1. University of Stockholm (1970)
7. Åström, H., Holmgren, A., Jonsson, B.: Blood volume in angina pectoris. Br. Heart J. In print (1978)
8. Carlens, P., Landou, C., Pehrsson, K.: Left ventricular pump function after aorto-coronary bypass surgery. In preparation (1978)
9. Ekelund, L.G., Holmgren, A.: Central haemodynamics during exercise. Circ. Res. *20*, 20-21 (1967)
10. Strandell, T.: Circulatory studies on healthy old men. Acta Med. Scand. *414*, [Suppl.] (1964)

Pulmonary Artery Pressure During Exercise and LV Diastolic Compliance Before and After Coronary Artery Surgery

J. Jehle, K. Bornikoel, K. L. Neuhaus, G. Sauer, and P. Spiller

The elevation in pulmonary artery pressure and in left ventricular enddiastolic pressure in ischemic heart disease is partially caused by an increased ventricular stiffness [1,3,5]. Nitroglycerin does not only immediately alleviate angina, it also induces a reduction of ventricular stiffness at rest (Fig. 1). We have previously shown that this improvement of ventricular stiffness could be due to a reduction of ischemia caused by a decrease in myocardial oxygen consumption [6]. We have now investigated whether improvement of ischemia after coronary bypass surgery would result in a similar change of ventricular stiffness.

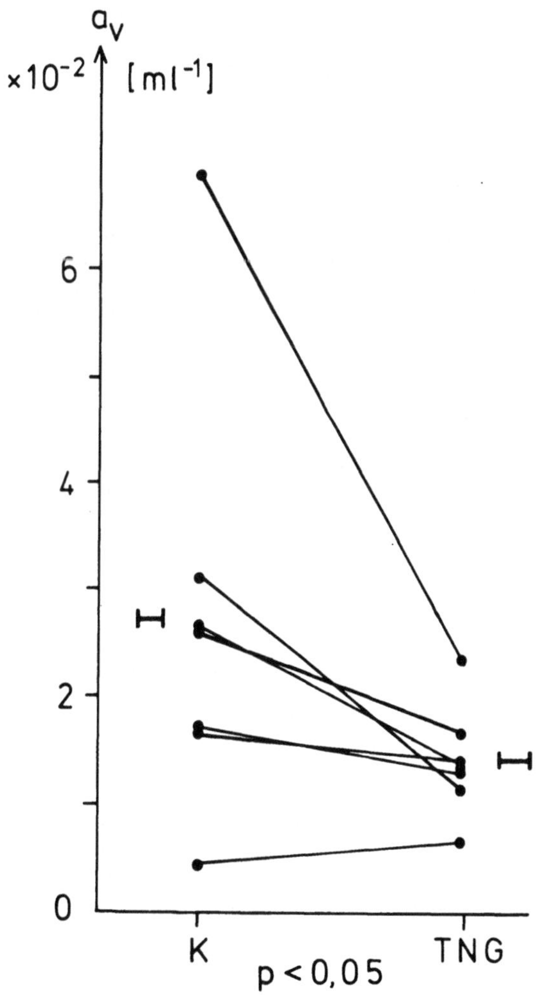

Fig. 1. The influence of nitroglycerin (*TNG*) on ventricular stiffness. The passive elastic modulus a_v is high before the administration of TNG (*K*) and significantly lower after TNG. The higher the initial value, the greater is the effect of TNG

A total of 19 patients with coronary artery disease were examined. Of these, 14 had previously suffered a myocardial infarction. The investigations were done before and on an average of 3.8 months after aortocoronary bypass. The mean age was 45.9 years, ranging from 30 to 64 years. A total of 33 grafts were implanted, 29 of these, i.e., 88% were patent. Biplane cineventriculograms in the RAO and LAO projections were recorded at 100 frames/s. Simultaneously, pressures were recorded by a catheter tip manometer. We determined: heart rate, maximal systolic and enddiastolic pressure, and enddiastolic, as well as, endsystolic volume. The volumes were measured at the time of opening and closing of the aortic valve. From this, we calculated stroke volume and ejection fraction. In addition, mean circumferential fiber shortening velocity of three diameters of the RAO projection was determined ($\overline{V_{CF}}$).

Three different physiologic expressions of compliance were used:

1) Total observed compliance, as $\frac{\Delta P}{\Delta V}$ /ESVI [5]
2) The reciprocal value, related to mean diastolic pressure, i.e., total diastolic stiffness, as $\frac{\Delta V}{\Delta P}$ /$\bar{P}$ [5]
3) The passive elastic modulus $a_v = \frac{dV}{dP}$ /P

This index is represented by the slope of the diastolic logarithm pressure-volume curve [6]. In ten patients, we obtained measurements of pulmonary artery pressures at rest and during exercise before and after surgery.

In the following, of the two pairs of figures in brackets, the former represent preoperative values, the latter postoperative. Statistical analysis was performed using Student's T-Test for paired values.

Maximal systolic pressure (131 ± 22 mmHg and 130 ± 23 mmHg) and enddiastolic pressure (19.1 ± 6.8 mmHg and 19.8 ± 6.2 mmHg) were unchanged before and after surgery. Heart rate, measured during angiography, increased significantly from 79 ± 18/min to 87 ± 17/min (Fig. 2). Enddiastolic (107 ± 23 ml/m^2 and 104 ± 25 ml/m^2) and endsystolic volumes (60 ± 19 ml/m^2 and 56 ± 23 ml/m^2) remained unaltered by surgery. Consequently, ejection fraction was unaltered as well (47 ± 11% pre- and postoperatively). In contrast to the ejection fraction, mean circumferential fiber shortening velocity increased significantly from 0.81 ± 0.23 circ·s^{-1} to 0.92 ± 0.22 circ·s^{-1} (Fig. 3). This was partially due to the decrease of ejection time postoperatively, and partially to an increase of circumferential fiber shortening velocity in the revascularized areas [2].

Figure 4 shows the results obtained with the three different expressions of ventricular compliance. Although the individual values behave differently, the mean values were not significantly different, when total observed compliance ($\frac{\Delta V}{\Delta P}$ /ESVI) or total diastolic stiffness ($\frac{\Delta P}{\Delta V}$ /$\bar{P}$) were used. No different results were found, if only patients with closed grafts (*broken lines*) or patients without infarction (*crosses*) were considered. However, the passive elastic modulus a_v increased significantly after surgery. The difference in results between the first two methods and the third method could be due to the different definitions of endsystolic and enddiastolic volume used in the calculation. In the first two methods, stroke volume and endsystolic volume were utilized as it is usually done [5]. In the third

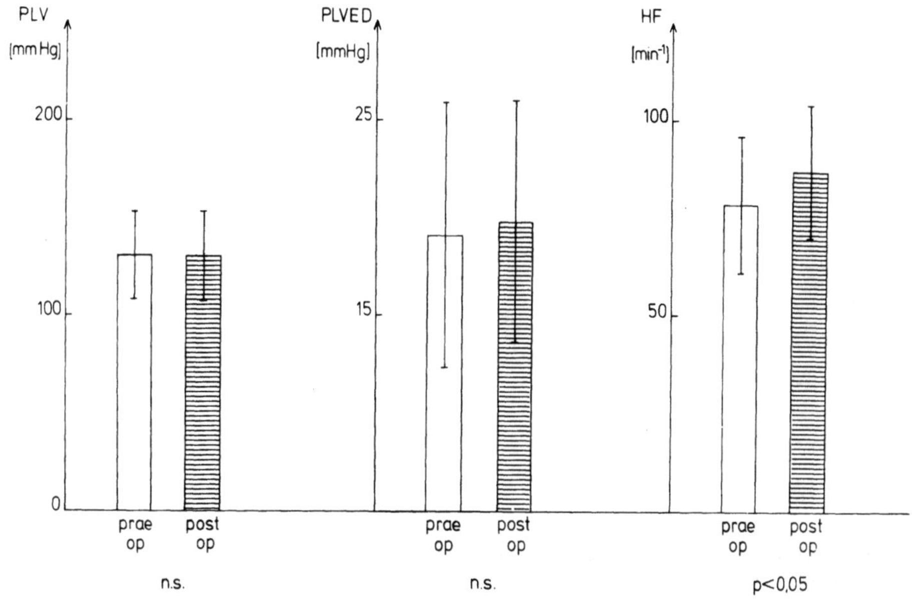

Fig. 2. Mean values of maximal systolic pressure (PLV), enddiastolic pressure (PLVED), and heart rate (HF) before (*white bars*) and after surgery (*striped bars*). Unchanged pressures before and after surgery, significant increase in postoperative heart rate

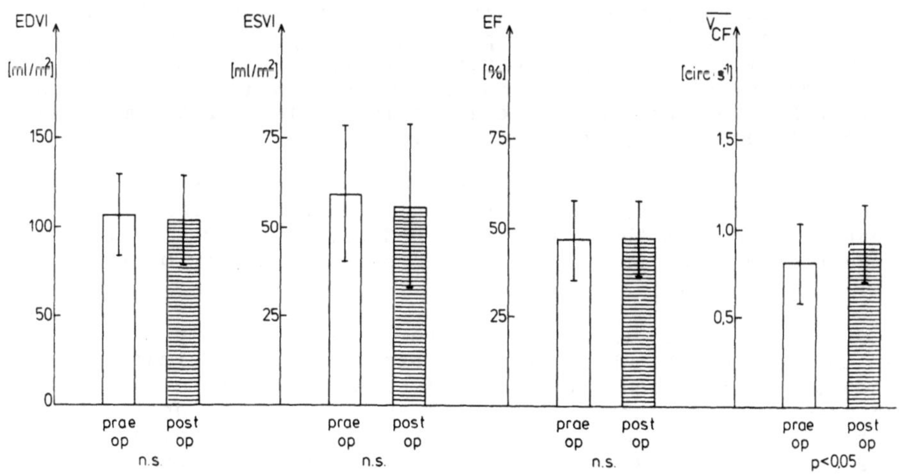

Fig. 3. Mean values of enddiastolic (EDVI) and endsystolic (ESVI) volume, ejection fraction (EF), and mean circumferential fiber shortening velocity ($\overline{V_{CF}}$) before (*white bars*) and after surgery (*striped bars*). No change was found pre- or postoperatively in EDVI, ESVI, or EF, whereas $\overline{V_{CF}}$ increased significantly postoperatively

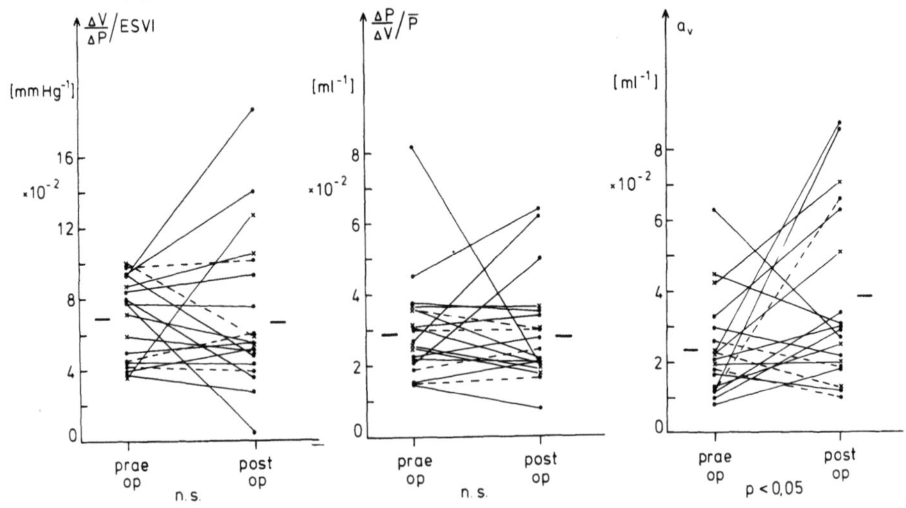

Fig. 4. The values of three different expressions of ventricular compliance pre- and postoperatively. *Crosses*: patients without myocardial infarction; *broken lines*: patients with closed grafts; *dash*: mean values. Further clarification in text

method, we determined the volumes when the diastolic pressure was at its lowest and highest value. The difference between these volumes did not correspond to the stroke volume used in methods one and two. In method three, the early diastolic volume is greater postoperatively. Since the enddiastolic pressures and volumes, as well as, the early diastolic pressures were the same pre- and postoperatively, the greater early diastolic volume postoperatively must be the reason for the increased stiffness that we measured with method three. From these results, it is apparent that there is no indication for an improvement of compliance by any of the three methods.

This is in contrast to the observations of Mason and his co-workers. These authors demonstrated that ventricular compliance improved in those patients in whom the grafts remained patent. These findings were independent of whether or not the patients had a history of infarction [3].

In ten of our patients, in whom the three indices of compliance were similar to those of the whole group, pressures in the pulmary artery were recorded at rest and during exercise. At rest, there was no difference pre- and postoperatively. Although exercise and angiography were not simultaneously performed, it is of interest to note that the unchanged mean pulmonary artery pressure corresponds to the unchanged enddiastolic pressure of the left ventricle.

Figure 5 shows heart rate and mean pulmonary pressure at a comparable exercise load. The increase in heart rate was greater postoperatively, from 108 ± 20/min to 118 ± 13/min. This could be due to the diminished physical fitness of these patients 4 months after surgery. Mean pulmonary artery pressure decreased from 34 ± 11 mmHg to 30 ± 6 mmHg. Among the ten patients, there was only one, in whom the pressure markedly increased (from 20 mmHg to 40 mmHg). In this patient, ejection fraction and $\overline{V_{CF}}$ decreased postoperatively, so that myocardial injury must be considered despite graft patency. However, there was no electrocardiographic indication for postoperative infarction.

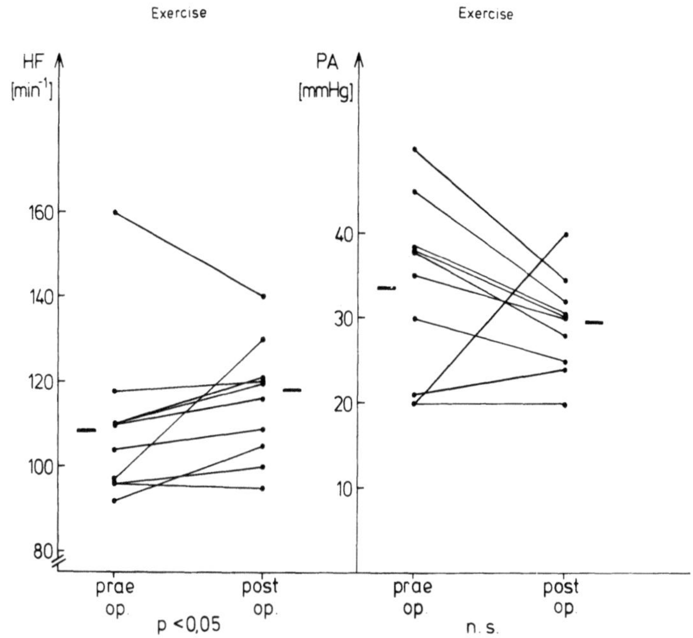

Fig. 5. Heart rate (HF) and mean pulmonary artery pressure (PA) at comparable exercise load pre- and postoperatively. *Dash*: mean values.
Further clarification in text

Thus, even in patients with considerably increased stiffness, there was during exercise a decrease in mean pulmonary artery pressure.

Conclusions

1) There was no improvement of systolic ventricular function at rest.
2) Although ventricular compliance is preoperatively reduced, there is no postoperative improvement. The results were independent of graft patency.
3) The postoperative decrease of mean pulmonary artery pressure during exercise is most likely due to improved systolic function and not to a change in compliance [4]. This is based on our findings that the compliance was unchanged at rest and therefore would probably not be changed during exercise. However, this statement remains to be proven by appropriate measurements.

References

1. Bardet, J., Rocha, P., Rigaud, M., Bourdarias, J.P., Mathivat, A.: Left ventricular compliance in acute myocardial infarction in man. Cardiovasc. Res. *11*, 122 (1977)
2. Bornikoel, K., Neuhaus, K.L., Niessen, H.W., Jehle, J., Rönsberg, D.: Änderungen der zirkumferentiellen Verkürzungsgeschwindigkeit und der lokalen Wandbewegung nach aortokoronarem Bypass. Verh. Dtsch. Ges. Inn. Med. *82*, 1215 (1976)
3. Diamond, G., Forrester, J.S.: Effect of coronary artery disease and acute myocardial infarction on left ventricular compliance in man. Circulation *45*, 11 (1972)

4. Lösse, B., Schicha, H., Jehle, J., Krönert, H., Becker, V., Feinendegen, L.E., Loogen, F.: Störungen der rechts- und linksventrikulären Funktion bei koronarer Herzerkrankung (KHK) und ihre Beeinflussung durch aorto-koronare Bypass-Operation. Verh. Dtsch. Ges. Kreislaufforsch. *43*, 323 (1977)
5. Miller, R.R., De Maria, A.N., Amsterdam, E.A., Mailander, M.M., Zelis, R., Lurie, A.J., Mason, D.T.: Improvement of reduced left ventricular diastolic compliance in ischemic heart disease after successful coronary artery bypass surgery. Am. J. Cardiol. *35*, 11 (1975)
6. Sauer, G., Jehle, J., Karsch, R., Kreuzer, H., Neuhaus, K.L., Spiller, P.: Der Einfluß von Nitroglycerin auf Hämodynamik, Wandspannung und Sauerstoffverbrauch des linken Ventrikels. Z. Kardiol. *65*, 753 (1976)

Factors Influencing Improvement of Hemodynamics During Exercise

P. Stürzenhofecker, H. Roskamm, and K. Schnellbacher

During our last conference in Geneva 1975, dealing with ventricular function at rest and during exercise, we could demonstrate that there is a rather good correlation between the size of the ischemic area of the left ventricle and the increase in mean pulmonary arterial wedge pressure (PCP) during exercise-induced angina. Thus the degree of PCP-rise is a semiquantitative indicator of the severity and size of ischemia. In this paper we would like to deliberate on the factors influencing improvement of hemodynamics during exercise after aorto-coronary bypass surgery. After subtracting the early deaths (3.57%), we were left with 693 patients operated on up until the end of 1977. In these patients 1,702 grafts were constructed, thus averaging 2.45 grafts per patient. Most patients had 3-vessel disease and 14% had left main stem disease. 16.9% of the patients received one graft and nearly 50% at least three grafts (Table 1).

Functional studies were performed preoperatively, 8 weeks, 1 year, and 2 years after surgery.

Preoperatively, 15% of the patients had no angina; 8 weeks postoperatively 74% of the patients were completely free from angina, even at a high exercise load. This frequency slightly decreased within 1-2 years. The percentage of patients who pre- and postoperatively had no ischemic ST-segment depression and those who had normal hemodynamics during exercise, is quite similar.

Inspite of increasing exercise tolerance, PCP-pressure and ischemic ST-segment depression decreased without showing significant changes within 1-2 years postoperatively.

Table 1. Number of vessels involved and grafts constructed in 693 patients. Age: x = 51 (24-70) years. 645 ♂, 48 ♀

	n =	%		n =	%
1-vessel	92	13.3	1 graft	117	16.9
2-vessel	216	31.2	2 grafts	237	34.2
3-vessel	385	55.5	3 grafts	254	36.7
			≥4 grafts	85	12.2
(LMCA	98	14.1)			
Total	693	100.0		693	100.0

Early mortality
3.57% (3 months)

Grafts/patient
2.45

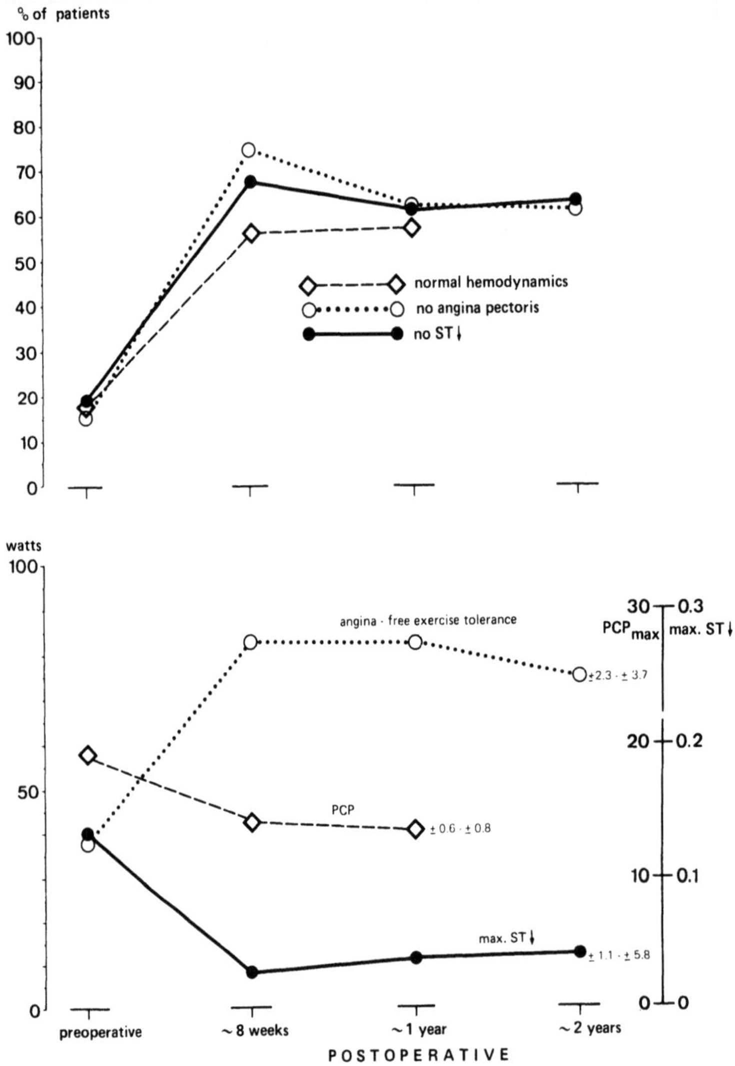

Fig. 1. a) Hemodynamics, angina pectoris, ST-segment depression preoperatively, 8 weeks, 1 year, and 2 years following coronary bypass graft surgery. b) Exercise tolerance, pulmonary wedge pressure, and maximum ST-segment depression preoperatively, 8 weeks, 1 year, and 2 years following coronary bypass graft surgery

Figure 2 shows that there are no significant differences between patients with 1-, 2-, or 3-vessel disease, also those with left main stem disease showed a quite similar increase of exercise tolerance after surgery.

One year after the operation of 490 patients, a second coronary angiography was performed in 403. These patients were divided into four groups (Table 2).

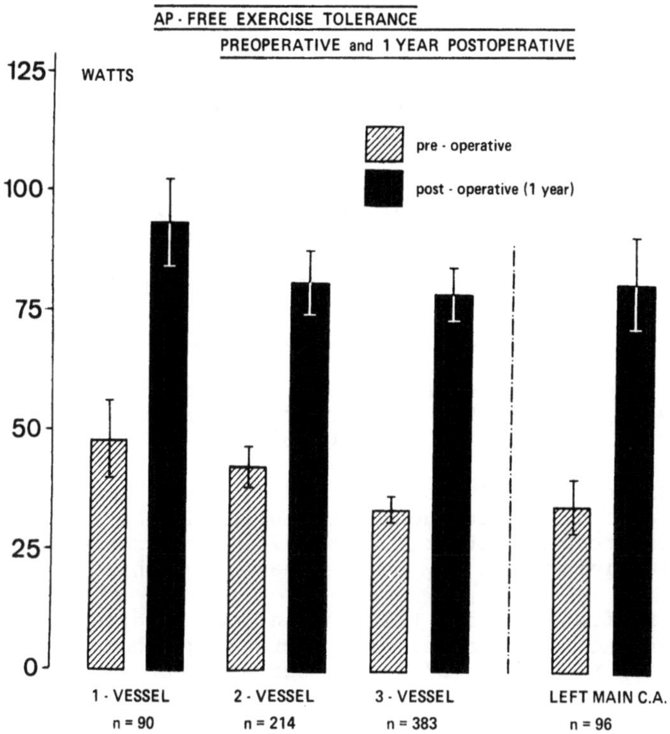

Fig. 2. AP - free exercise tolerance preoperative and 1 year postoperative

Table 2. Extent of revascularization and graft patency in 403 patients

Group	A *n* = 189	B *n* = 107	C *n* = 82	D *n* = 25
Revascular-ization	Complete	Sufficient	Insufficient	All grafts occluded
Definition	All arteries with ≥50% stenosis successfully bypassed	1 graft oc-cluded (LAD-graft patent)	At least 1 graft open (LAD-graft oc-cluded)	All grafts occluded
Vessel disease	2.2	2.6	2.4	2.4
No. of grafts	2.2	2.9	2.6	2.8
Patent grafts per patient	2.2	2.0	1.1	0

Group A: Complete revascularization (*n* = 189): (all arteries with more than 50% stenosis were provided with a patent graft).

Group B: Sufficient revascularization (*n* = 107). One graft was occluded but not that to the left anterior descending artery (LAD).

Group C: Insufficient revascularization (*n* = 82). There was at least one open graft, LAD-graft was occluded.

Group D: No surgical success: (All grafts were occluded). (n = 25)

This, of course, is a rather subjective classification, but it corresponds quite well with the average number of open grafts in each group. All four groups were quite similar in the average number of vessels involved and the average number of grafts constructed:

Group A (189 patients) had an average of 2.2 open grafts. By definition this figure is identical with the number of grafts constructed.
In Group B (107 patients) there was an average of two patent grafts of 2.9 grafts constructed.
In Group C (82 patients) there was an average of 1.1 open grafts of 2.6 grafts constructed.
In Group D (25 patients) by definition all grafts were occluded.

With increasing incompleteness of revascularization from group A to group C, the frequency of patients being postoperatively totally free from angina had decreased from 70% to 50% (Fig. 3).

Unexpectedly, in the group with all grafts occluded, 60% of the patients were free from angina. But it should be mentioned that the number of patients in this group is rather low (n = 25). Occurrance of perioperative myocardial infarction may be one reason for this.

Quantification of angina-free exercise tolerance allows a better differentiation between the four groups. With increasing incompleness of revascularization the effect of bypass surgery becomes smaller.

The number of patients without ischemic ST-segment depression after surgery decreases from group A to C. Unexpectedly, there is again a high number of patients without ST-segment depression in the group with all grafts occluded. The occurrance of perioperative infarction may have some influence.

The number of patients with normal PCP and cardiac output at rest and during exercise decreases from 75% in group A to 45% in group C.

In the group with all grafts occluded there was no change after surgery. It should be mentioned that in this group the number of patients with normal hemodynamics *preoperatively* was the highest in spite of multiple-vessel disease. This may be explained by diffuse scarring which might lead to a lower rise of PCP during exercise.

Perhaps this should be a factor to be considered if indications for bypass surgery are discussed: a low rise of PCP indicates only small amounts of viable myocardium. Thus, the degree of PCP could be an indicator of a high occlusion rate. Differences between the groups were more pronounced when ST-segment depression and PCP pressure during exercise were considered. With increasing incompleteness of revascularization the postoperative decrease becomes smaller (Fig. 5)

In group D, with all grafts occluded, there is no change of PCP postoperatively.

The most striking differences were found between the groups when ST-segment depression and PCP pressure were related to the maximum work load.

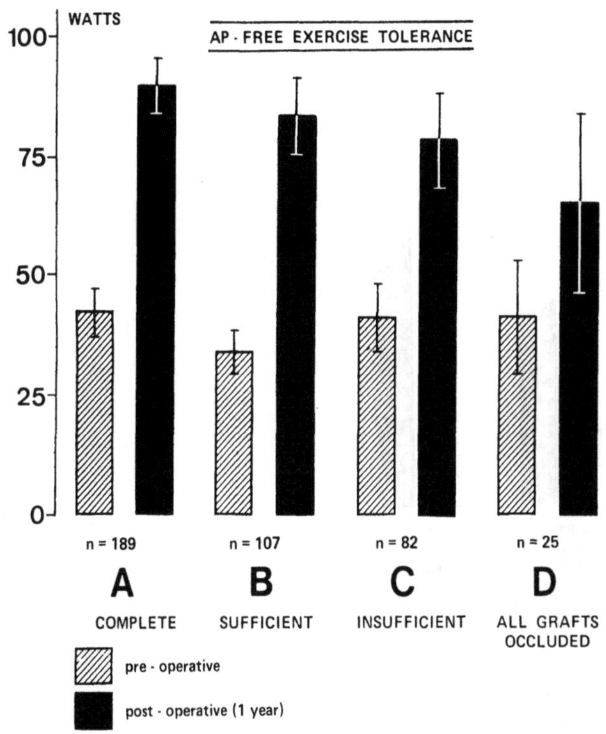

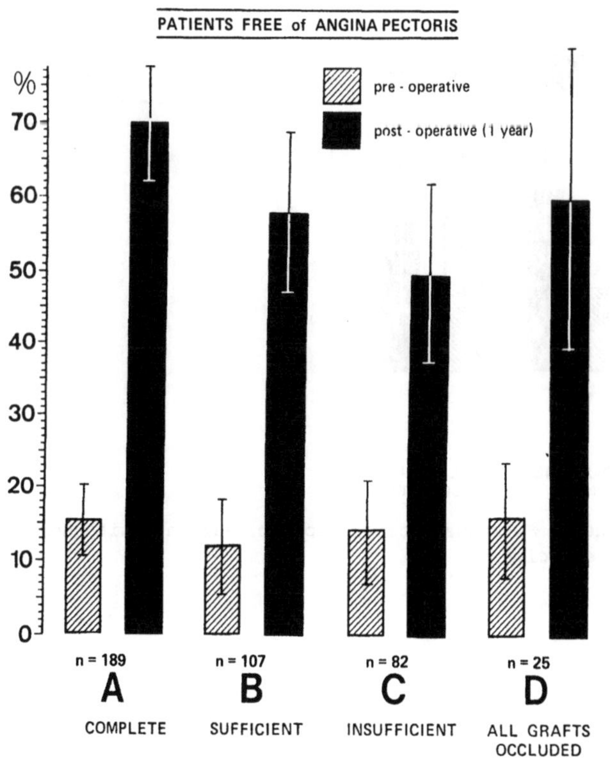

Fig. 3. a) Percentage of patients postoperatively free from angina. b) AP - Free exercise tolerance

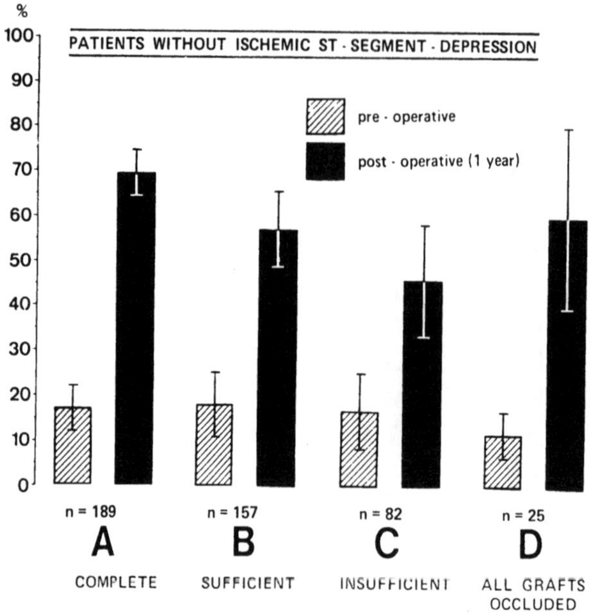

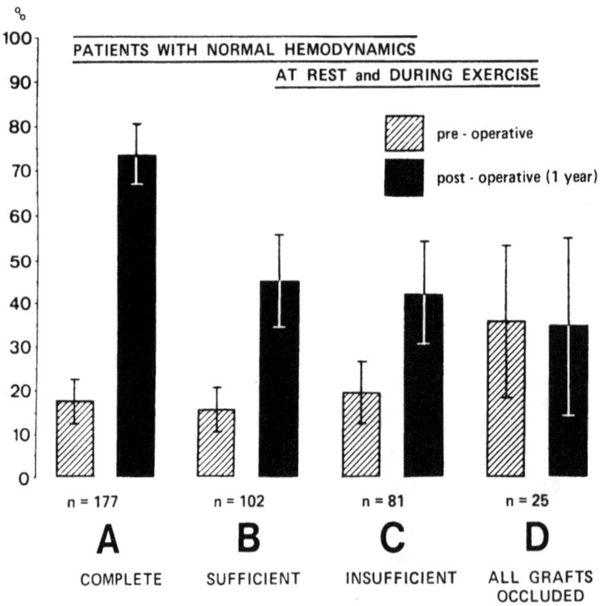

Fig. 4. a) Patients without ischemic ST-segment depression. b) Patients with normal hemodynamics at rest and during exercise

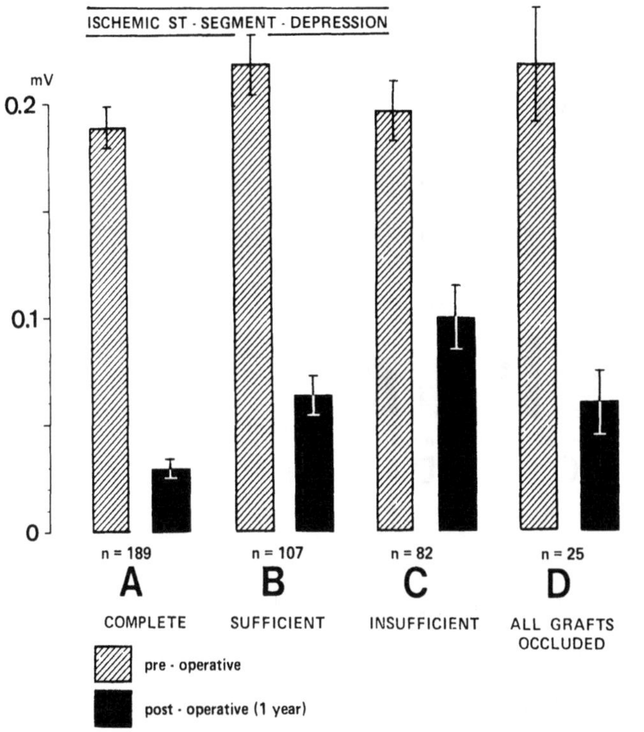

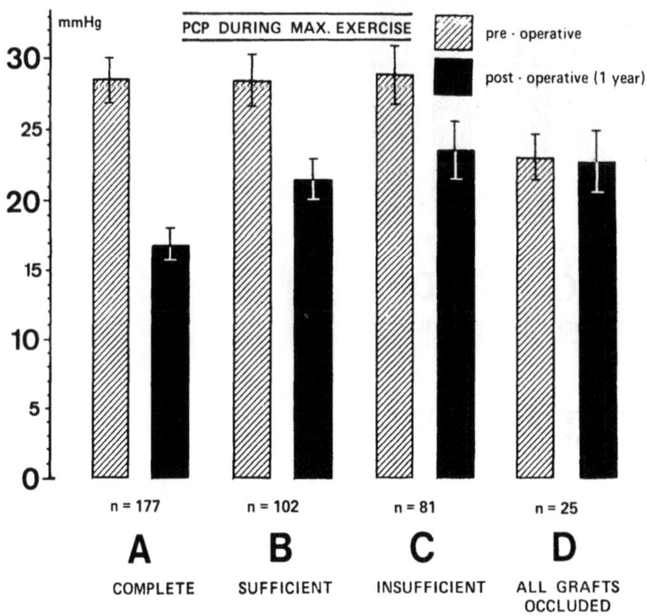

Fig. 5. a) ST-segment depression pre- and postoperatively. b) Pulmonary wedge pressure during exercise pre- and postoperatively

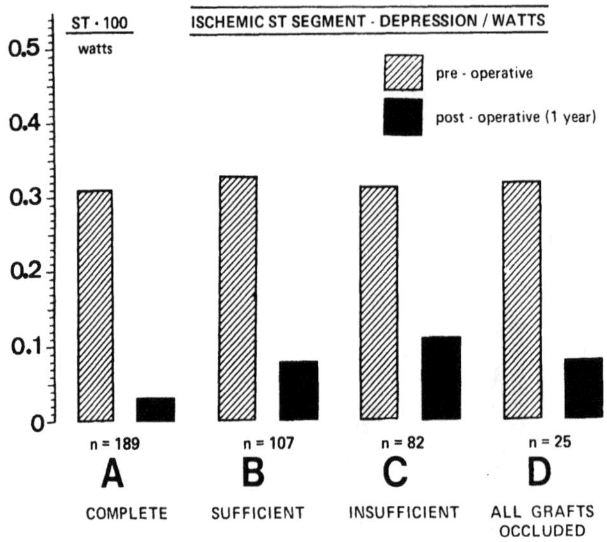

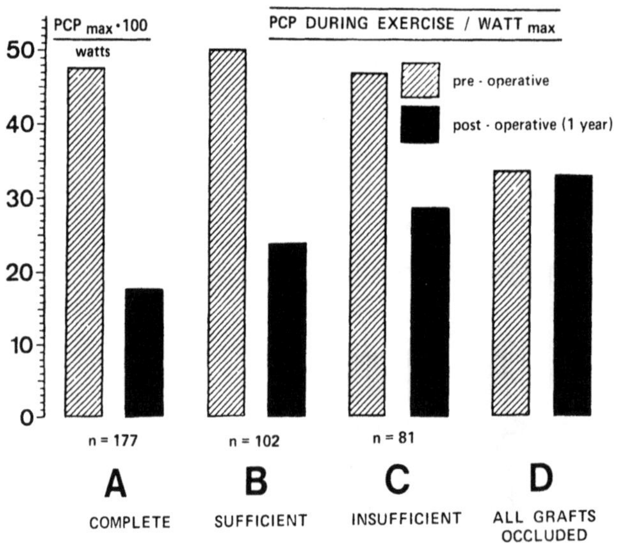

Fig. 6. a) Ischemic ST-segment depression/Watts,
b) PCP during exercise/$Watt_{max}$

In conclusion, hemodynamic improvement after aortocoronary bypass surgery mainly depends on the completeness of revascularization. High PCP-rise preoperatively is combined with good postoperative results. Thus, hemodynamic studies during exercise can be used as an additional indicator for adequate and successful revascularization.

Thallium^{201} Myocardial Perfusion Scintigraphy for the Evaluation of Post Coronary Bypass Patients

B. H. Greenberg, R. Hart, E. H. Botvinick, J. A. Werner, B. H. Brundage, D. M. Shames, K. Chatterjee, and W. W. Parmley

Abstract

To determine the utility of thallium-201 stress scintigraphy for the assessment of coronary bypass surgery, we evaluated chest pain, stress electrocardiograms, and scintigrams in 27 patients following surgery. These findings were compared with those of coronary angiography where ≥ 75% stenosis in a graft, its distal vessel, or in an ungrafted native vessel, represented significant postoperative lesions. Chest pain lacked sensitivity (60%) and was nonspecific (20%) for the identification of postoperative coronary lesions. Stress electrocardiography had low sensitivity (60%) and good specificity (86%) for the diagnosis of coronary lesions. However, electrocardiography was not helpful in six patients who had equivocal or suboptimal tests. The scintigram had good sensitivity (77%) and was highly specific for the diagnosis of coronary stenosis. The scintigram was significantly more specific than chest pain ($P < 0.01$), gave excellent localizing information, and added to the accuracy of both conclusive and inconclusive stress tests. In nine patients in whom preoperative stress scintigrams had also been obtained, comparison of pre- and postoperative studies reflected the effects of bypass surgery on coronary perfusion. Scintigraphy is a useful technique for the noninvasive evaluation of the postcoronary bypass patient and postoperative scintigraphy alone is of great value in documenting surgical results.

Introduction

Each year in the United States an estimated 50,000 coronary artery bypass procedures are performed [1]. As a result a large group of postbypass patients will require follow-up evaluation for the presence of myocardial ischemia in the future. Although useful information in the post-bypass patient is obtained from a history of symptomatic improvement, resting electrocardiogram, and the functional and electrocardiographic response to graded exercise, evaluation of the extent of revascularization and graft patency relies on repeat coronary angiography. Since this procedure is costly, time consuming, and subjects the patient to a small, but definite risk [2,3], the use of angiography in the follow-up of bypass patients has been limited.

Thallium-201 (201 Tl) stress scintigraphy is a noninvasive method used to assess regional myocardial perfusion and indirectly to identify significant coronary stenosis [4-6]. It has been successfully used to evaluate patients with coronary artery disease [4-6]. We sought to determine the value of this method for the follow-up evaluation of post-bypass patients. Further, we wished to determine whether comparison with preoperative scintigraphy was necessary for interpreting postoperative studies or whether a postoperative study alone would suffice.

Methods

Patient Population
The 27 patients studied represent all patients who underwent 201 Tl stress scintigraphy at this institution as part of follow-up evaluation after coronary bypass surgery. Nine of these patients had undergone stress scintigraphy preoperatively. Twenty-five of these patients also underwent postoperative selective coronary angiography. The 23 males and 4 females averaged 52.5 years (33-69 years). Postoperative evaluation was undertaken in 17 patients because of recurrent chest pain. Eleven of these patients had typical angina pectoris. Ten patients who were free of chest pain were studied because either the individual or the physician desired information regarding graft patency. Two patients were experiencing rest pain. Four patients were receiving propranolol and 7 patients were receiving digoxin at the time of study. Two patients had single grafts, 9 had double, 12 had triple, and 5 had quadruple bypass grafts with an average of 2.7 grafts per subject. Thirty-two grafts were placed to the left anterior descending coronary artery, or diagonal vessels (LAD), 23 to the circumflex or marginal vessels (LCX), and 17 to the right coronary artery (RCA). With the exception of three internal mammary to LAD grafts, saphenous veins were used in all instances.

Stress Testing
In 25 patients stress perfusion scintigraphy was performed in conjunction with graded treadmill exercise according to the method of Bruce [7]. A 12-lead electrocardiogram was taken at rest and an intravenous catheter was placed in an antecubital vein to facilitate administration of 201 Tl. The blood pressure and CM5 electrocardiogram lead were monitored during standing, hyperventilation, exercise, and a 6-8 min recovery period. The treadmill electrocardiogram was abnormal and considered positive for ischemia if there was ≥1 mm horizontal or downsloping ST segment depression beyond an isoelectric baseline, 0.08 from the J-point during exercise or during recovery. The treadmill electrocardiogram was called equivocal for ischemia, regardless of the degree of exercise induced ST segment depression, if the baseline ST segment was depressed more than 1 mm. Negative treadmill tests that failed to reach 85% of the maximal predicted heart rate for that age-group were classified as suboptimal studies.

In two patients with rest pain thought to be cardiac in origin stress perfusion scintigraphy was performed in conjunction with atrial pacing [8]. A # 7 French bipolar pacing catheter was positioned in the upper right atrium. Pacing was begun at 20 beats/min above the sinus rate and increased by 10-15 beats/min at 2 min intervals until limited by the patients' symptoms or block at the atrioventricular node. Electrocardiogram monitoring and evaluation were the same as during exercise.

Electrocardiograms were interpreted by two independent observers who had no knowledge of the patients' identity, coronary anatomy, or scintigraphic findings. There was complete agreement in 96% of the studies and minor disagreements in 4%, the latter being decided by concensus with the aid of a third observer.

Perfusion Scintigraphy
All scintigrams were performed with the patient in a fasting state. 201 Tl was administered in a dose of 1.5-2.0 mCi intravenously at peak stress and, when indicated, at rest (see below). Exercise or pacing was continued for 60 s after the administration of 201 Tl. Imaging was begun within 10 min of administration of the tracer and

was generally completed within 30 min. Scintigraphy was performed using either a portable[1] or stationary[2] 37 phototube camera equipped with a converging collimator and employing a 20% window centered at 75 KeV. Hepatic and splenic radioactivity was shielded when significant. To ensure adequate evaluation of relative myocardial radioactivity, an image was taken to 200,000 counts in the anterior projection and the time noted. This was followed by images in the 45° left anterior oblique and left lateral projections taken to equal time. Unprocessed images printed on Polaroid film were obtained for the initial 15 studies. In 12 patients studied thereafter, images were also acquired on a PDP 11/40 computer and image enhancement performed by spreading the gray scale between peak cardiac radioactivity (upper threshold) and a mean background level (lower threshold). While computer processing made defects seen in the analog images more prominent and occasionally increased the security of interpretation, all defects were identified from the analog image.

Patients with normal stress scintigrams were not restudied. Patients wit abnormal stress scintigrams were restudied at rest in all three projections using the same camera and imaging technique one week after the initial study. After initiation of this study if became apparent that a delayed rest image, obtained 4 h after the stress study, would accurately depict resting perfusion [9]. In patients currently studied at this institution the latter method is now used. Scintigraphy was performed at an average of 16.3 months (range of 2-70) after surgery. Among 25 patients who underwent postoperative coronary angiography, scintigraphy was performed within 1 month of angiography in 21 patients, and within 4 months in all patients. There was no history of an ischemic event between the two tests in any patient. The results of preoperative 201 Tl stress scintigraphy were available for comparison with postoperative studies in nine patients.

Stress scintigrams which showed new or enlargerd defects compared to the rest image indicated segments of relative hypoperfusion and were considered positive for stress induced myocardial ischemia. Scintigraphic defects at rest were interpreted as evidence of prior infarction. The findings of postoperative scintigrams were compared to those obtained preoperatively and changes in perfusion noted. Scintigrams were evaluated by two independent observers without knowledge of the patients' identity, coronary anatomy, or the results of stress testing. Observer agreement was complete in 92% of images. Minor observer disagreement concerning the location or extent of abnormalities was seen in 8% of images and was decided by concensus with the aid of a third independent observer.

Scintigraphic defects were localized to regions of coronary perfusion according to the known coronary anatomy. Each scintigraphic projection was divided into three left ventricular segments. The anterior projection was divided into anterior wall, apex, and inferior wall; the left anterior oblique projection into posterolateral wall, inferior wall, and septum; and the left lateral projection into the anterolateral or free wall, apex, and inferior wall. Hypoperfusion in the distribution of the LAD was diagnosed by scintigraphic defects involving the septum with or without the involvement of the anterolateral wall, while hypoperfusion in the distribution of the LCX was diagnosed by defects involving the posterolateral wall and hypoperfusion in the distribution of the RCA was diagnosed by defects in-

---

[1] Ohio Nuclear, Solon, Ohio

[2] Pho Gamma IV, Searle Radiographics, Inc., DesPlains, Illinois

volving the inferior wall. Since apical abnormalities could result from hypoperfusion in the distribution of any of the three vessls, localization depended on the presence of accompanying scintigraphic abnormalities.

Coronary Angiography

Selective coronary angiography with visualization of grafts and native coronary circulation was performed in multiple projections by the Judkins technique in 25 patients. If a graft could not be demonstrated by selective angiography und definite evidence of graft closure at the aortic anastomosis was not found, aortic root biplane angiography was performed in the 60° left anterior oblique and the 30° right anterior oblique projections. The degree of coronary and graft stenosis was determined by agreement of two independent observers who were unaware of the results of scintigraphy or stress testing. Narrowing of ≥75% by diameter in either a graft, the coronary artery distal to the graft, or a major coronary artery that had not been grafted was considered significant.

Results

Coronary Anatomy

Significant stenosis existed in the native vessel proximal to the site of graft insertion in all grafted vessels with a single exception so that perfusion was dependent on the integrity of the graft. Complete revascularization was thought to be present in nine patients, in whom all grafts, distal vessels, and major native ungrafted vessels were free of significant stenosis, and in a tenth patient, who had an occluded RCA graft but was without significant stenosis in the native RCA. Three patients, in whom all grafts were patent, had stenosis either distal to a patent graft or in ungrafted native vessel. Twelve patients were found to have stenosis in one or more grafts.

Chest Pain

Among those 25 patients who underwent angiography, 17 patients had chest pain. Nine of these patients had stenosis of either a graft or native vessel, while eight were considered to be completely revascularized. In none of these patients did the history, examination, or laboratory evaluation suggest postcardiotomy syndrome. Among the 11 patients with a history of typical angina, seven had stenosis in either a graft or native vessel. However, four were considered to be completely revascularized. Among eight catheterized patients without chest pain, only two were completely revascularized. Overall, chest pain was present in 9 of 15 patients with a significant postoperative coronary abnormality, a sensitivity of 60%. Chest pain was absent in only two of ten patients with angiographic evidence of complete revascularization, a specificity of only 20%.

Postoperative Stress Testing

In the group of 23 patients undergoing postoperative graded exercise testing who also had followup coronary angiograms. Six tests were inconclusive; two due to suboptimal stress, three because of baseline ST segment changes, and one because of rate related left bundle branch block. Five of these patients had significant stenosis in either a graft or a native vessel. Among the remaining 17 patients, angiographic evidence of significant narrowing in either a graft or native vessel was seen in six of the seven patients with a positive stress test, but also in four of the ten with a negative stress test. When the euqivocal tests were excluded, a positive stress electrocardiogram was present in six of ten patients with significant postoperative coronary abnormalities, a sensitivity of 60%, and a negative stress electrocardiogram was present in six of seven patients with angiographic evidence of complete revascularization, a specificity of 86%.

Patients with complete revascularization exercised for a slightly longer time, 8.2 versus 7.0 min, than did those with graft or native vessel stenosis. However, the difference was not significant and could not reliably predict the extent of revascularization in an individual patient.

Two patients with rest pain underwent atrial pacing stress. Both had negative ST responses for ischemia and both were considered to be completely revascularized on angiography.

Postoperative Stress Scintigrams

In patients undergoing postoperative coronary angiography, 201 Tl scintigraphy was performed during atrial pacing in two patients and in association with treadmill testing in 23 patients. Overall, stress scintigraphy was negative in 15 patients. In ten patients, no scintigraphic defect was seen and in five patients, the defect seen during stress was unchanged from the rest study. Two patients had suboptimal stress and both had graft stenosis on angiography. Of the patients with negative scintigrams during optimal stress testing, 10 of 13 (77%) were considered to be completely revascularized. Of the three patients with negative scintigrams and vessel stenosis, two had stenosis in the distribution of all three coronary vessels. Patient 18 also had a large defect at rest. Neither patient had well developed collaterals on angiography. The other patient with negative stress scintigraphy had a fixed defect during rest and exercise in a region supplied by an occluded graft. The distal native vessel received considerable collateral flow from an adjacent successfully grafted vessel. Of the ten patients with positive stress scintigraphy, all had significant angiographic lesions in vessels perfusing the region of scintigraphic abnormality. Eight patients had stenosis of one or more grafts. Two patients with positive scintigrams had fully patent grafts, however, stenosis in ungrafted native vessel and/or stenosis distal to graft insertion was noted on angiography. A positive scintigram was present in 10 fo 13 optimally stressed patients with significant postoperative coronary abnormalities, a sensitivity of 77% and a negative scintigram was present in each of ten patients with angiographic evidence of complete revascularization, a specificity of 100%.

Positive stress scintigraphy in the vascular distribution of the LAD was seen in 6 of the 25 patients. All had significant narrowing of the graft or of the distal native vessel.

Positive stress scintigraphy with defects in the distribution of the LCX was seen in five patients. Three of these patients had significant graft stenoses and two others had patent grafts but significant stenosis in a major ungrafted branch of the circumflex system.

Three patients had positive stress scintigraphy in the distribution of the RCA. Each of these had RCA graft stenosis.

Overall, the perfusion pattern involving the distribution of 75 vessels in 25 patients was assessed. In all cases, a positive scintigram correctly localized stenosis to the distribution of the appropriate vessel. When all vessels with stenosis were considered, 14 of 28, or 50%, were identified by stress scintigraphy. Of the 14 stenotic vessels not identified by stress scintigraphy, 5 were distributed to segments with rest defects which did not change during exercise. 201 Tl imaging thus localized 19 of 28 vessels, or 68% of those with significant stenoses. Stress scintigraphy was totally specific and in no instance did stress scintigraphy demonstrate hypoperfusion of the segment without a corresponding stenosis in the vascular supply.

Comparison of Pre- and Postoperative Scintigrams
Nine patients were evaluated with stress scintigraphy both pre- and postoperatively. In six patients who exercised postoperatively to the same or greater levels than they had exercised preoperatively, there was scintigraphic evidence of improved perfusion. Four of these patients, three with persistent pain, were shown to be completely revascularized. The other two did not have a postoperative angiogram. In three patients, all of whom were free of chest pain, postoperative stress scintigraphy was unchanged from the preoperative study. In all three patients, significant stenosis was seen on angiography. Since the postoperative scintigram successfully predicted revascularization in the seven patients who underwent repeated angiography, preoperative scintigraphy did not contribute to the predictive accuracy of the method.

Stress Scintigraphy Compared to Chest Pain and Stress Electrocardiography
The sensitivity of postoperative chest pain (60%), stress electrocardiographic (60%), or scintigraphic abnormalities (77%) for the presence of postoperative coronary abnormalities showed no significant difference and were each moderately successful in identifying patients with incomplete revascularization. However, the scintigram was 100% specific for postoperative coronary abnormalities, and was signficantly better than chest pain ($P < 0.01$) for the identification of such abnormalities. Although the specificity of the stress electrocardiogram was not significantly different from that of scintigraphy, the latter study did occasionally identify patients with false positive as well as false negative stress tests.

Exercise testing was inconclusive in six patients. Scintigraphy was positive in three of these patients, all of whom had significant stenosis on angiography. Scintigraphy was negative in three patients, one of whom was completely revascularized. The two patients with negative scintigrams and stenosis on angiography had suboptimal stress tests.

Prior Infarction
Among the 27 patients included in the study, nine had abnormal rest scintigrams. Seven of these subjects had Q waves on the electrocardiogram in the distribution corresponding to the perfusion defect. An additional defect was seen on stress scintigraphy in three of these patients, all with a related graft or native vessel stenosis. Of the six patients who had negative stress scintigrams with a fixed defect, three had stenosis of a vessel in addition to that which supplied the segment of myocardium in which the rest defect was found.

Discussion

Thallium-201 is a monovalent cation, the myocardial uptake of which in viable tissue is proportional to regional coronary blood flow. Of the radionuclides currently available to noninvasively evaluate myocardial perfusion, 201 Tl appears to have the best physical properties in order to obtain high resolution perfusion images [10]. Perfusion defects during 201 Tl imaging appear to correlate well with coronary stenosis [4-6]. This study was designed to assess the use of 201 Tl stress scintigraphy in the follow-up evaluation of coronary bypass patients and to correlate the scintigraphic findings with coronary anatomy.

201 Tl stress scintigraphy was positive in 10 of 25 patients who underwent repeated angiography. All ten had ≥75% narrowing of at least one vessel. Stenosis was found in the grafts of eight of these patients and in a site distal to the graft insertion or in an ungrafted vessel in the other two patients. Had angiographic evaluation been confined to examination of the grafts, these latter two patients might have been considered examples of a false positive scintigram. Their presence in this series helps underscore the complexity of the vascular supply in the post-bypass patient, and to point out conditions, other than graft stenosis, that could lead to hypoperfusion and result in poor postoperative results.

201 Tl stress scintigraphy was negative in 15 patients who underwent repeated angiography. Ten of these patients were considered to be completely revascularized. Two patients with graft stenosis had negative 201 Tl scintigraphy during suboptimal stress testing. McLaughlin and coworkers have shown that the ability of stress scintigraphy to identify critical stenosis increases with the level of exercise [11], and it is possible that these patients did not develop perfusion defects due to insufficient stress. In patients with optimal stress, 10 of 13 (77%) who had negative scintigrams were considered to be fully revascularized. Combined sensitivity and specificity, overall scintigraphic accuracy was 85%, a level similar to that achieved in patients with coronary artery disease who had not undergone bypass surgery [4-6]. Since the accuracy of scintigraphy was assessed by comparing it to angiography, three patients appeared to have false negative scintigrams. An alternative possibility in these patients is that despite the presence of what was felt to be significant stenosis, hypoperfusion did not develop. Flow to a segment of myocardium which is apparently perfused by a stenotic graft or native vessel may not depend exclusively on this single coronary vessel. Collateral flow, possibly originating from a successfully grafted adjacent vessel, may be of sufficient magnitude to protect against stress induced hypoperfusion. Significant collateral flow to a region served by a stenotic graft was noted in one of our patients.

Other possible reasons for negative scintigraphy with coronary stenosis were sought. In two patients, a large rest defect representing prior infarction likely served to decrease our ability to recognize stress induced hypoperfusion. Since scintigraphic defects depend on relative hypoperfusion of a segment of myocardium, a region may be hypoperfused during stress, but still have greater perfusion than an infarcted region, and thus not be recognized. In two patients with triple vessel disease it is possible that stress induced hypoperfusion developed in a homogeneous pattern so that localized relative perfusion defects were not seen [12].

Although many of our patients were receiving inderal and/or digoxin, drugs which could affect the distribution of 201 Tl, the good results noted in this study, as well as those reported previously in patients evaluated for the presence of coronary disease [6], suggest that these drugs have a minimal effect on the scintigram.

While positive 201 Tl stress scintigraphy accurately localized the presence of a stenotic vessel in each case, the test did not identify all stenotic vessels. In this series, 50% of all stenotic grafts and/or native vessels were identified by stress scintigraphy. When defects seen in the rest study were combined with those brought out by stress, 69% of stenotic vessels were identified. This lack of overall sensitivity in relating stenosis to perfusion may again in part be due to the possible role of collateral vessels. In addition, several of the patients had multivessel disease and positive scintigraphy successfully localized perfusion defects to some but not all of the involved vessels. Since the test detects relative perfusion it is probable that patients with multiple areas of hypoperfusion develop defects only in the most severely affected regions.

It should be noted that perfusion defects often were subtle and considerable experience is necessary to accurately identify such abnormalities. In this study all scintigraphic defects were identified from the analog images by blinded observers. As suggested by Berger and co-workers computer enhancement of images may facilitate interpretation and further increase the diagnostic yield of the procedure [13].

Zaret and co-workers [14] compared pre- and post-bypass K-43 scintigrams to evaluate graft patency and found the method specific, but far less sensitive than seen here. They showed that patients with normal or improved scintigraphy had at least one patent graft, while those whose scintigrams were worse or unchanged following surgery had all grafts occluded. Lurie and co-workers [15] showed an improvement in the perfusion pattern of 15 patients studied pre- and post-bypass with Rubidium 81 stress scintigraphy. However, angiographic confirmation of surgical results was not obtained.

Recent reports have suggested that comparison of pre- and postoperative 201 Tl stress scintigraphy can be used as a reliable predictor of graft patency [16-18], and Ritchie and co-workers concluded that the presence of an exercise defect in the postoperative study was associated with lowered graft patency rates [18]. Our results confirm that postoperative imaging alone can be used to predict the extent of revascularization and graft patency and that accurate postoperative evaluation is possible in bypass patients who had not been evaluated preoperatively.

In cases where scintigraphy was performed both pre- and postoperatively, evidence of improved perfusion was seen in patients with successful revascularization. These results are consistent with previous reports which showed that scintigraphic improvement was associated with graft patency while scintigraphic deterioration or lack of scintigraphic change was consistent with graft closure or incomplete revascularization [14-18].

Although patient history, exercise capacity, and electrocardiographic response to exercise are helpful in the evaluation and management of post-bypass patients, they are relatively poor indicators of revascularization and graft patency. In the patients included in this report, chest pain was a particularly unreliable parameter by which to assess the results of surgery and could not discriminate patients with recurrent vascular stenosis from those who were completely revascularized. Although the relief of chest pain has been shown to correlate with graft patency [19,21] additional factors, including the placebo effect of surgery, perioperative infarction, and possibly surgical denervation, complicate the interpretation of symptom relief [22-24]. In the reports of both Sheldon [20] and Kouchoukos [21], a significant number of patients with graft closure experienced relief of chest pain. The poor discriminating quality of chest pain, even when described as typical angina, in this group of patients differs considerably from the experience in unoperated patients where angina is reliably correlated with coronary disease [25].

Although improved exercise tolerance has been associated with revascularization [26-27], individual variation is great and prediction of graft patency is hazardous, particularly when a preoperative test is not available for comparison [28]. In our patients the slight trend toward greater exercise tolerance in completely revascularized patients was a poor indicator of the status of coronary anatomy in an individual patient.

When 201 Tl stress scintigraphy was compared to stress electrocardiography, scintigraphy appeared to be of greatest value in patients whose electrocardiograms were inconclusive. Scintigraphy also added to the diagnostic accuracy of stress testing by identifying occasional patients with false positive and false negative electrocardiograms. Similar results using stress scintigraphy have been reported in the evaluation of ungrafted patients [4-6,12]. Additionally, the scintigram offered localizing information which could be quite useful in the evaluation of coronary stenosis following bypass graft surgery.

We monitored only a single CM5 electrocardiographic lead. The use of multiple leads during stress testing would likely result in increased sensitivity of the stress test to ischemic changes, however it is probable that the number of false positives would also increase leading to a fall in specificity. Multiple leads would probably not resolve the equivocal tests.

The patients in this study constitute a selective group and do not represent the coronary bypass population as a whole. Close to two-thirds of these patients were studied because of recurrent chest pain. A less selective study population would likely result in a lower incidence of graft occlusion and a somewhat different scintigraphic accuracy. This population, however, does appear to be representative of patients who require followup evaluation postoperatively for clinical indications.

In summary, the effectiveness of 201 Tl myocardial perfusion scintigraphy in post-bypass patients appears similar to that in ungrafted patients. Factors influencing image sensitivity and specificity also appear similar in the two groups. 201 Tl scintigraphy appears to be an important noninvasive method by which myocardial perfusion can be assessed in the post-bypass patient. Although comparison of pre- and postoperative studies can be used to document the effects of surgery, postoperative scintigraphy alone can sensitively and specifically detect and localize significant stenosis in grafts or native vessels. This method should serve as a useful noninvasive technique for the future evaluation of the postcoronary bypass patient.

References

1. Mundth, E.D., Austen, W.G.: Surgical measures for coronary heart disease. N. Engl. J. Med. *293*, 13-19, 75-80, 124-130 (1975)
2. Bourassa, M.G., Noble, J.: Complication rate of coronary arteriography. Circulation *53*, 106-114 (1976)
3. Shah, A., Gnoj, J., Fisher, V.J.: Complications of selective coronary ateriography by the Judkins technique and their prevention. Am. Heart. J. *90*, 353-359 (1975)

4. Bailey, I.K., Griffith, L.S.C., Roulau, G., Strauss, H.W., Pitt, B.: Thallium 201 myocardial perfusion imaging at rest and during exercise. Circulation *55*, 79-87 (1977)
5. Ritchie, J.L., Zaret, B.L., Strauss, H.W., Pitt, B., Berman, D.S., Schelbert, H.R., Ashburn, W.L., Hamilton, G.W.: Myocardial imaging with thallium 201 at rest and exercise. A multicenter study: Coronary angographic and electrocardiographic correlation. Am. J. Cardiol. *39*, 321, (1977) (Abs)
6. Botvinick, E.H., Taradash, M.R., Shames, D.M., Parmley, W.W.: Thallium 201 myocardial perfusion scintigraphy for the clinical clarification of normal, abnormal and equivocal electrocardiographic stress tests. Am. J. Cardiol. *41*, 43-51 (1978)
7. Bruce, R.A.: Exercise testing of patients with coronary heart disease: Principles and normal standards for evaluation. Ann. Clin. Res. *3*, 323-332 (1971)
8. Botvinick, E.H., Shames, D.A., Ratshin, R.A., Chatterjee, K., Parmley, W.W.: The physiologic assessment of critical coronary stenosis by relative myocardial perfusion imaging with atrial pacing. Am. J. Cardiol. *37*, 122 (1976) (Abs.)
9. Pohost, G.M., Zir, L.M., Moore, R.H., McKusick, K.A., Guiney, T.E., Beller, G.A.: Differentiation of transiently ischemic from infarcted myocardium by serial imaging after a single dose of thallium 201. Circulation *55*, 294-302 (1977)
10. Strauss, H.W., Harrison, K., Langan, J.K., Lebowits, E., Pitt, B.: Thallium 201 for myocardial imaging. Relation of thallium 201 to regional myocardial perfusion. Circulation *51*, 641-645 (1975)
11. McLaughlin, P.R., Martin, R.P., Dohergy, P., Daspit, S., Goric, M., Haskell, W., Lewis, S., Icriss, J.P., Harrison, D.C.: Reproducibility of thallium 201 myocardial imaging. Circulation *55*, 497-503 (1977)
12. Botvinick, E.H., Shames, D.H., Gershengorn, K.M., Carlsson, E., Ratshin, R.A., Parmley, W.W.: Myocardial stress perfusion scintigraphy with rubidium-81 versus stress electrocardiography. Am. J. Cardiol. *39*, 364-371 (1977)
13. Berger, H.J., Gottschalk, A., Zaret, B.L.: Dual radionuclide study of acute myocardial infarction. Ann. Int. Med. *88*, 145-154 (1978)
14. Zaret, B.L., Martin, N.D., McGowan, R.L., Strauss, H.W., Wells, N.P. (Jr), Flamm, M.D.: Rest and exercise potassium-43 myocardial perfusion imaging for the noninvasive evaluation of aortocoronary bypass surgery. Circulation *49*, 688-695 (1974)
15. Lurie, A.J., Salel, A.F., Berman, D.S., DeNardo, G.L., Hurley, E.J., Mason, D.T.: Determination of improved myocardial perfusion after aortocoronary bypass surgery by exercise rubidium-81 scintigraphy. Circulation *52* [Suppl. 2], 141 (1975)
16. Ormond, J., Platt, M., Mills, L., Shapiro, W., Pugh, B., Blomquist, C.G., Parkey, R.W., Willerson, J.T.: Thallium-201 scintigraphy and exercise testing in evaluating patients prior to and after coronary bypass surgery. Circulation *55/56* [Suppl. 3], 131 (1977) (Abs.)
17. Sbarbaro, J.A., Harischandra, K., Cantez, S., Harper, P., Resnekov, L.: Tl-201 imaging in the assessment of coronary artery bypass graft (CABG) patency. Circulation *55/56* [Suppl. 3], 231 (1977) (Abs.)
18. Ritchie, J.L., Narahara, K.A., Trobaugh, G.B., Williams, D.L., Hamilton, G.A.: Thallium-201 myocardial imaging before and after coronary revascularization: assessment of regional myocardial blood flow and graft patency. Circulation *56*, 830-836 (1977)
19. Alderman, E.L., Matloff, H.J., Wexler, L., Shumway, N.E., Harrison, D.C.: Results of direct coronary artery surgery for the treatment of angina pectoris. N. Engl. J. Med. *288*, 535-539 (1973)
20. Sheldon, W.C., Rincon, G., Effler, D.B., Proudfit, W.L., Sones, S.M. (Jr): Vein graft surgery for coronary artery disease: Survival and angiographic results in 1,000 patients. Circulation *48* [Suppl. 3], 184-189 (1973)
21. Kouchoukos, N.T., Kirklin, J.W., Oberman, A.: An appraisal of coronary bypass grafting. Circulation *50*, 11-16 (1974)
22. Cobb, L.A., Thomas, G.I., Dillard, D.H., Merendino, K.A., Bruce, R.A.: An evaluation of internal mammary ligation by a double blind technic. N. Engl. J. Med. *260*, 115-118 (1959)

23. Dimond, E.G., Kittle, C.G., Crockett, J.E.: Comparison of internal mammary artery ligation and sham operation for angina pectoris. Am. J. Cardiol. *5*, 483-486 (1960)
24. Ross, R.S.: Ischemic heart disease: An overview. Am J. Cardiol. *36*, 496-505 (1975)
25. Humphries, J.O., Kuller, L., Ross, R.S., Freisinger, G.C., Page, E.E.: Natural history of ischemic heart disease in relation to arteriographic findings. Circulation *49*, 489-497 (1974)

Regional Ventricular Function at Rest, During Leg Raising and Physical Exercise Before and After Aortocoronary Bypass Surgery

W.-D. Bussmann, V. Mayer, G. Kober, and M. Kaltenbach

Summary

In nine patients with coronary heart disease isometric contractility indices and ejection phase parameters were measured simultaneously using an angiographic catheter with a manometer at the tip (MILLAR). Regional wall motion at rest, after leg raising, and during physical exercise (bicycle ergometer) was analyzed applying the hemiaxis method. Five weeks after aortocoronary bypass surgery these examinations were repeated.

Preoperatively left ventricular enddiastolic pressure (LVEDP) increased from 21 to 37 mmHg following leg raising. The velocity of mean circumferential fiber shortening (Vcf) and of regional shortening in the anterior wall decreased significantly. All patients discontinued physical exercise due to angina pectoris. LVEDP increased from 21 to 39 mmHg. Large hypokinetic and akinetic areas developed especially in the anterior wall. Velocity of fiber shortening of the anterior wall decreased from 1.43 to 0.76/s. Enddiastolic volume remained unchanged while endsystolic volume increased significantly.

In six patients with patent grafts surgery had a beneficial effect. Comparing angiograms at rest no significant changes were found. After leg raising and physical exercise, however, marked improvement in ventricular function occurred compared to the preoperative performance. All six patients were exercised without having complaints at a load of 100 W for 8 min. Velocity of fiber shortening in the anterior wall increased significantly from 0.76 to 2.56/s, mean Vcf from 1.11 to 2.12 circ/s, max dP/dt from 2302 to 4280 mmHg/s and Vpm from 27.8 to 55.7/s.

Functional improvement in individual wall segments amounted to 500% in the mean. Ejection fraction increased from 54% to 76%. Enddiastolic volume remained unchanged while endsystolic volume decreased from 67 to 33 ml/1.73 m^2 ($P < 0.002$).

In three patients the bypass occluded or myocardial infarction occurred intraoperatively. Postoperative findings at rest and during exercise were unchanged as compared to preoperative values.

Following successful bypass surgery ventricular function at rest did not change. During exercise, however, a marked improvement in overall and in regional ventricular function was found.

Introduction

In patients with coronary heart disease left ventricular wall motion disturbances should be normalized following revascularization of ischemic areas after aortocoronary bypass surgery. Recent studies, however, do not report an improvement of ejection fraction following bypass surgery [1-3]. In these investigations only ventriculograms at rest were compared in the evaluation of pre- and postoperative function.

The beneficial effect of surgery can only be assessed in ventriculograms during exercise. As there have been no such reports in the literature, pre- and postoperative angiograms were done in nine patients. Stress consisted of leg raising and physical work on a bicycle ergometer. The extent of regional wall motion disturbance was assessed quantitatively and pre- and postoperative findings were compared [4-8].

Patients and Methods

Nine patients with angina pectoris were studied pre- and postoperatively at rest, after leg raising, and physical exercise. All patients had severe stenosis in the left anterior descending branch (LAD more than 80%). Two patients had an occlusion and three patients a severe stenosis of the right coronary artery. In two patients the circumflex branch was markedly narrowed (more than 90%), in seven patients it was diffusely stenosed. Three patients had a minor infarction in the inferior wall, two had a small nontransmural infarction of the anterior wall.

In nine patients an aortocoronary bypass was implanted to the LAD. Four patients received an additional bypass to one of the diagonal branches and one patient to the right coronary artery. Postoperative examinations were done 4-8 weeks, with a mean of 5 weeks, following surgery. Patients were divided into two groups according to postoperative findings:

Group I: Six patients with well functioning, open bypasses without intraoperative myocardial infarction.
Group II: Three patients with occluded bypasses and intraoperative myocardial infarction, respectively.

Protocol

Following diagnostic coronary arteriography, an angiographic catheter with a manometer at the tip and four side openings for injection of contrast medium was used (Millar-Instruments Inc., 8 F, type PC 481). Measuring hemodynamic parameters at rest, a ventriculogram in right anterior oblique position (RAO 40°) was performed. Then,

1) Volume load was induced by raising the patients legs to about 45 cm, i.e., patients feet were connected to the peddles of the ergometer. Three minutes following leg raising contrast medium was injected again into the left ventricle (RAO 40°). Hemodynamic parameters were measured simultaneously.
2) Patients were exercised in supine position on the bicycle ergometer at a load of 50-100 W for 3-8 min. Exercise was discontinued

when angina pectoris occurred. Within 20-30 sec following physical exercise ventriculography was done in RAO 40° position.

In all cases the following time schedule was strictly adhered to: Ventriculogram at rest 15 min following coronary angiography, 10-15 min later ventriculogram during leg raising, and again 10-15 min later ventriculogram during exercise. For each ventriculogram 25-35 ml of renographin 76% were injected at 20 atm via the Cordis pump. The film had 50 frames/s.

Parameters

Only ventriculograms of good quality were evaluated. Using the 8 F Millar catheter, premature ventricular beats occurred rarely. In cases where extrasystolic beats did occur the following second or third normal beat was evaluated.

After each angiogram the magnification factor was assessed with the displacement method [9]. Enddiastolic (EDV) and endsystolic (ESV) volumes were computed from one plane RAO ventriculograms with the area-length method using a semi-automatic device (Volumat, Siemens, Erlangen). An overestimation up to 25% of EDV and of stroke volume in monoplane as compared to biplane technique had to be considered [10]. A correction factor was not used since only monoplane angiograms were compared.

Velocity of mean circumferential fiber shortening and hemiaxis velocity of contractile elements (dP/dt/P = Vpm) were determined by the tip-manometer [11-14]. Statistical analysis was done using Student's t-test for paired comparison.

Results

Group I

Preoperatively all patients developed mild to severe angina pectoris, some with dyspnea. Physical exercise, therefore, had to be discontinued by all patients except one. Two patients developed mild angina upon leg raising, as documented by ST-segment depression in the ECG. Patient N.G. had severe angina upon raising his legs and was not exercised.

Postoperatively patients had no complaints after leg raising or physical exercise. The preoperative work load was well tolerated in all cases. Moreover, the work load was increased to 100 W with a duration up to 8 min (Table 1).
The velocity of mean circumferential fiber shortening markedly decreased slightly during physical exercise. Postoperatively mean Vcf at rest was slightly higher as compared to the preoperative value. After leg raising, however, mean Vcf increased markedly as compared to the preoperative value. The increase in mean Vcf during physical exercise was even more pronounced (Fig. 1, Table 1).

Control patients had no or only mild coronary artery disease and normal ventricular function. There was no significant difference in overall left ventricular function between postoperative findings and performance of the control group (Fig. 1).

Table 1. Pre- and postoperative parameters at rest, after leg raising, and during physical exercise (group 1)

At rest preop.	HR /min	LVP mmHg	LVEDP mmHg	Vpm /s	max dP/dt mmHg/s	$\overline{Vcf}$ circ/s	EDV $ml/1.73m^2$	ESV $ml/1.73m^2$	EF %
N.G.	83	182	37.0	19.0	1960	0.80	220	91	59
S.O.	89	137	10.5	51.2	2180	2.27	127	10	92
B.E.	56	127	30.2	24.5	1590	1.32	141	40	71
N.J.	81	189	31.0	28.0	1910	1.00	108	45	58
L.W.	78	193	12.3	43.3	2190	0.93	141	60	57
H.W.	78	143	16.8	33.3	1830	1.31	119	37	69
$\bar{X} \pm 1$ SD	77.5±11	162±29	21.3±11	33.2±12	1943±226	1.27±0.5	143±40	47±27	68±23
n	6	6	6	6	6	6	6	6	6
At rest postop.									
N.G.	81	139	6.5	62.1	1880	0.89	176	81	53
S.O.	96	122	18.2	33.8	2000	1.90	128	25	80
B.E.	83	141	21.9	31.5	3510	1.62	177	46	74
N.J.	96	123	7.2	78.6	2000	0.95	111	57	49
L.W.	105	126	22.1	33.7	2060	1.61	150	35	76
H.W.	103	146	15.7	44.7	2540	1.37	121	36	70
$\bar{X} \pm 1$ SD	94±10	133±11	15.2±7	45.7±18	2331±621	1.39±0.4	143±28	47±20	68±13
n	6	6	6	6	6	6	6	6	6
P preop. vs. postop.	<0.0125	<0.05	ns	ns	ns	ns	ns	ns	ns

Table 1. Continued

Preop. after leg raising	HR /min	LVP mmHg	LVEDP mmHg	Vpm /s	max dP/dt mmHg/s	$\overline{Vcf}$ circ/s	EDV ml/1.73m²	ESV ml/1.73m²	EF %
N.G.	99	207	57.0	18.3	2460	0.19	192	155	19
S.O.	91	122	24.9	29.3	1940	1.49	126	25	80
B.E.	76	145	37.1	24.8	1940	1.03	150	39	74
N.J.	77	199	30.2	31.0	2020	1.03	143	50	65
L.W.	82	220	50.8	23.8	2430	0.76	149	71	53
H.W.	74	134	22.6	30.0	1820	1.48	177	51	71
n	6	6	6	6	6	6	6	6	6
$\bar{X} \pm 1$ SD	83±10	171±43	37.1±14	26.2±4.8	2101±273	0.99±0.5	156±24	65±46	60±10
Postop. after leg raising									
N.G.	84	154	15.6	38.6	2500	0.96	190	94	50
S.O.	103	122	22.4	30.2	2100	1.99	121	21	82
B.E.	86	132	33.9	25.6	3540	1.67	146	35	75
N.J.	99	147	18.9	39.0	2160	1.60	142	30	78
L.W.	105	130	25.6	27.1	2440	1.57	183	45	75
H.W.	99	134	18.7	34.6	2350	1.43	120	31	74
n	6	6	6	6	6	6	6	6	6
$\bar{X} \pm 1$ SD	96.9±9	137±12	22.5±7	32.5±6	2515±525	1.53±0.3	150±30	43±26	72±11
P preop. vs postop.	<0.05	<0.05	<0.05	<0.05	<0.10	<0.005	ns	<0.025	<0.05

Table 1. Continued

Preop. after physical exercise	HR /min	LVP mmHg	LVEDP mmHg	Vpm /s	max dP/dt mmHg/s	$\overline{Vcf}$ circ/s	EDV ml/1.73m^2	ESV ml/1.73m^2	EF %	load watts	D s
S.O.	98	130	33.2	28.3	1850	1.50	148	49	67	50	300
B.E.	81	137	44.8	20.0	1710	1.10	170	59	65	30	40
N.J.	163	169	26.1	37.3	3070	1.05	123	75	39	100	420
L.W.	93	248	65.6	23.0	2880	0.74	144	82	43	75	300
H.W.	101	134	28.3	30.6	2000	1.16	162	68	58	75	270
n	5	5	5	5	5	5	5	5	5	5	5
$\bar{X} \pm 1$ SD	107 32	164 49	39.6 16	27.8 7	2302 626	1.11 0.3	149 18	67 13	54 13	66 26	226 138
Postop. after physical exercise											
S.O.	115	154	27.0	42.9	3000	2.01	119	23	80	100	480
B.E.	143	144	12.1	77.1	5000	2.66	165	30	81	100	480
N.J.	139	174	20.0	74.4	5030	2.58	120	25	79	100	480
L.W.	135	183	39.6	35.7	4345	1.90	169	47	72	100	480
H.W.	129	161	20.0	48.2	4025	1.49	117	39	67	100	480
n	5	5	5	5	5	5	5	5	5	5	5
$\bar{X} \pm 1$ SD	132±11	163±15	23.7±10	55.7±19	4280±835	2.12±0.5	138±26	32.8±10	75.8±6	100±0	480±0
P preop. vs. postop.	<0.10	ns	<0.025	<0.025	<0.005	<0.01	ns	<0.0025	<0.0125	<0.025	<0.01

Abbreviations:

HR	heart rate (min^{-1})
LVEDP	left ventricular enddiastolic pressure (mmHg)
LVP	left ventricular systolic pressure (mmHg)
Vpm	peak measured velocity of contractile elements (/s)
max dP/dt	maximum rate of pressure rise (mmHg/s)
$\overline{Vcf}$	velocity of mean circumferential fiber shortening (circ/s)
EDV	enddiastolic volume (ml/1.73 m^2 body surface area)
ESV	endsystolic volume (ml/1.73 m^2 body surface area)
EF	ejection fraction (%)
load	work load (watts)
D	duration of exercise (s)
n	number of patients
$X \pm 1$ SD	mean value, standard deviation
P preop. vs postop.	significance of postoperative findings as compared to preoperative values

Table 2. Pre- and postoperative velocity of fiber shortening of hemiaxes m1 through m6 at rest, after leg raising, and during physical exercise (group I)

Preop. at rest	Vm1 /s	Vms /s	Vm3 /s	$\overline{Vma}$ /s	Vm4 /s	Vm5 /s	Vm6 /s	$\overline{Vmi}$ /s	m1 %	m2 %	m3 %	$\overline{ma}$ %	m4 %	m5 %	m6 %	$\overline{mi}$ %
N.G.	1.27	1.40	1.70	1.46	-2.80	0.00	1.10	-0.56	33	36	44	38	-73	0	29	-15
S.O.	2.44	3.13	2.70	2.80	1.96	2.00	1.38	1.78	71	91	78	82	57	58	40	52
B.E.	2.10	1.76	1.71	1.86	1.24	0.39	0.39	0.67	74	62	60	65	43	14	14	24
N.J.	0.24	0.64	1.27	0.72	1.39	1.33	1.09	1.27	8	21	42	24	46	44	36	42
L.W.	1.01	0.59	0.63	0.74	1.35	0.74	1.25	1.11	34	20	21	25	46	25	43	38
H.W.	0.95	0.71	1.39	1.02	1.75	2.10	1.20	1.67	34	26	50	37	63	75	42	60
n	6	6	6	6	6	6	6	6	6	6	6	6	6	6	6	6
$\bar{X} \pm 1$ SD	1.33 ±0.80	1.37 ±0.93	1.56 ±0.68	1.43 ±0.80	0.82 ±1.8	1.10 ±0.85	1.07 ±0.35	0.99 ±0.85	42 ±25	43 ±28	49 ±19	45 ±23	30 ±50	36 ±28	34 ±11	34 ±26
Postop. at rest																
N.G.	0.77	0.85	1.20	0.94	0.59	1.03	0.86	0.83	21	23	32	25	16	28	23	22
S.O.	2.96	3.20	2.20	2.80	1.00	1.10	0.60	0.90	83	88	61	77	28	32	18	26
B.E.	2.10	2.00	1.58	1.89	2.24	1.10	1.03	1.45	61	58	46	55	65	31	30	42
N.J.	0.65	0.76	0.90	0.77	1.37	1.20	0.93	1.16	19	22	26	22	40	34	27	34
L.W.	2.30	2.03	1.97	2.10	0.83	0.94	1.44	1.07	67	59	57	61	24	27	42	31
H.W.	1.76	1.03	0.64	1.14	2.03	1.94	1.21	1.73	58	34	21	38	67	64	40	57
n	6	6	6	6	6	6	6	6	6	6	6	6	6	6	6	6
$\bar{X} \pm 1$ SD	1.75 ±0.90	1.64 ±0.95	1.41 ±0.61	1.60 ±0.80	1.34 ±0.65	1.22 ±0.36	1.00 ±0.29	1.19 ±0.34	52 ±28	47 ±25	41 ±16	46 ±21	40 ±21	36 ±13	30 ±9	35 ±12
P preop.vs. postop.	<0.10	ns	ns	ns	ns	ns	ns	ns	ns	ns	ns	ns	ns	ns	ns	ns

Table 2. Continued

Preop. after leg raising	Vm1 /s	Vm2 /s	Vm3 /s	$\overline{Vma}$ /s	Vm4 /s	Vm5 /s	Vm6 /s	$\overline{Vmi}$ /s	m1 %	m2 %	m3 %	$\overline{ma}$ %	m4 %	m5 %	m6 %	$\overline{mi}$ %
N.G.	0.20	0.20	0.12	0.17	-1.60	0.56	1.20	0.05	5	5	3	4	-40	14	30	1.3
S.O.	2.12	1.26	1.13	1.52	1.20	1.96	1.39	1.52	66	39	35	47	37	61	43	47
B.E.	1.60	1.14	1.22	1.32	1.06	0.95	0.56	0.86	55	39	41	45	36	32	19	29
N.J.	0.76	0.82	0.91	0.82	1.33	1.30	1.03	1.22	25	27	30	27	44	43	34	40
L.W.	0.98	0.82	0.83	0.88	0.95	0.50	0.48	0.64	34	29	29	31	33	17	17	22
H.W.	1.24	0.53	1.33	1.04	1.92	2.22	1.44	1.86	45	19	48	37	69	80	52	67
n	6	6	6	6	6	6	6	6	6	6	6	6	6	6	6	6
$\bar{X} \pm 1$ SD	1.15 ±0.66	0.79 ±0.39	0.92 ±0.43	0.96 ±0.46	0.81 ±1.22	1.27 ±0.55	1.01 ±0.41	1.03 ±0.65	38 ±21	26 ±12	31 ±15	32 ±15	30 ±35	41 ±25	33 ±13	34 ±22
Postop. after leg raising																
N.G.	1.24	1.12	1.52	1.28	0.00	0.34	1.00	0.45	36	32	44	37	0	10	29	13
S.O.	2.90	2.60	2.00	2.50	1.80	1.80	0.96	1.50	81	72	57	70	50	50	27	42
B.E.	2.10	1.80	1.55	1.82	2.19	1.32	1.13	1.55	64	56	48	56	68	41	35	48
N.J.	1.77	1.48	1.74	1.66	1.52	1.55	1.71	1.58	55	46	54	52	47	48	53	49
L.W.	2.01	2.02	1.66	1.90	1.43	1.15	1.38	1.32	58	59	48	55	41	33	40	38
H.W.	2.15	1.42	0.61	1.39	2.00	1.15	1.24	1.46	71	47	20	46	66	38	41	48
n	6	6	6	6	6	6	6	6	6	6	6	6	6	6	6	6
$\bar{X} \pm 1$ SD	2.03 ±0.50	1.74 ±0.50	1.51 ±0.47	1.75 ±0.43	1.49 ±0.78	1.21 ±0.49	1.23 ±0.27	1.31 ±0.43	60 ±15	52 ±23	45 ±13	53 ±11	45 ±25	37 ±15	38 ±9	40 ±13
P preop. vs. postop.	<0.0005	<0.0125	<0.10	<0.0025	<0.025	ns	ns	<0.10	<0.0025	<0.005	<0.10	<0.0025	<0.05	ns	ns	ns

Table 2. Continued

Preop. during physical exercise	Vm1 /s	Vm2 /s	Vm3 /s	$\overline{Vma}$ /s	Vm4 /s	Vm5 /s	Vm6 /s	$\overline{Vmi}$ /s	m1 %	m2 %	m3 %	$\overline{ma}$ %	m4 %	m5 %	m6 %	$\overline{mi}$ %
S.O.	1.40	0.70	0.60	0.90	1.70	2.20	1.70	1.90	39	20	17	25	48	61	47	52
B.E.	1.56	0.64	1.25	1.15	1.50	1.04	0.72	1.09	50	21	40	37	48	33	23	35
N.J.	0.80	0.00	0.00	0.25	1.10	1.80	2.80	1.94	13	0	0	4	18	29	45	31
L.W.	0.93	0.65	0.67	0.75	0.54	0.76	0.95	0.75	31	21	22	25	18	25	31	25
H.W.	1.00	0.71	0.61	0.77	1.29	2.16	1.42	1.62	31	22	19	24	40	67	44	50
n	5	5	5	5	5	5	5	5	5	5	5	5	5	5	5	5
$\bar{X} \pm 1$ SD	1.13 ±0.33	0.54 ±0.30	0.64 ±0.44	0.76 ±0.35	1.22 ±0.44	1.59 ±0.65	1.52 ±0.81	1.25 ±0.69	33 ±13	17 ±9	20 ±14	23 ±11	34 ±15	43 ±19	38 ±10	39 ±11
Postop. during physical exercise																
S.O.	3.50	3.10	2.70	3.10	1.90	1.00	0.30	1.10	91	81	70	81	50	26	7	28
B.E.	3.66	3.70	2.90	3.40	2.14	1.62	1.57	1.77	77	78	61	72	45	34	33	37
N.J.	2.95	1.95	1.50	2.15	3.50	3.30	2.47	3.11	56	37	29	41	67	63	47	59
L.W.	2.84	3.37	3.11	3.11	0.31	0.85	1.38	0.85	65	77	71	71	7	19	32	19
H.W.	1.88	1.12	0.12	1.04	3.40	1.88	1.44	2.24	47	28	3	26	89	47	36	56
n	5	5	5	5	5	5	5	5	5	5	5	5	5	5	5	5
$\bar{X} \pm 1$ SD	2.96 0.70	2.64 1.1	2.06 1.25	2.56 0.97	2.25 1.30	1.73 0.98	1.43 0.77	1.81 0.90	67 17	60 25	47 30	58 23	51 29	38 17	31 14	40 17
P preop. vs. postop.	<0.0025	<0.01	<0.025	<0.005	<0.005	ns	ns	ns	<0.005	<0.01	<0.05	<0.01	ns	ns	ns	ns

Abbreviations:

Vml - Vm6	velocity of fiber shortening of hemiaxes ml to m6 (/s)
vma	mean velocity of fiber shortening in the anterior wall (/s)
Vmi	mean velocity of fiber shortening in the inferior wall (/s)
ml - m6	percentual fiber shortening in hemiaxes ml - m6 (%)
ma	mean percentual fiber shortening in the anterior wall (%)
mi	mean percentual fiber shortening in the inferior wall (%)
n	number of patients
X ± 1 SD	mean value, standard deviation
P preop. vs postop.	significance of postoperative findings compared to preoperative values

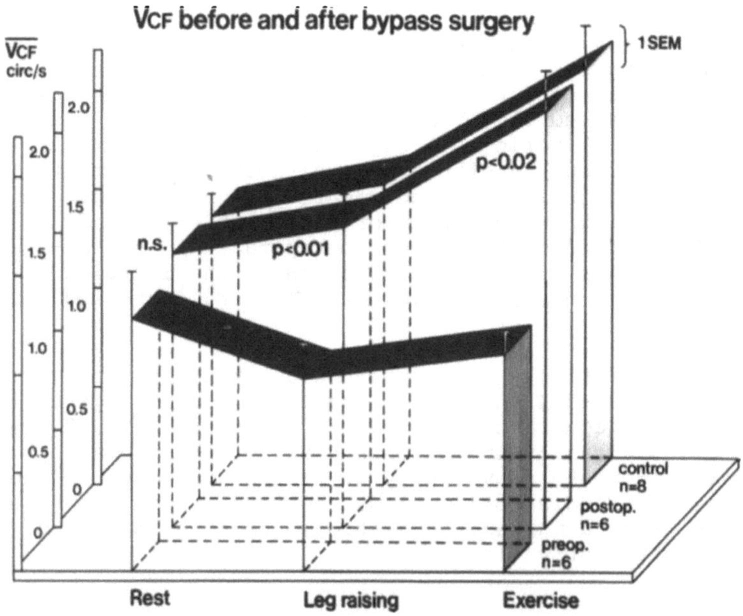

Fig. 1. Velocity of mean circumferential fiber shortening ($\overline{Vcf}$) at rest, after leg raising, and during physical exercise before and after bypass surgery as compared to a control group. Preoperative: decrease of mean Vcf after leg raising, insufficient increase during physical exercise. Postoperative: significant increase of mean Vcf after leg raising and during physical exercise as compared to preoperative values; performance almost as in control group

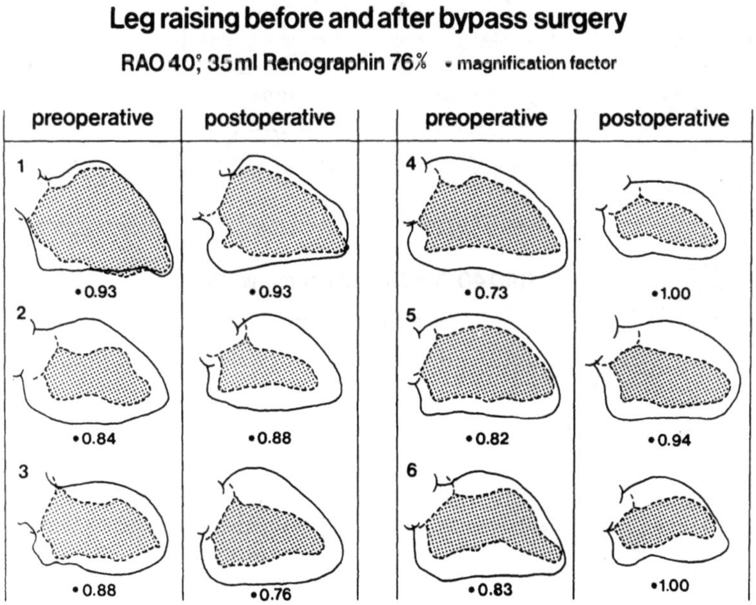

Fig. 2. Pre- and postoperative ventriculograms after leg raising. The magnification factor is indicated below each ventriculogram. Preoperatively all patients developed hypokinesis or akinesis, especially in the anterior wall and in the apex, as well as in the apical area of the inferior wall. Postoperatively left ventricular function improved markedly in all patients. Previous hypokinetic and akinetic areas contract normally in some patients

Regional Function

Leg Raising. Preoperatively all patients developed regional hypokinesis or akinesis during leg raising, especially in the anterior wall and in the apex as well as in apical areas of the inferior wall. Postoperatively ventricular function improved significantly in all patients. Hypokinetic and akinetic wall segments contracted almost normally in some patients, and in others a significant improvement was noted (Fig. 2). These findings are documented in the increase in velocity of fiber shortening in the anterior wall (Table 2). Enddiastolic pressure was significantly lower postoperatively as compared to preoperative values (37 mmHg vs 22.5 mmHg). Enddiastolic volume remained unchanged, endsystolic volume, however, decreased significantly (Table 1).

Physical Exercise. Preoperatively new hypokinetic, akinetic, or dyskinetic areas (case 1, 3, and 4 in Fig. 3) developed during angina pectoris. Postoperatively contraction normalized in patients 1, 2, and 3 and improved significantly in patients 4 and 5. These findings are documented in the increase of velocity in fiber shortening in the anterior wall (Table 2). Enddiastolic volume remained unchanged while endsystolic volume decreased markedly. Ejection, fraction, max dP/dt and Vpm increased significantly (Table 1).

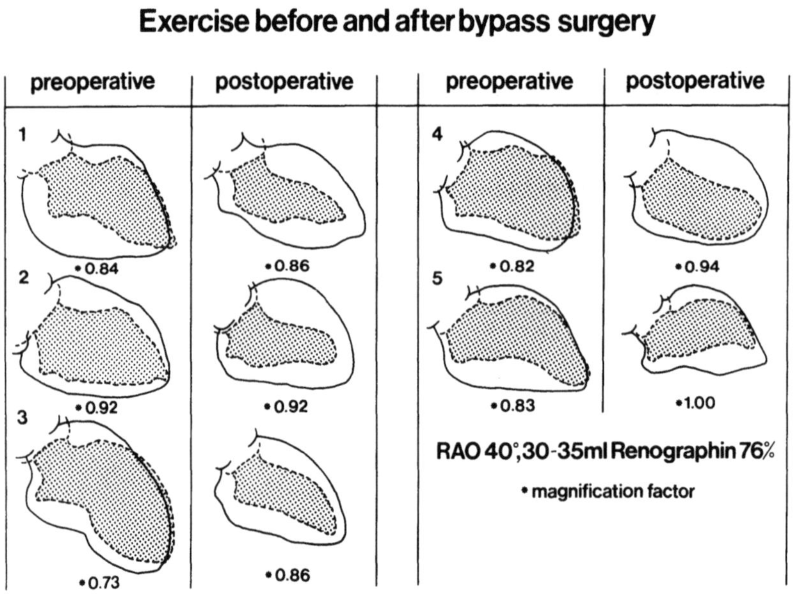

Fig. 3. Pre- and postoperative ventriculograms during physical exercise. The magnification factor is indicated below each ventriculogram. Preoperatively hypokinetic and sometimes akinetic (example 1, 3, and 4) areas were present. Postoperatively regional wall motion normalized in patients 1 through 3, and was markedly improved in patients 4 and 5

Anterior Wall - Inferior Wall
Preoperatively the velocity of fiber shortening in the anterior wall decreased after leg raising and physical exercise. Fiber shortening in the inferior wall remained unchanged after leg raising as opposed to values at rest, but increased during physical exercise. Hence, the impaired contraction in the anterior wall was partially compensated by the inferior wall. Postoperatively the velocity of fiber shortening in the anterior wall increased after leg raising and physical exercise. Fiber shortening of the inferior wall was relatively less pronounced as compared to the preoperative findings (Table 2).

Middle Hemiaxis in the Anterior Wall (Vm2)
The velocity of fiber shortening in the middle anterior hemiaxis (Vm2) preoperatively decreased more than half after leg raising and physical exercise (Fig. 4, Table 2). Postoperatively velocity of fiber shortening increased by 200% after leg raising and by 500% during physical exercise. Comparison with a control group of 4 patients [6] revealed a postoperative performance in Vm2 comparable to that in patients with normal coronary angiograms (Fig. 4).

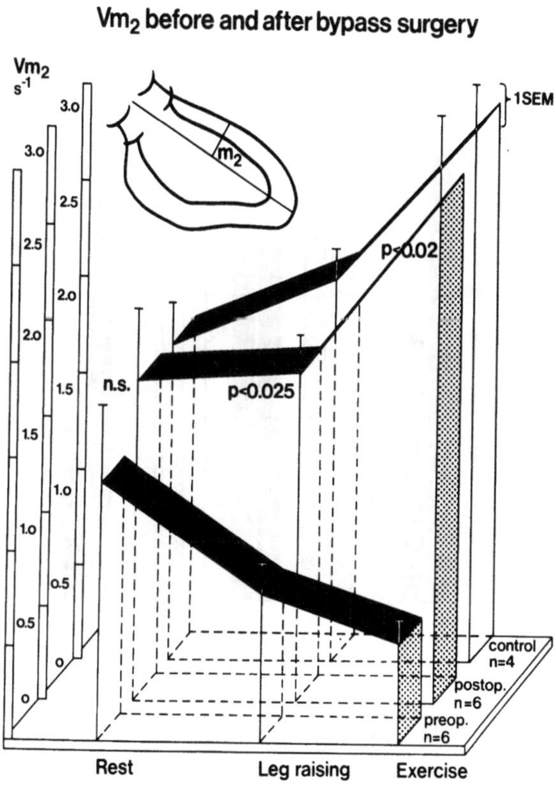

Fig. 4. Velocity of fiber shortening in the middle anterior hemiaxis (Vm2) before and after bypass surgery as compared to control group. Preoperatively Vm2 significantly decreases after leg raising and physical exercise. Postoperatively the increase in Vm2 was highly significant. Postoperative Vm2 values are comparable to those in control group with normal left ventricles

Additional Parameters

Isometric parameters (max dP/dt, Vpm) changed similarly as mean Vcf. LVEDP decreased significantly postoperatively. Enddiastolic volume did not change markedly. Endsystolic volume, however, decreased significantly (Fig. 5, Table 1).

The heart rate at rest increased postoperatively as compared to preoperatively as compared to preoperative values (94/min versus 77.5/min). Heart rate was also markedly increased after leg raising and physical exercise. Correspondingly ejection time was shorter. By a shorter ejection time, velocity parameters (mean Vcf, Vm1 - Vm6) increased. Ejection fraction (EF) and percent shortening in the hemiaxis (m1 - m6), parameters independent of ejection time, however, increased significantly during leg raising and exercise as compared to preoperative values (Tables 1 and 2).

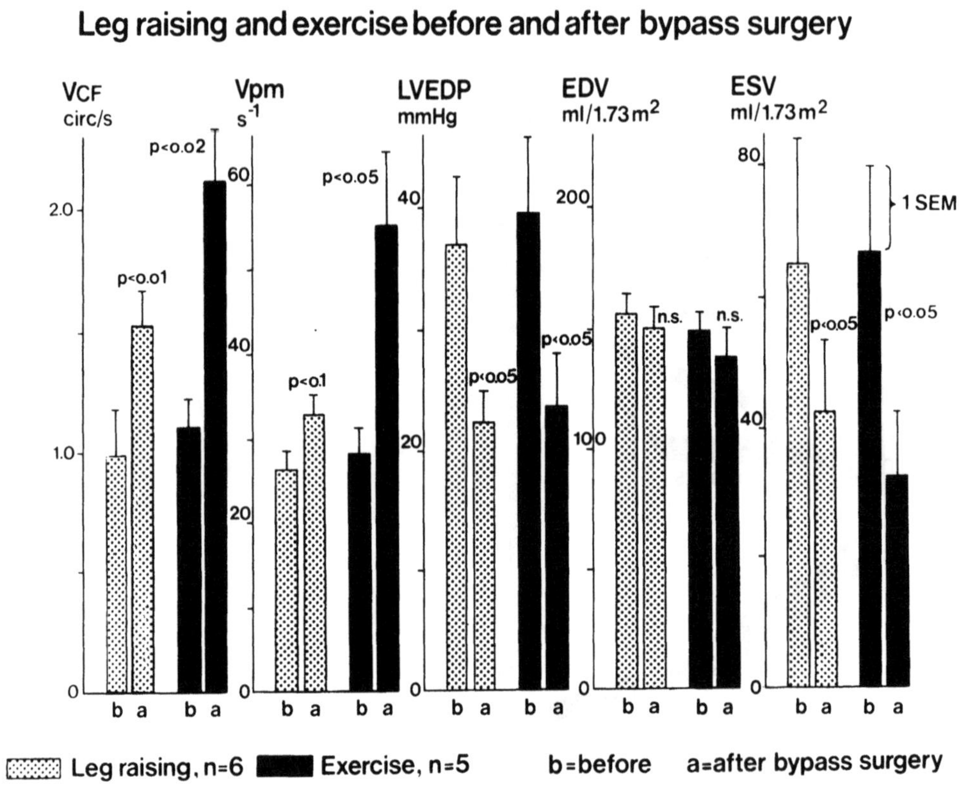

Fig. 5. Hemodynamic parameters after leg raising and physical exercise before and after bypass surgery. Postoperatively mean Vcf and Vpm increased significantly. Left ventricular enddiastolic pressure (LVEDP) decreased significantly postoperatively after leg raising and physical exercise. Enddiastolic volume (EDV) remained unchanged while endsystolic volume (ESV) decreased markedly

Group II
In three patients the grafts occluded or myocardial infarction occurred during operation. There were no significant differences between pre- and postoperative values. Mean Vcf increased during leg raising only slightly preoperatively from 0.85 to 1.01 circ/s postoperatively, and after physical exercise from 1.05 to 1.29 circ/s (Fig. 6). Enddiastolic and endsystolic volume increased as compared to values before surgery.

Discussion

Preoperative Findings
In patients with severe coronary heart disease regional ventricular function can be normal at rest. However, during exercise hypokinesis or akinesis developed in poststenotic areas [4,6,8,15]. Corresponding to the preponderant affection of LAD, regional wall motion disturbances were especially marked in the anterior wall and in the apex. The decrease in amplitude of contraction and in velocity of fiber shortening are especially pronounced in this segment Vm2 (Fig. 4).

Leg Raising
Wall motion disturbances during physical exercise in poststenotic areas are due to underperfusion. However, ventricular dysfunction after leg raising cannot be easily explained. After leg raising, i.e., acute volume load, left ventricular enddiastolic pressure increases markedly. Other parameters such as heart rate or systolic pressure do not change significantly. Enddiastolic volume increased only

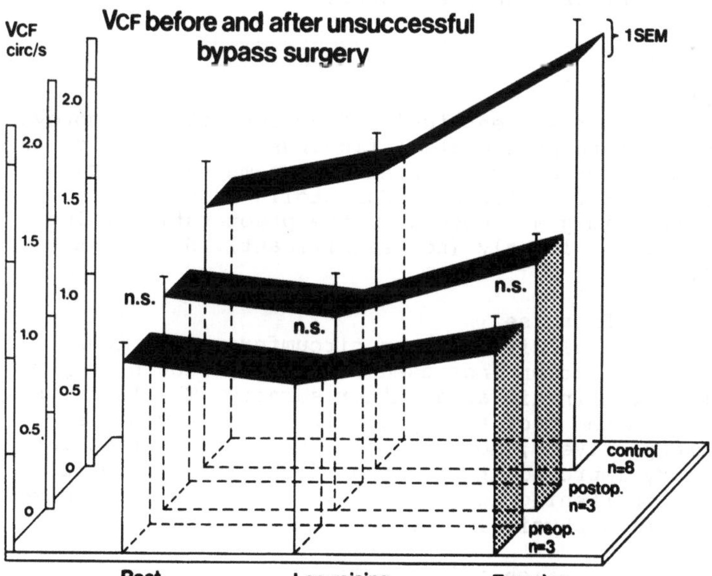

Fig. 6. Velocity of mean circumferential fiber shortening (mean Vcf) at rest, after leg raising, and physical exercise before and after unseccessful bypass surgery as compared to a control group (normal left ventricle). Preoperative: decrease in velocity of fiber shortening after leg raising and insufficient increase during physical exercise. Postoperative: no significant difference to preoperative values

slightly and not significantly, whereas endsystolic volume in correspondence to hypokinesis increased significantly. Therefore, it seems obvious that the increase in left ventricular enddiastolic pressure may be the cause of regional wall motion disturbances.

Two mechanisms are involved:

1) According to Raff et al. [16] an increase of left ventricular enddiastolic pressure by 10 mmHg results in an increase of coronary resistance by 11%. After leg raising the increase in left ventricular diastolic pressure passively results in a reduction of perfusion of poststenotic areas and especially to the endocardial layers.
2) The increase in diastolic wall tension due to an increased enddiastolic pressure results in an increase in myocardial oxygen consumption [17].

Both mechanisms, i.e., the increase in the extravascular component of coronary resistance and the increase in oxygen consumption due to the increased diastolic wall tension may explain ischemia and hypokinesis due to leg raising.

Clinical signs also point to the fact that leg raising causes ischemia. In one patient leg raising induced severe angina pectoris. In two other patients mild angina and ST-depression were observed.

Physical Exercise
While leg raising resulted in an increase of preload and in some cases caused angina pectoris, physical exercise induced in all patients severe angina pectoris and hypokinesis. The increased pre- and afterload and exercise tachycardia induced a marked increase in oxygen consumption and hypokinesis due to ischemia.

Postoperative Findings

Hemodynamics at Rest
It should be noted that at rest ventricular function did not improve significantly as compared to preoperative findings. Enddiastolic and endsystolic volume and ejection fraction had the same values pre- and postoperatively. Only left ventricular enddiastolic pressure decreased in the mean by 6 mmHg as opposed to the preoperative value. Mean Vcf and Vpm increased slightly (not significant). Heart rate increased significantly.

Leg Raising and Physical Exercise
In both stress conditions velocity of mean circumferential fiber shortening and ejection fraction increased markedly following reperfusion of hypokinetic or akinetic areas after surgery. The functional improvement results from the fact that postoperatively angina pectoris or ischemia, respectively, do not occur. Regional ventricular function is particulary improved in the area of the anterior wall. The velocity of fiber shortening in the anterior wall (Vm2) increases in the mean by 500% during physical exercise.

The increase in ejection fraction and in velocity of mean circumferential fiber shortening is due to the reduction in endsystolic volume and the nearly unchanged enddiastolic volume. Left ventricular enddiastolic pressure decreased markedly. These changes are combined with a marked improvement of left ventricular contractility:
In accordance with ejection phase parameters (mean Vcf, EF) isometric contractility indices improved significantly after successful bypass surgery. Postoperatively max dP/dt and Vpm increased significantly

due to the abolition of ischemia. A higher workload was tolerated as compared to preoperative exercise capacity.

When comparing postoperative findings with performance of a control group no significant difference was found. Hence, following bypass surgery, patients with coronary heart disease performed similarly to a healthy control group under stress conditions.

Pressure-Volume Relation

Preoperatively enddiastolic volume did not increase, either after leg raising or during physical exercise, while enddiastolic pressure increased significantly. After successful bypass surgery findings were reversed: Under stress conditions enddiastolic volume remained unchanged while enddiastolic pressure was reduced by more than 15 mmHg. These findings document a steep pressure-volume relation. Unchanged ventricular volumes can be found with extremely high (preoperatively up to 40 mmHg) and low (postoperatively down to 22 mmHg) ventricular pressure values. In dog experiments Böttcher et al. [18] found similar steep pressure-volume relations.

Increase of Mean Vcf After Leg Raising

After leg raising regional function and velocity of mean circumferential fiber shortening increased after leg raising in control patients and in postoperative patients with coronary heart disease. These findings partially contradict those of Mahler et al. [19] who did not find an increase of velocity of mean circumferential fiber shortening following intravenous volume load in animal experiments. However, volume load also increased afterload. In the patients studied leg raising resulted in an increase in preload but not in an increase of afterload (see Table 1).

Heart Rate

Heart rate at reast, after leg raising, and during physical exercise was significantly higher postoperatively as compared to preoperative values. The increase in heart rate is probably due to a hyperkinetic reaction or an increased sympathetic stimulation which decreases with time elapsing after surgery. The increase in heart rate is combined with a reduction in ejection time. Since the ejection time is a parameter in the calculation of mean Vcf and velocity of regional shortening postoperative values of velocity of fiber shortening are relatively too high. Therefore, tables also indicate ejection fraction and percentual fiber shortening. These data represent functional improvement as well as the velocity values. Hence, the improvement in left ventricular performance is only to a small degree due to the postoperatively increased heart rate. The same applies to the unproportionally high increase of max dP/dt.

This assumption is also supported by the fact that in patients with unsuccessful bypass surgery an increase in heart rate without improvement in left ventricular function was found.

Collaterals

Comparison of pre- and postoperative coronary angiograms revealed that collaterals were not present following successful bypass surgery. It may be concluded that preoperatively functioning collaterals do not suffice to avoid regional wall motion function disturbances during stress. Smith et al. [20] found in tests with Xenon-133 that myocardial blood flow is not significantly improved by collaterals. Helfant et al. [21,22] reported that collaterals do not prevent asynergy, abnormal hemodynamics, or ischemia in exercise ECGs. Carroll et al. [23] found no improvement in ventricular function in the presence of good collaterals. It is concluded, that the postoperative increase in blood supply normalizes ventricular function during stress conditions irrespective of the presence of collaterals.

Compensation in the Inferior Wall
Ischemic dysfunction of the anterior wall preoperatively is compensated by a marked increase in shortening of nonischemic myocardial areas of the inferior wall. Postoperatively this phenomenon disappeared since the anterior wall regained adequate function.

Unsuccessful Surgery
In patients of group II ventricular function did not improve. LVEDP was not reduced postoperatively either at rest or after stress, and overall left ventricular function did not improve.

The present results indicate that left ventricular function does not improve at rest following bypass surgery. During exercise, however, a marked improvement was found. Improvement of regional wall motion is most pronounced in those areas which preoperatively are most impaired. This effect occurs during leg raising and more so during physical.

References

1. Kong, Y., Behar, V.S., Peter, R.H., Morris, J.J.: Early effect of aorto-coronary bypass surgery on epicardial segment shortening. Circulation *41,42,* 175 (1970)
2. Kouchoukos, N.T., Doty, D.B., Beuttner, L.E., Kirlin, J.W.: Treatment of postinfarction cardiac failure by myocardial excision and revascularization. Circulation *43,44,* 108 (1971)
3. Chatterjee, K., Swan, H.J.C., Parmley, W.W., Sustaita, H., Marcus, H.S., Matloff, J.: Influence of direkt myocardial revascularization on left ventricular asynergy and function in patients with coronary heart disease with and without previous myocardial infarction. Circulation *47*, 276-286 (1973)
4. Bussmann, W.D., Thaler, R., Heeger, J., Kober, G., Hopf, R., Kaltenbach, M.: Angiographische und hämodynamische Befunde des linken Ventrikels nach Volumenbelastung und körperlicher Arbeit bei Patienten mit koronarer Herzkrankheit (KHK). Verh. Dtsch. Ges. Kreislaufforsch. *41*, 168-171 (1975)
5. Bussmann, W.D., Heeger, J., Thaler, R., Kober, G., Hopf, R., Kaltenbach, M.: Comparison of velocity parameters of the isovolumic and ejection phase in man. In: Coronary angiography and angina pectoris. Lichtlen, P.R., pp. 122-132. Stuttgart: Thieme 1975
6. Bussmann, W.D., Thaler, R., Kober, G., Hopf, R., Kaltenbach, M.: Angiographie des linken Ventrikels nach Volumenbelastung und körperlicher Arbeit bei koronarer Herzkrankheit. Z. Kardiol. *65*, 693-707 (1976)
7. Krayenbühl, H.P., Schönbeck, M., Rutishauser, W., Wirz, P.: Abnormal segmental contraction velocity in coronary artery disease produced by isometric exercise and atrial pacing. Am. J. Cardiol. *35*, 785-794 (1975)
8. Sharma, B., Raphael, M.J., Thadani, U., Taylor, S.H., Steiner, R.E., Goodwin, J.F.: Left ventricular pressure-volume changes during exercise induced pain in patients with angina pectoris. Br. Heart J. *36*, 1038 (1974) (Abs.)
9. Kaltenbach, M., Schulz, W.: Kineangiographische Bestimmung von Ventrikelvolumina mit Rechnerhilfe. Dtsch. Med. Wochenschr. *100*, 590-593 (1975)
10. Cohn, P,F., Gorlin, R., Adams, D.F., Chahine, R.A., Vokonas, P.S., Herman, M.V.: Comparison of biplane and single plane left ventriculograms in patients with coronary artery disease. Am. J. Cardiol. *33*, 1-6 (1974)
11. Bussmann, W.D.: Kontraktilitätsreserve des linken Ventrikels unter körperlicher und pharmakologischer Belastung bei verschiedenen Herzerkrankungen. Frankfurt, Thesis 1974
12. Bussmann, W.D., Joss, B., Kaltenbach, M.: Recheneinheit zur Bestimmung der größten gemessenen Verkürzungsgeschwindigkeit der kontraktilen Elemente. Z. Kardiol. *64*, 289-299 (1975)

13. Krayenbühl, H.P., Rutishauser, W., Wirz, P., Amende, I., Mehmel, H.: High fidelity left ventricular pressure measurements for the assessment of cardiac contractility in man. Am. J. Cardiol. *31*, 415-427 (1973)
14. Mehmel, H., Krayenbühl, H.P., Wirz, P.: Isovolumic contraction dynamics in man according to two different muscle models. J. Appl. Physiol. *33*, 409-414 (1972)
15. Schönbeck, M., Krayenbühl, H.P., Rutishauser, W., Wirz, P., Wellauer, J.: Quantitative angiocardiographische Haemodynamik bei Herzgesunden und bei Patienten mit einer Koronarsklerose (CAD) in Ruhe und während Belastung. Verh. Dtsch. Ges. Inn. Med. *80*, 1056-1060 (1974)
16. Raff, W.K., Kosche, F., Lochner, W.: Extravascular coronary resistance and its relation to microcurculation. Influence of heart rate, end-diastolic pressure and maximal rate of rise of intraventricular pressure. Am. J. Cardiol. *29*, 598-603 (1972)
17. Greenberg, H., Dweyer, E.M., (Jr.), Jameson, A.G., Pinkernell, B.H.: Effects of nitroglycerin on the major determinants of myocardial oxygen consumption. An angiographic and hemodynamic assessment. Am. J. Cardiol. *36*, 426-432 (1975)
18. Boettcher, D., Vatner, S., Heyndrick, G., Millard, R., Braunwald, E.: Role of frank-starling mechanism in control of cardiac function in normal conscious dogs.
19. Mahler, F., Ross, J., (Jr.), O'Rourke, R.A., Covell, J.W.: Effects of changes in preload, afterload and inotropic state on ejection and isovolumic phase measures of contractility in conscious dog. Am. J. Cardiol. *35*, 626-634 (1975)
20. Smith, S.C., Gorlin, R., Herman, M.V., Taylor, W.J., Collins, J.J., (Jr.): Myocardial blood flow in man: effect of coronary collateral circulation and coronary artery bypass surgery. J. Clin. Invest. *51*, 2556-2565 (1972)
21. Helfant, R.H., Kemp, H.G., Gorlin, R.: Coronary atherosclerosis, coronary collaterals and their relation to cardiac function. Ann. Intern. Med. *73*, 189-193 (1970)
22. Helfant, R.H., Gorlin, R.: The coronary collateral circulation. Ann. Intern. Med. *77*, 995-997 (1972)
23. Carroll, R.J., Verani, M.S., Falsetti, H.L.: The effect of collateral circulation on segmental left ventricular contraction. Circulation *50*, 709-713 (1974)

Global and Regional Postoperative Left Ventricular Function in Relation to Preoperative Function and Degree of Revascularization

I. Amende, R. Simon, W. Hood, W. Liese, H. G. Borst, and P. Lichtlen

The effects of coronary artery bypass grafting on resting global and regional left ventricular (LV) function were studied from single plane cineangiograms performed in the 40° RAO projection before and 12 days to 6 months after bypass surgery. Sixteen patients were selected to study the relationship between revascularization of the left anterior decending coronary artery (LAD) and right coronary artery (RCA) and changes in regional motion of the respective LV wall segments.

In a group of 14 patients, myocardial markers were used to analyze the effects of LAD grafting on anterior wall motion. The degree of myocardial revascularization was assessed by comparison of pre- and postoperative coronary angiograms. A functional revascularization index was derived from graft patency and preoperative anatomy. For each patient the ratio of patent grafts to the number of coronary vessels with significant obstructive lesions (>75%) supplying viable myocardium was scored in percent [1].

Global systolic function was evaluated in terms of ejection fraction and mean normalized systolic ejection rate. Regional systolic function was evaluated in terms of percentage shortening of basal, middle, and apical transverse diameters and hemiaxes. Diameters and hemiaxes were measured at 26%, 50% and 76% increments of the long axes at both enddiastole and endsystole, by use of a computer-assisted video system. Additionally, regional function was evaluated in terms of segmental ejection fraction. A computerized system superimposed enddiastolic and endsystolic LV silhouettes by aligning the long axes and fixing their midpoints. Five angular segments were defined from the midpoint on each silhouette beginning at the left aortic valve margin and ending at the right aortic valve margin. Segmental ejection fraction represented the percentage change in area of each segment.

Figure 1 summarizes the effects of bypass grafting on global LV function in the selected 16 patients. Ejection fraction did not change, whereas mean normalized systolic ejection rate increased significantly. Figure 2 illustrates the effects of bypass grafting on regional function. Percentage shortening of transverse diameters showed no change in any segment. Percentage shortening of transverse diameters showed no change in any segment. Percentage shortening of hemiaxes did not change in the anterobasal and apical segment, but increased significantly in the anteromiddle segment. Analysis of segmental ejection fraction, as shown in Fig. 3, revealed no significant change in any segment. The overall functional revascularization index of these patients was 83%. Six had incomplete revascularization with an index of 50%-66%. Analysis of LV performance in this subgroup revealed a significant increase in mean normalized systolic ejection rate, but the ejection fraction remained unaltered. These changes were identical to the alterations in global function of the whole group. Thus, an improvement of global function does not depend on the completeness

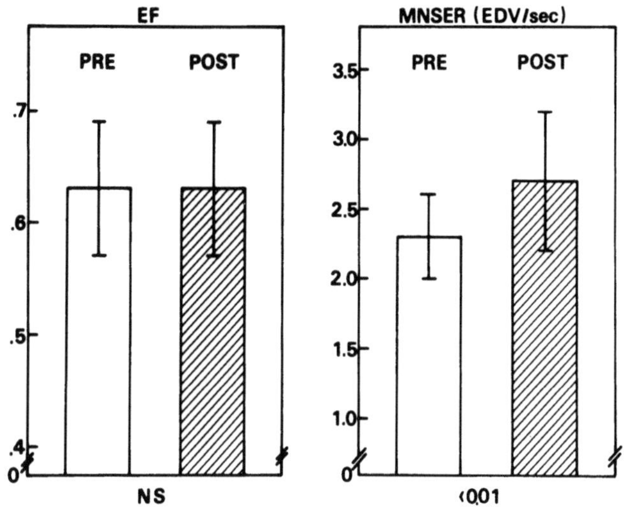

Fig. 1. Global left ventricular function before and after bypass grafting. Effect on ejection fraction (*EF*) and mean normalized systolic ejection rate (*MNSER*). n = 16 pts. mean ± 1 S.D.

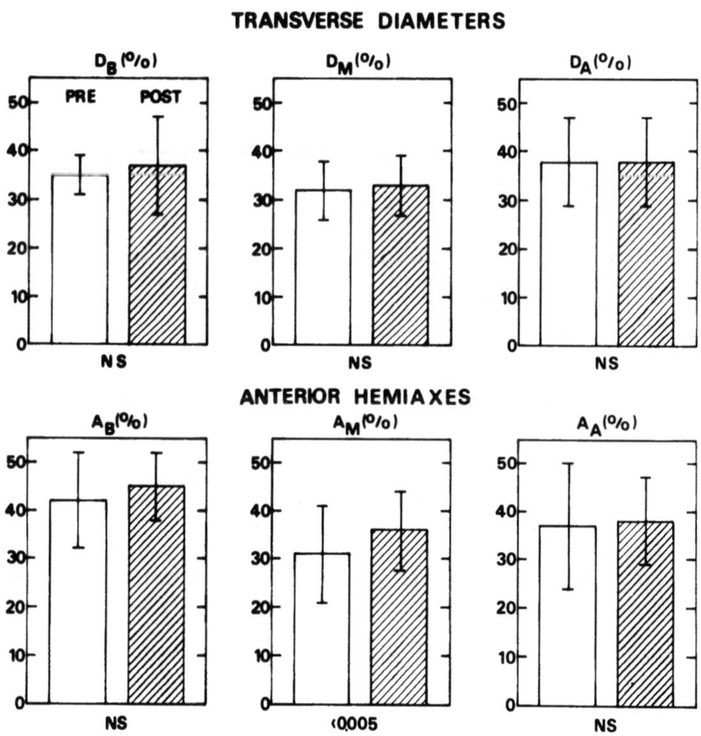

Fig. 2. Regional left ventricular function before and after bypass grafting. Effect on percentage shortening of transverse diameters and anterior hemiaxes. n = 16 mean ± 1 S.D. *B* basal; *M* middle; *A* apical

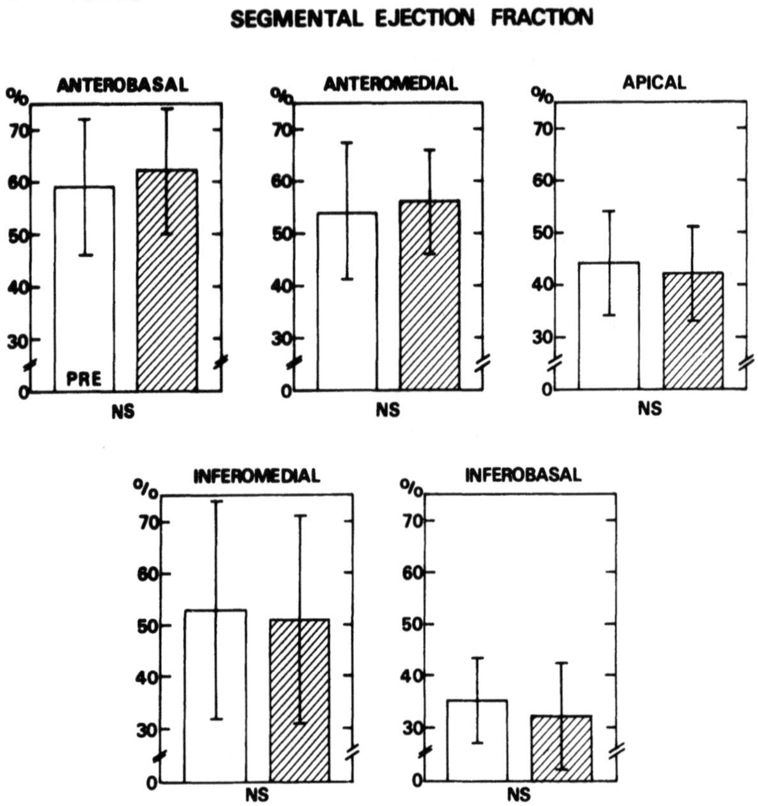

Fig. 3. Regional left ventricular function before and after bypass grafting. Effect on segmental ejection fraction. n = 16 mean ± 1 S.D.

of revascularization. This is illustrated by Fig. 4, which shows the pre- and postoperative coronary angiograms from a patient with RCA and LAD occlusion. There was retrograde filling of both vessels from the circumflex artery. The functional revascularization index was 50%.

Figures 5 and 6 show the effects of RCA grafting on global LV function in the same patient. After operation there was a marked decrease in enddiastolic volume (230 to 147 ml), an increase in ejection fraction (54% to 61%, and an increase in mean normalized systolic ejection rate (1.90 to 2.71 EDV/s). These results were accompanied by a considerable improvement in regional function. Both percentage shortening of transverse diameters and anterior hemiaxes increased in the basal and middle segments. Segmental ejection fraction showed an increase in the anterobasal and apical areas.

Parameters of regional LV function determined from only enddiastolic and endsystolic silhouettes may not accurately reflect regional wall motion abnormalities. A more sensitive approach to analysis of regional wall motion after bypass grafting is the use of myocardial markers implanted in revascularized segments [2]. Figure 7 illustrates the position of anterior myoardial markers in a patient after grafting of the LAD. Markers were filmed in a slight LAO projection at 80 or 150 frames/sec. A computer-assisted video system was used to determine changes in marker distance frame-by-fram during one heart cycle. The distances were normalized for enddiastolic distance.

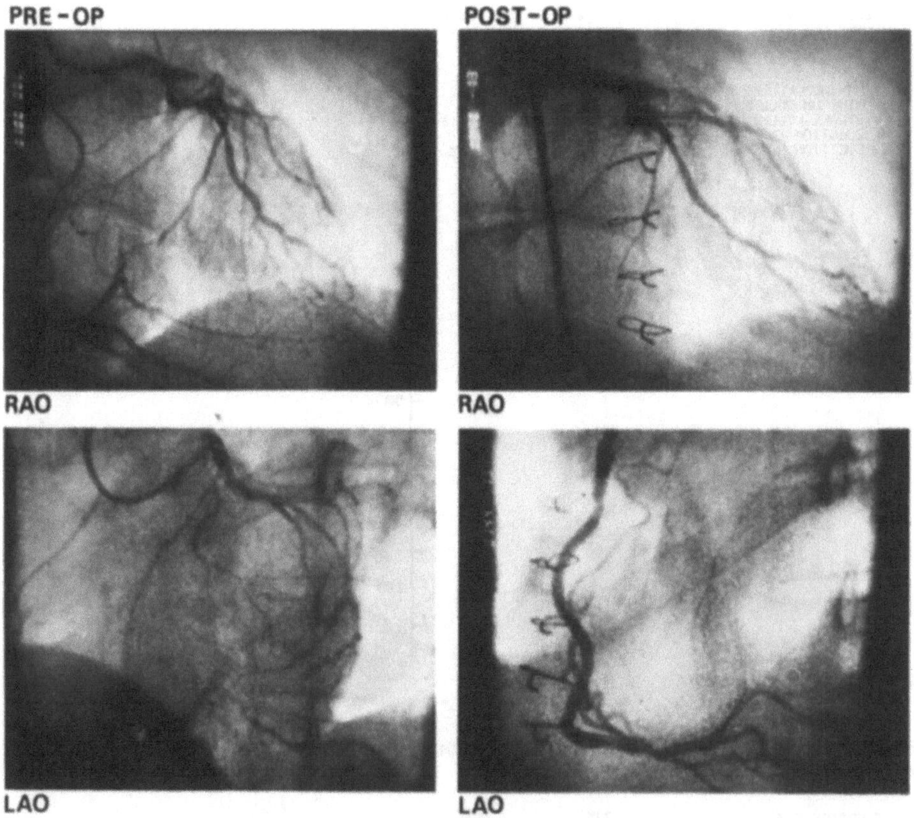

Fig. 4. Coronary angiograms before and after RCA-grafting. Functional revascularization index 50%. (M.R., 34 years, 2-vessel disease)

Figure 8 depicts anterior wall motion before and after bypass grafting in 14 patients. Preoperative distances were obtained from coronary bifurcations and postoperatively from myocardial markers. The figure illustrates that significant obstruction of the LAD is associated in some patients with marked regional contraction abnormalities, and that successful revascularization can normalize these anterior wall motion disorders at rest [3]. Figure 9 demonstrates the sensitivity of the marker method. In this paitent stressing of the myocardium by handgrip revealed early relaxation of the anterior wall not present at rest. This patient's coronary angiogram showed a patent LAD graft, but there was a significant obstruction distal do its implantation.

Conclusions

Following successful bypass grafting, mean normalized systolic ejection rate may reveal improvement in global LV function when ejection fraction does not.

Percentage shortening of hemiaxes may reflect improvement in regional LV function when that of transverse diameters or when segmental ejection fraction does not.

EJECTION TIME........... :	204		MSEC
MEAN VCF................ :	0.923		/SEC
	A-L	SIMPSON	
* MAXIMUM VOLUME......... :	230	248	ML
* MINIMUM VOLUME......... :	106	117	ML
* STROKE VOLUME.......... :	124	131	ML
EJECTION FRACTION...... :	54	53	%
EJECTION RATE.......... :	1.90	1.87	/SEC

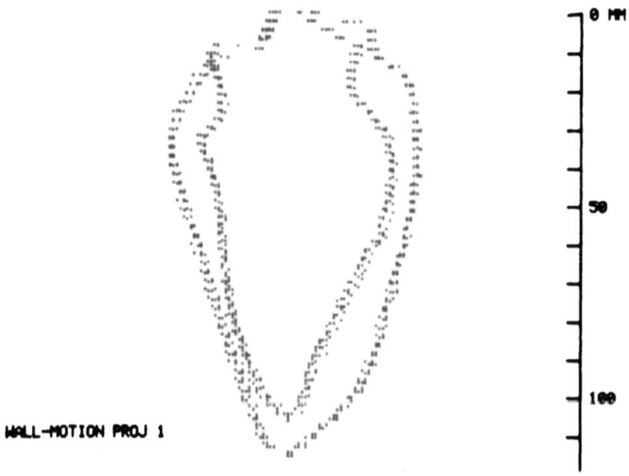

2: A=0.255 S/A= 3.20 2.21.1978 8.12.1976 565/076
VC-A= 1.00 VC-S= 2.32 MEYER R PRAE OP CAD

Fig. 5. Left ventricular function before bypass surgery in the same patient as in Fig. 4

EJECTION TIME........... :	225		MSEC
MEAN VCF................ :	1.535		/SEC
	A-L	SIMPSON	
* MAXIMUM VOLUME......... :	147	163	ML
* MINIMUM VOLUME......... :	57	64	ML
* STROKE VOLUME.......... :	90	99	ML
EJECTION FRACTION...... :	61	61	%
EJECTION RATE.......... :	2.71	2.71	/SEC

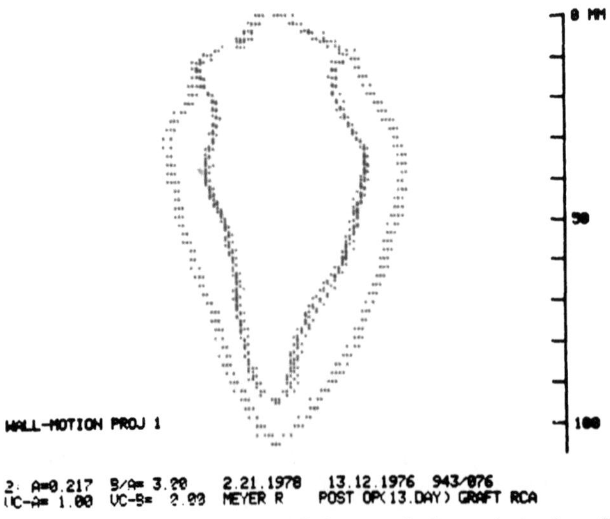

2: A=0.217 S/A= 3.20 2.21.1978 13.12.1976 943/076
VC-A= 1.00 VC-S= 2.03 MEYER R POST OP(13.DAY) GRAFT RCA

Fig. 6. Effect of RCA-grafting on left ventricular function in the same patient as in Fig. 4

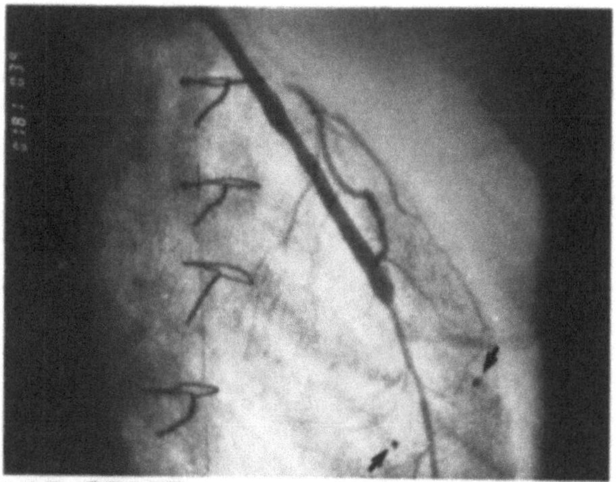

LAD GRAFT

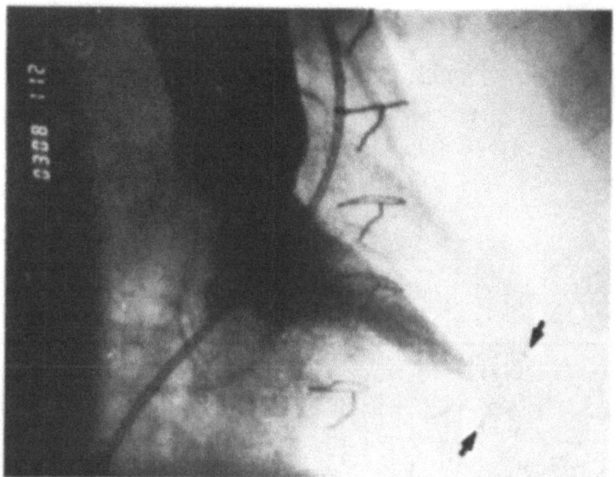

END-SYSTOLE

Fig. 7. Position of anterior myocardial markers in a patient after LAD-grafting. (V.E., 66 years, 872/75)

Analysis of wall motion by myocardial markers confirms the improvement in regional LV function within the grafted area.

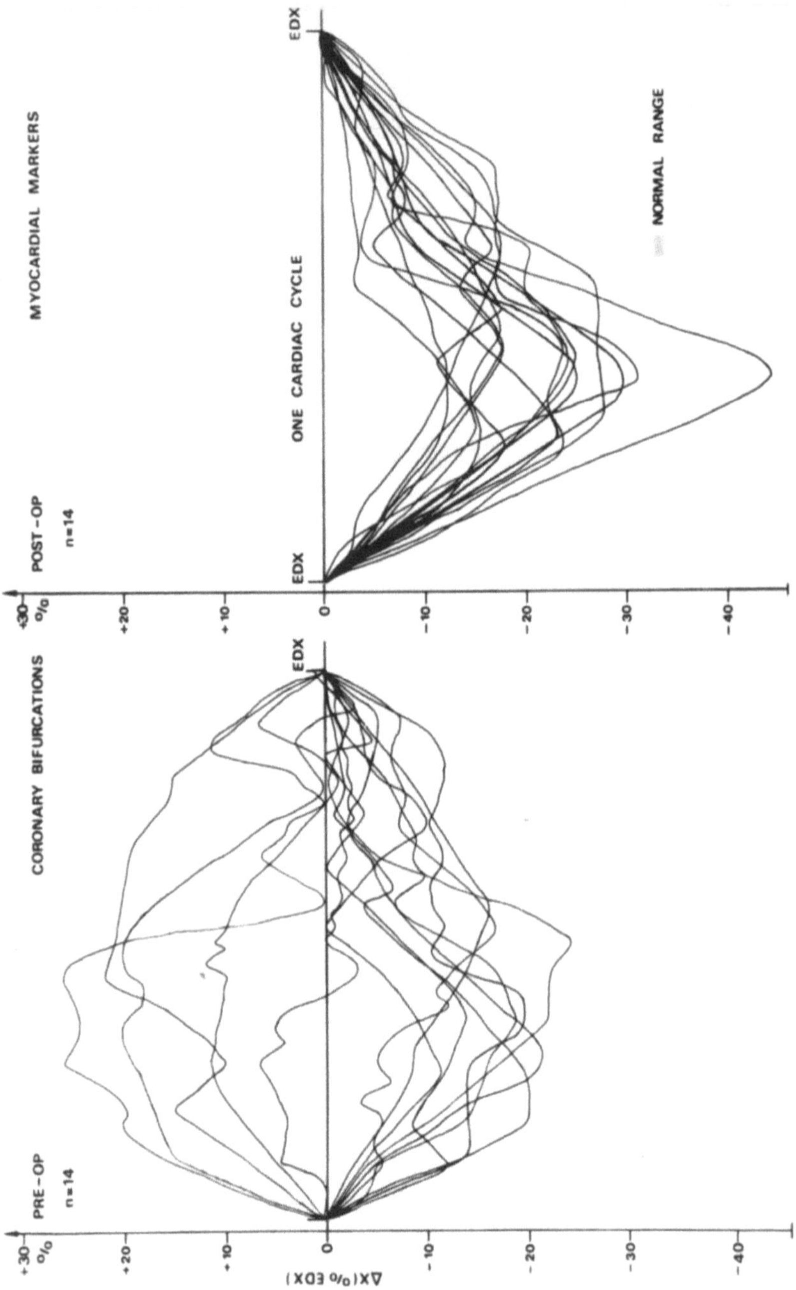

Fig. 8. Anterior wall motion before and after bypass grafting. Preoperative measurements of distances were obtained from coronary bifurcations. The changes in distance were normalized for the enddiastolic distance and plotted frame-by-frame during one heart cycle

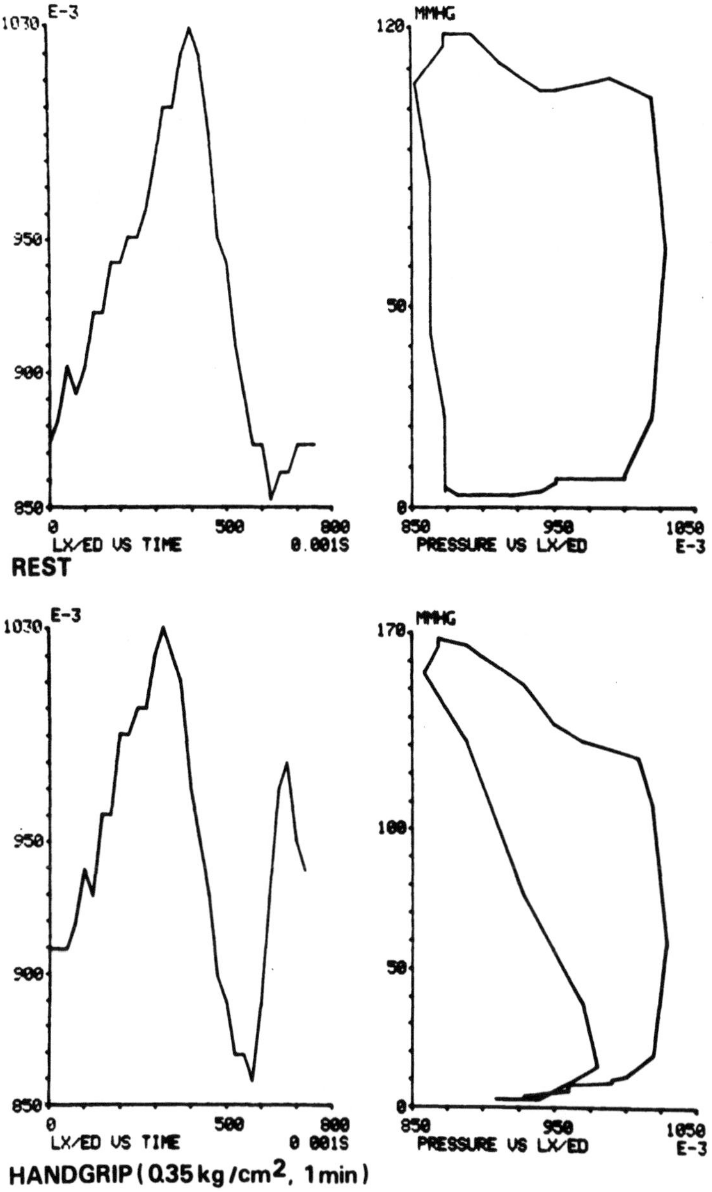

Fig. 9. Effect of handgrip on anterior wall motion after LAD-grafting. Marker distance, normalized for enddiastolic distance, is plotted versus time and high-fidelity left ventricular pressure. (V.E., 66 years, 872/75 myocardial markers)

References

1. Levine, J.A., Bechtel, D.J., Cohn, P.F., Herman, M.V., Gorlin, R., Cohn, L.H., Collins, J.J. (Jr.): Ventricular function before and after direct revascularization surgery. A proposal for an index of vascularization to correlate angiographic and ventriculographic findings. Circulation *51*, 1071 (1975)
2. Hetzer, R., Heim, K., Borst, H.G., Amende, I., Sigwart, U.: Cineradiographical studies of local ventricular motility before and after aorto-coronary bypass. Thoraxchirurgie *24*, 296 (1976)
3. Kong, Y., Morris, J.J., McIntosh, H.D.: Assessment of regional myocardial performance from biplane coronary cineangiograms. Am. J. Cardiol. *27*, 529 (1971)

Early Myocardial Depression After Coronary Artery Bypass Surgery

P. W. Serruys, R. W. Brower, H. J. ten Katen, M. v. d. Brand, and P. G. Hugenholtz

Introduction

In the majority of reports describing surgical mortality and its correlates, the greatest single step in the survival curves occurs in the first month after surgery. Thus, this early postoperative period takes on a relatively greater significance and represents a period which, if well controlled, could do much to further reduce the overall surgical mortality. Even in the absence of preoperative myocardial infarctions some clinical, hemodynamic, electrocardiographic, echocardiographic, and enzymatic data suggest that myocardial injury occurs as a result of the direct traumatic effects of the operative procedure, whether it be extracorporeal perfusion, the anesthetic, thoracotomy, or myocardial surgery itself. Nevertheless, there continues to be controversy over the effects of coronary bypass grafting on left ventricular function in the early and late postoperative period, which is due in large part to the difficulties involved in obtaining direct and accurate measurements of function during this period.

Several questions arise concerning these results:

1) Is there some specific evidence corroborating the clinical findings of postoperative depression?
2) What is the time course of the recovery from this myocardial injury?
3) Are the normal and the grafted regions differently affected by the operative procedure?

With the recent development of a new method [1-4] to measure regional shortening in the bypassed regions, using radiopaque epicardial markers implanted during surgery, these different questions can be answered in some detail.

Methods

Coronary artery bypass grafting (end to side) was performed on 56 consecutive patients scheduled for elective surgery, age range 41 to 62 years, 52 men and 4 women. Four patients had an aneurysmectomy. Topical hypothermia with 4° saline was employed. Radiopaque marker pairs were sutured to the epicardium 0-3 cm distal to the coronary anastomosis, 2 cm apart, and aligned transverse to the major axis of the heart (Fig. 1). Markers were not placed in aneurysmatic or infarcted myocardium as observed at surgery. A total of 120 marker pairs were placed in bypass regions and 31 pairs in apparently normally perfused control regions on the anterior surface near the base of the heart.

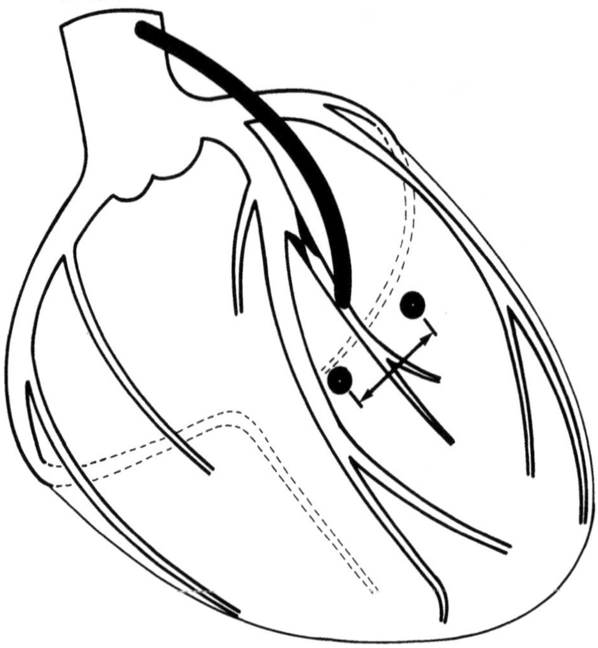

Fig. 1. Radiopaque markers were placed circa 2 cm apart transverse to the major axis and 0-3 cm distal to the coronary anastomosis. Where possible an additional marker pair (not shown) was placed in normally perfused control regions on the anterior surface near the base of the heart. Marker pairs were filmed for minimal foreshortening, and pair separation measured from the projected images

Marker motion was recorded with a conventional monoplane ciné angiographic apparatus at 50 frames/s. The procedure was to position the C-arm perpendicular to the shortening axis of the marker pair being recorded (minimal foreshortening), and this was repeated for all marker pairs sequentially. For follow-up recordings the previously recorded C-arm postion for each marker pair was used. Patients were examined at 1 week, 1 month, 3 months, 6 months, 9 months, and 1 year after surgery. The films were projected and marker pair separation measured with a conventional Vernier caliper. Marker pair separation for at least four heart beats was measured starting from the frame prior to onset of the Q wave of the ECG to the minimum separation (Fig. 2). The results of the measurements of these beats were averaged. Shortening fraction (SF) and time to onset of shortening (T = time from onset of the Q wave of the ECG to maximum marker separation) were determined.

Cardiac catheterization was performed 3 months before surgery and 1 year after surgery. Relevant clinical information including cardiothoracic ratio, heart rate, systolic and diastolic blood pressure were obtained 3 months and 1 day prior to surgery, and at 1 week, 1 month, and every 3 months after surgery up to 1 year.

Results

The results of the cardiac catheterization (3 months preoperative and 1 year postoperative) are summarized in Fig. 3. Heart rate during both investigations are identical: 72 beats/min versus 74 beats/min. Ejec-

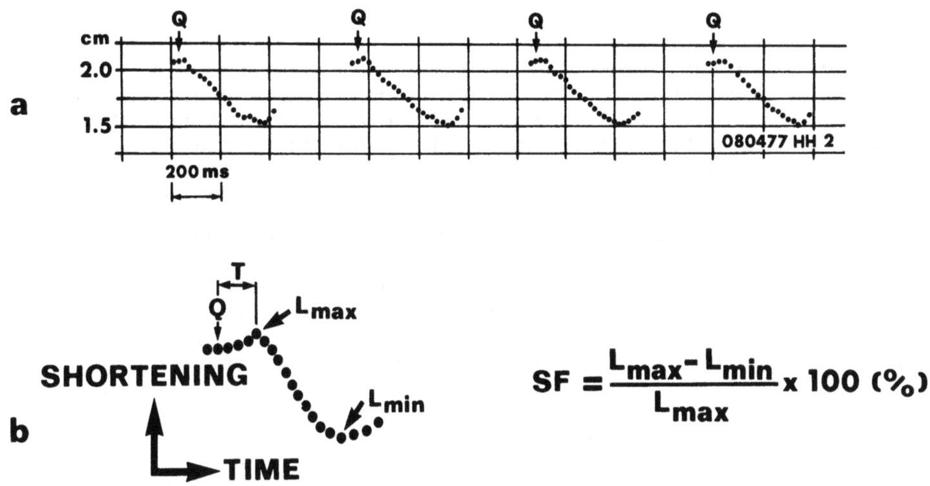

Fig. 2. a) Marker pair separation is plotted from the frame prior to the Q wave of the ECG to after minimal marker separation. b) This information is quantified by measuring the onset of shortening (T), and the shortening fraction (SF)

	HAEMODYNAMICS preop	vs 1yr postop	
HR	72 ± 12	74 ± 12	beat min^{-1}
EF	55 ± 10	55 ± 13	%
Vmax	49 ± 9	48 ± 9	sec^{-1}
LVEDP	14 ± 7	18 ± 7 *	mmHg
LVEDV	74 ± 16	89 ± 26 *	ml m^{-2}
mean Ao P	106 ± 17	115 ± 21 *	mmHg
CI	3.19 ± 0.63	2.90 ± 0.54 *	l min^{-1}
syst. resist.	1432 ± 344	1701 ± 464 *	dynes sec cm^{-5}

* significant $p < 0.0025$ paired t test

Fig. 3. Results of the 3 months preoperative and 1 year postoperative catheterization.: heart rate (HR), ejection fraction (EF), maximal rate of change of normalized left ventricular pressure under zero loading (Vmax), left ventricular end diastolic pressure (LVEDP), left ventricular end diastolic volume (LVEDV), mean aortic pressure (AoP), cardiac indec (CI), and systemic resistance tion fraction (EF) and maximum rate of change of pressure divided by instantaneous pressure and extrapolated to zero loading (Vmax) also remain unchanged and within the normal range. However, a significant (P = 0.0025) change was found in left ventricular end diastolic pressure (LVEDP increased by 4 mmHg or 28%) and in left ventricular end-diastolic volume (LVEDV increased by 15 ml or 20%). Angiographic volumes were calculated by the area-length method using the correction formula of Heintzen: $V_{true} = .72\ V_{meas.} - 4.7$. There was also a significant (P = 0.0025) increase in mean aortic pressure (AoP) of 8.4% and a decrease in cardiac index (CI) of 9.0%. This resulted in an increase in the calculated systemic peripheral resistance of 270 $dyn \cdot s \cdot cm^{-5}$, or 18% (Rp = AoP/(BSA·CI)). In view of the increase in volume, and especially the increase in aortic pressure, an increase in the afterload can be inferred. Thus, there was little change in overall left ventricular function from the preoperative measurements to that seen at 1 year postoperative, but there were changes in systemic resistance and a small left ventricular dilation.

The conventional clinical measurements such as cardiothoracic ratio (CT ratio) and diastolic blood pressure provide only a crude approximation to the pre- and afterload (Fig. 4). Nevertheless, they can not be ignored in this respect and do reveal the general trend of the loading conditions during the early and late postoperative periods. This trend of postoperative recovery is clearly illustrated in Fig. 4. In the early postoperative period a consistent enlargement of heart size was observed. CT ratio was significantly increased from mean value of 46% preoperative to 53% at 1 week after the operation. At 1 month the CT ratio remains abnormally large, but only after 3 months does it return to the preoperative level. Simultaneously, the average heart rate is considerably higher at the first preoperative evaluation with a mean difference of 22 beats/min and returns to the preoperative heart rate only 6-9 months after surgery. Finally, the cuff blood pressures also show a significant decline of diastolic and systolic values at 1 week. The diastolic pressure is still low at 1 month and is only normalized at 3 months.

The follow-up of epicardial shortening is shown in Fig. 5: the dashed line for the control region and the solid line for the bypassed regions. In the first week shortening fraction (SF) in the control regions is greater than in bypassed regions: 11.5% versus 9.8%. At 1 month the original difference has disappeared. However, over a period of 6 months both groups show a steady and significant (P = 0.0001 from 1 week to 6 months) increase in SF. After 6 months SF of both groups remain stable at the value of 13.7% at 1 year postoperative and no further increase is manifest.

This initial depression and later improvement of shortening fraction can be interpreted as a recovery from myocardial injury incurred as part of the operative procudure. In this connection changes due to other variables such as heart rate, preload, and afterload have to be considered.

Discussion

Regional myocardial shortening is a complex indicator of ventricular performance and regional blood supply. Changes in shortening fraction are directionally related to loading conditions under which the ventricle is operating as well as to changes in the inotropic state of the myocardium. Compared with the preoperative state, the first post-

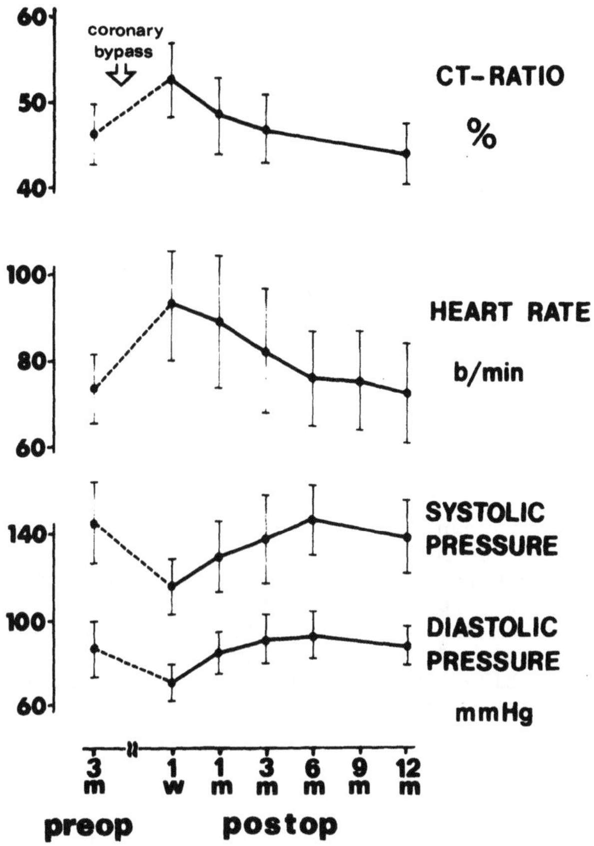

Fig. 4. Conventional clinical measurements from 3 months preoperative to 12 months postoperative

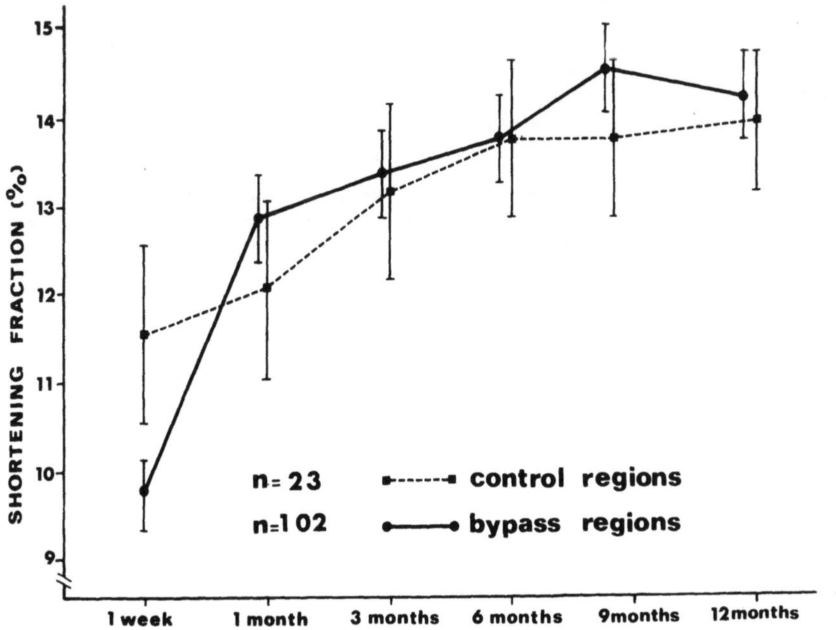

Fig. 5. Regional shortening fraction over the follow-up period

operative evaluation shows an increase in preload reflected by heart size enlargement and a decrease in afterload suggested by the low diastolic blood pressures. These combined changes in loading conditions would enhance the ejection fraction and consequently the regional shortening fraction. Conversely, between the first week and the first month the decrease in preload by the reduction of heart size and the increase in afterload by the rise in diastolic arterial pressure would cause a decrease in ejection fraction and shortening fraction. Thus, the postoperative increase in shortening fraction is not directionally related to changes in loading conditions or in chronotropic state. Thus, the slow increase in regional shortening most likely is due to recovery of the myocardium from the perioperative injury.

The use of cardiothoracic ratio in this context is questionable. Howver, we have excluded those cases where pericardial effusion could be proven by echocardiography.

In summary, early postoperative depression following coronary artery bypass grafting, its recovery, and stabilization at 3-6 months is now clearly established. This recovery can not be explained simply by the changes in loading conditions on the myocardium, which in fact if operating in isolation, would have resulted in changes in a direction opposite to those seen here. In the future this method provides us with a means whereby the mechanism may be better defined, whether a premedication program may be developed to reduce this depression to a minimum, or whether cardioprotective agents or procedures can reduce or eliminate this early postoperative depression.

References

1. Brower, R.W., Katen, H.J.ten, Serruys, P., Meester, G.T.: Regional ventricular shortening in man from juxtaposed radiopaque markers. Circulation *56*, III-19 (1977) (Abs.)
2. Brower, R.W., Meester, G.T., Katen, H.J.ten, Bos, E.: Correlation of saphenous vein bypass flow, reactive hyperemia, and regional shortening in the postoperative period. Circulation *56*, (1977) (Abs.)
3. Brower, R.W., Katen, H.J.ten, Meester, G.T.: A direct method for determining regional shortening after bypass surgery from radiopaque markers in man. Am. J. Cardiol. *41*, 1222-1229 (1978)
4. Brower, R.W., Serruys, P., Bos, E., Nauta, J.: Regional myocardial shortening in relation to graft reactive hyperemia and flow after coronary bypass surgery. J. Thorac. Cardiov. Surg. *77*, 92-100 (1979)

Indications for and Results of Reoperation

W. J. Keon

In the past few years, the surgical treatment of coronary artery disease has met with great enthusiasm. The saphenous vein bypass procedure has become the most widely used form of myocardial revascularization resulting in symptomatic improvement and return to normal activity [1-3]. Nevertheless, recently there have been reports of reoperation necessitated by residual or recurring angina resulting from failure of the original procedure, progression of disease, or inadequate primary revascularization [4-7].

We reported on our initial experience with reoperation in 1977 [8]. At that time we had completed reoperations on 34 men with no early or late mortality, and with complete relief from angina in 25 (73%) cases. Studies from other centers have reported acceptably low early mortality ranging from 2.8% [5]-12% [6]. However, the clinical results have varied considerably. Norwood and colleagues found that there was symptomatic improvement in only 48% of 23 patients, 30% of which were asymptomatic [7]. The Cleveland Clinic group reported an 87% improvement on follow-up of 202 patients with 65% asymptomatic [4]. Whereas, Allen and colleagues reported a 68% improvement in 62 patients with 31% asymptomatic [5].

The present study updates the results at the University of Ottawa Cardiac Unit.

Clinical Material and Methods

Of 2124 coronary artery bypass operations done at the University of Ottawa Cardiac Unit up until 31 December 1977, 77 (3.6%) have been reoperations. Three patients had their initial surgery at other centers. Seventy-four patients had two operations and three have had three operations. There were 74 men and 3 women with a mean age of 45.6 years at second operation. The mean duration between surgical episodes was 28.4 months with a range of 2 weeks to 108 months.

At the time of reoperation single-vessel disease was documented in two cases, double-vessel disease in 21 cases and triple-vessel disease in 54 cases. Table 1 illustrates the procedures performed in addition to direct coronary artery bypass grafting. There was an overall decrease in the number of additional procedures performed at second surgery (30) than at first surgery (44) but, left mammary implants and endarterectomies were the procedures most often performed in both series.

Table 2 summarizes the pre-OR # 1 ventricular classifications and change in ventricular classifications between the two operative procedures. Classification of left ventricular function is determined by a joint decision of cardiologists, cardiac surgeons, and radiologists, bases on a four segment

Table 1. Surgical procedures performed on patients undergoing reoperation

Procedures	O.R. #1	O.R. #2	O.R. #3
Coronary artery bypass grafts[a]	187	147	6
Exploration of graft	-	2	-
Left mammary implant	19	9	-
Double implant	3	-	-
LV resection	4	6	
Endarterectomy			
Single	15	8	-
Double	1	4	-
Aortic valve replacement[b]	1	1	-
Removal of mural thrombus and closure of LV perforation	-	1	-

[a] 1 saphenous vein graft to anterior descending vein

[b] AVR was done on the same patient at both operations

Table 2.

	N	I	II	III	IV
Prior to OR # 1	27	21	19	6	0
Prior to OR # 2	21	15	21	13	3
Change	↓6	↓6	↑2	↑7	↑3

assessment of the ventricle in the right anterior oblique view: Class I, one hypokinetic segment; Class II, two segments; Class III, three segments; and Class IV, four malfunctioning segments. Table 2 indicates that there was a general trend towards increased ventricular dysfunction between operations. Figure 1, a more detailed representation of the change in ventricular function, indicates six of the patients demonstrated improved ventricular function: two from Class I to normal; two from Class II to I and two from Class III to Class II. Eight of those patients originally classed as normal had increased dysfunction, three patients progressed to Class I: four progressed to Class II, four progressed to Class III and one progressed to Class IV. Only one patient in Class III progressed to Class IV.

At first surgery, 12 (15.5%) of the patients were classified as emergencies, nine as unstable angina, and five as acute myocardial infarction. At second surgery, only 6.5% were classed as emergencies, three with unstable angina and two with myocardial infarction.

Indications for Reoperation

The clinical indication for reoperation in most other studies has been severe, incapacitating angina [4,5,7]. This is not the case at the Ottawa Cardiac Unit where only 58 of 77 patients presenting for reoperation had angina. Table 3 presents a summary for the indications for reoperation in this patient population as defined in our unit. The two patients presenting with angiographic demonstration of technical operative failure did not have angina. In one case, the distal anastomosis of the circumflex graft was inadvertently made above the area of stenosis (Fig. 1). In another patient, the anatomy

Table 3. Indications for reoperation

Indication	Symptomatology With angina	Symptomatology without angina	Duration between operations
Angiographic demonstration of technical operative failure	0	2	1 months
Occlusion or several stenosis of grafts	20	12	9.2 months
Progression of disease	12	1	55.2 months
Occlusion or stenosis of grafts and progression of disease	29	4	36.8 months

was mistaken and two diagonal grafts were performed instead of two marginal grafts. The mean time between operations for these patients was 1 month and the technical errors were demonstrated at routine angiography performed 3 weeks after the first operation.

Of the 32 patients requiring operation because of occlusion or severe stenosis of one or more of the existing grafts, only 20 presented with angina. In the remaining 12 patients, the indication for reoperation was discovered at routine postoperative angiography (Fig. 3). The mean duration between operations for this group of patients was 9.2 months.

Thirteen patients required reoperation because of progression of disease in the native coronary vessels (angiographic illustration, Fig. 4). Twelve of these patients presented with angina and the mean duration of time between operations for this group of patients was 55.2 months.

Reoperation in the final group of patients was indicated by both occlusion of one or more grafts and progression of disease (Fig. 5). Only 4 of 33 patients in this group were without angina and the mean duration between operations was 36.8 months.

Operative Procedures

Two of the patients at reoperation did not have new vein grafts and were not put on cardiopulmonary bypass. One patient had a local occlusion of the distal anastomosis through which a probe could be easily passed restoring good graft flow (75 ml/min). In the other patient with an anterior descending graft occlusion, the saphenous vein was found to be severely diseased and the mammary artery to anterior descending artery anastomosis was performed.

In five patients, the previous graft, now occluded, was resected with a new piece of vein bypassing the stenosed section. Three of these patients did not require cardiopulmonary bypass. In yet another case, an arteriotomy was performed followed by a vein angioplasty.

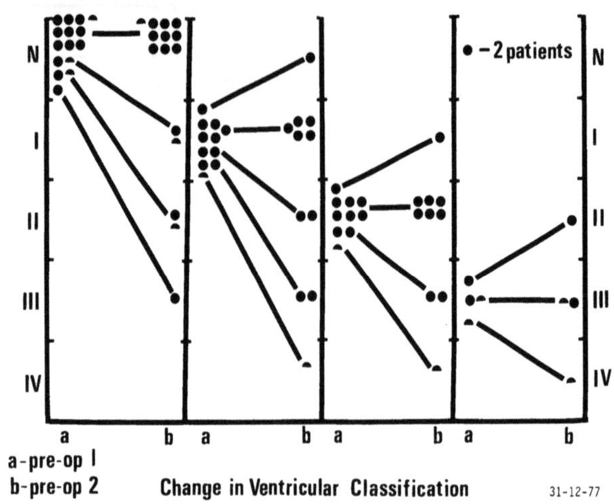

Fig. 1. Change in ventricular classifications between operations

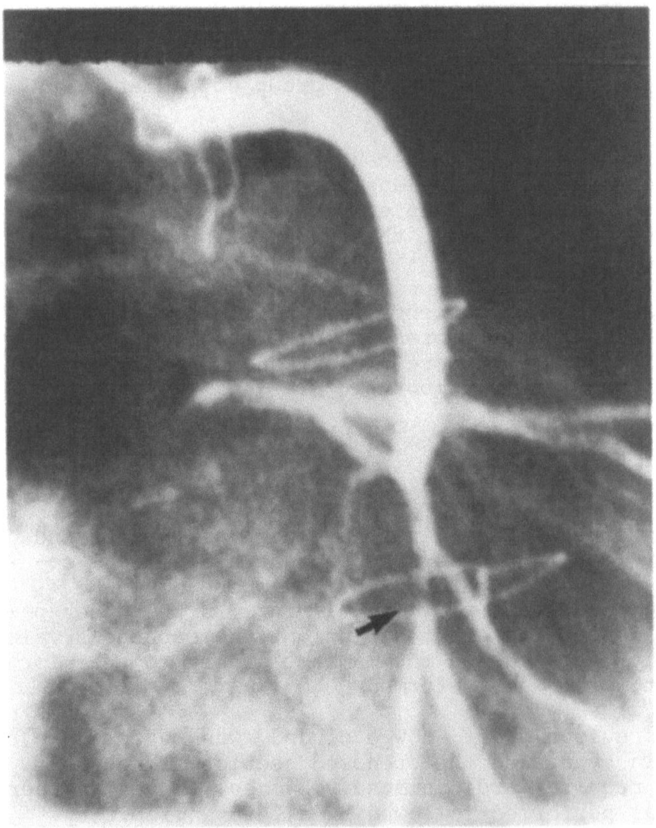

Fig. 2. Angiogram 3 weeks post-op # 1. Technical error at first operation. The graft has been placed proximal to the stenosis (arrow)

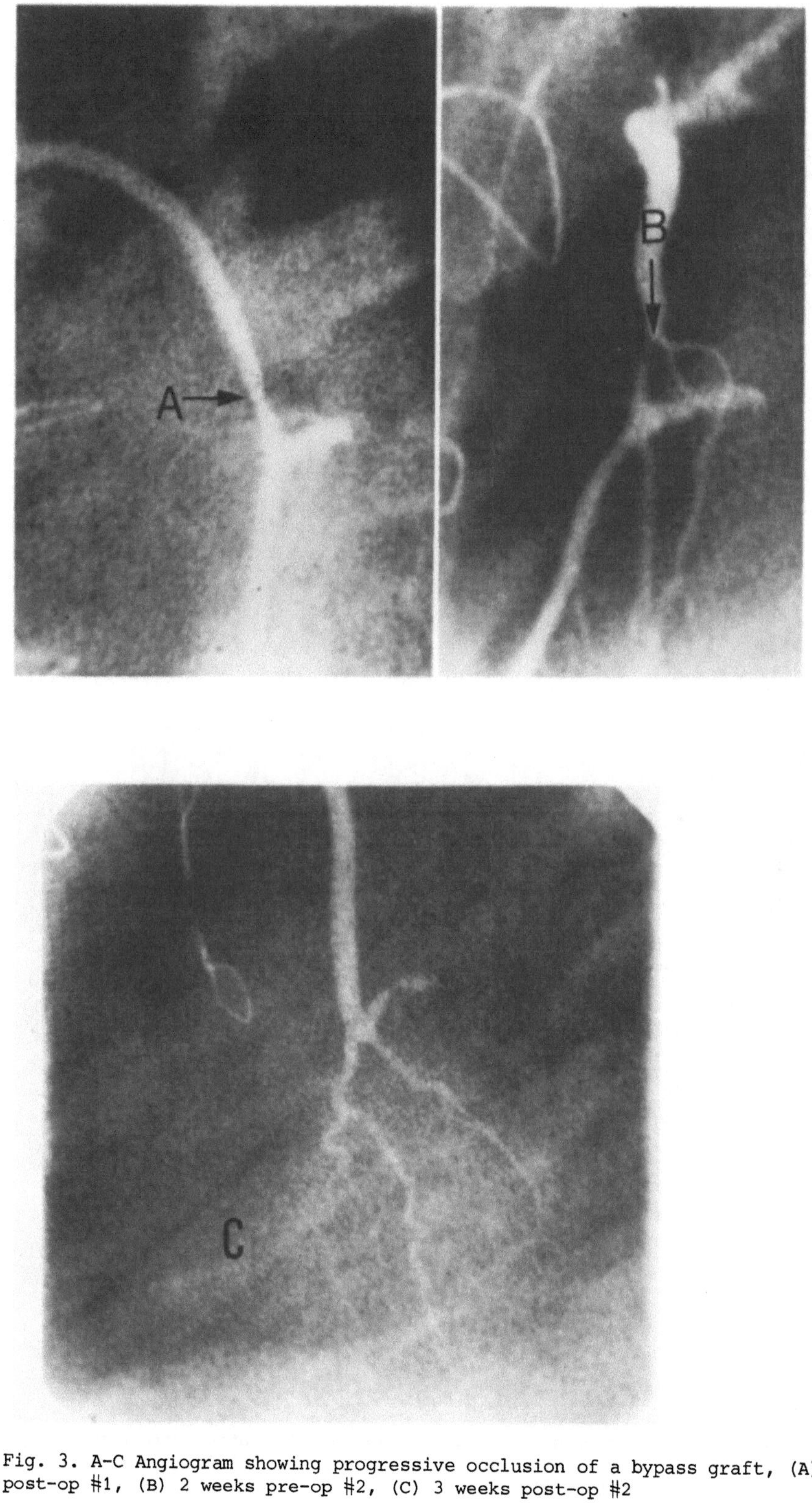

Fig. 3. A-C Angiogram showing progressive occlusion of a bypass graft, (A) early post-op #1, (B) 2 weeks pre-op #2, (C) 3 weeks post-op #2

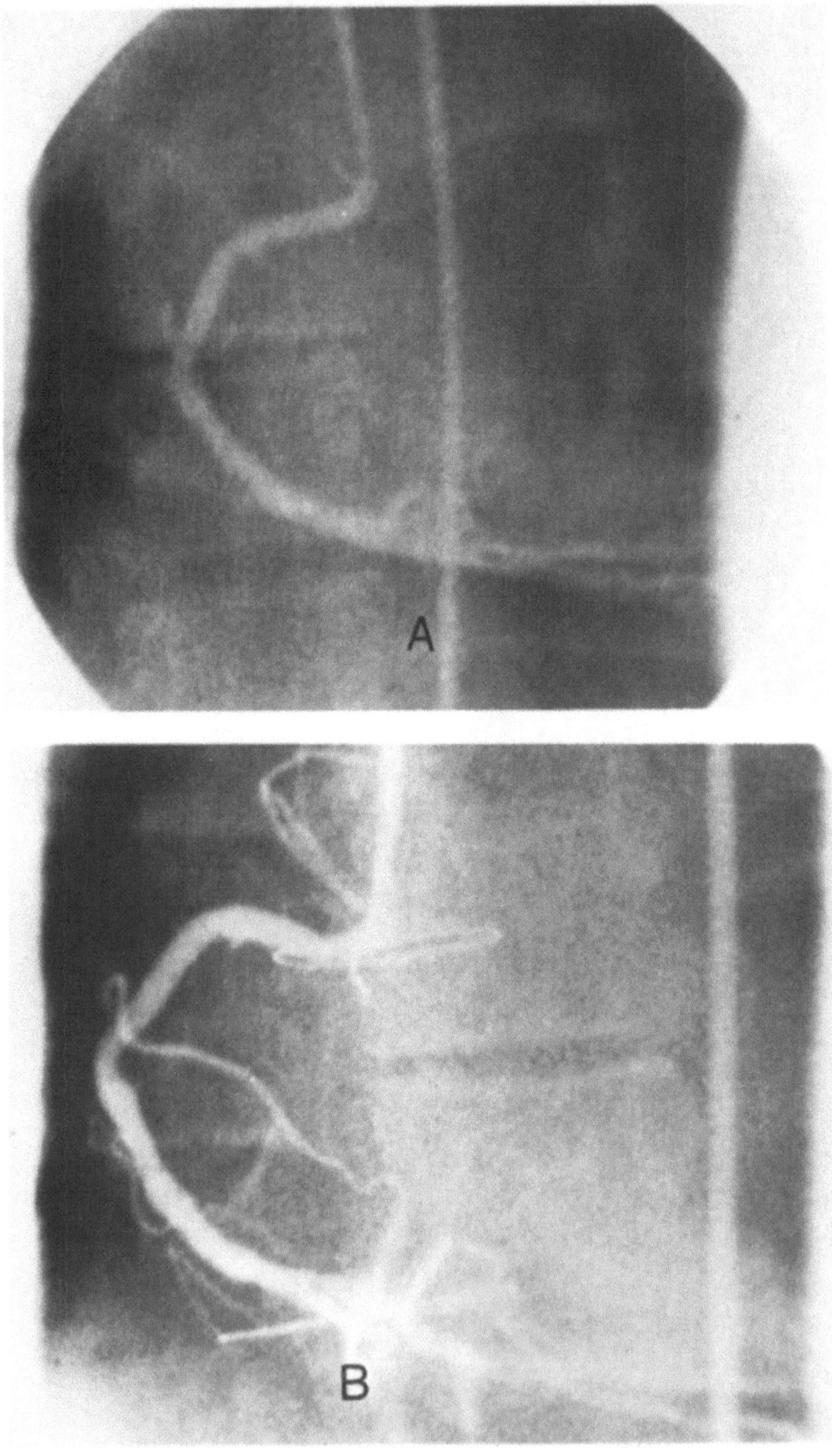

Fig. 4 A-D. Angiogram showing progression of disease in the native coronary artery; (A) pre-op #1, right coronary artery; (B) early post-op #1; (C) 23 months later, pre-op #2 and (D) 3 weeks post-op #2

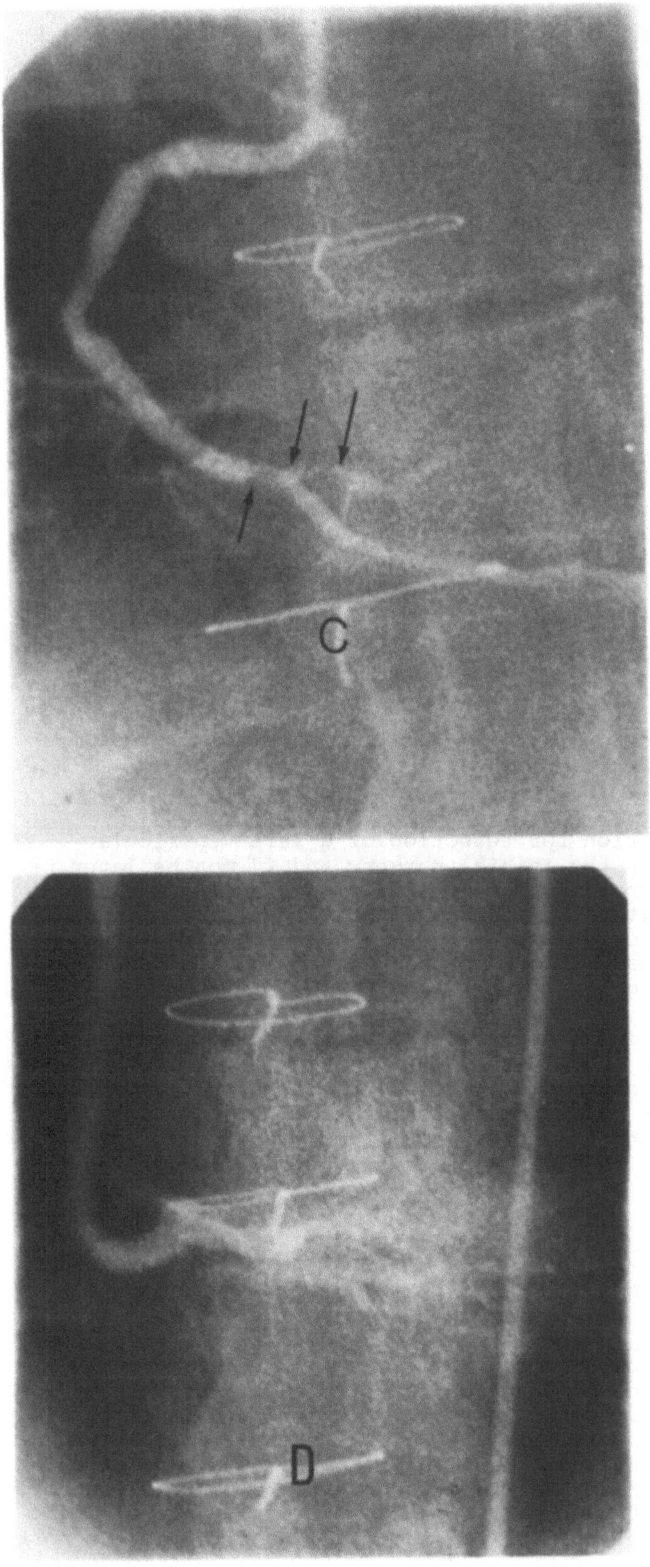

Fig. 4. Continued

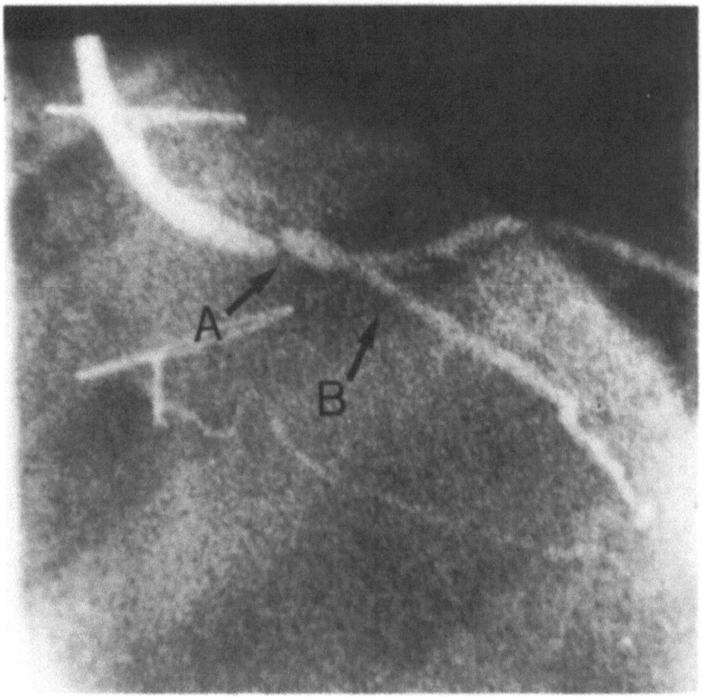

Fig. 5. Angiogram showing right coronary graft occlusion (A) and progression of disease (B) at 23 months postoperatively #1

One patient had reoperation for resection of a left ventricular aneurysm 46 months after the initial surgery and 17 months later he then required a third operation because of stenosis of the right graft. This was done without putting the patient on cardiopulmonary bypass. There were two other patients who did not require bypass at second operation; one had a right coronary graft and the other had a left anterior descending graft.

In most patients requiring reoperation for graft occlusion no new grafts were replaced in exactly the same position. Most of these were anstomosed a few millimeters distal to the previous anastomosis. One patient had a saphenous bypass graft to an anterior descending vein rather than an artery and this graft was found to be occluded at follow-up angiography despite an intra-operative blood flow of 260 ml/min.

Technical Considerations

There have been reports in the literature concerning technical complications encountered on reoperation. Stiles et al. reported in 1976 [6] that in five cases of reoperation functioning grafts were divided as the sternum was being opened and that the right and left ventricle were perforated on one occasion. Three of these individuals died. Allen et al. [5] reported that technical complications were uncommon with only one laceration of the right ventricle and one division of a patent graft. Neither of these complications adversely affected the outcome of the operation. Most of the technical complications reported occurred during the opening of the sternum. In our series of patients we had one patient with a functional graft divided on reopening the sternum and a second patient who had a perforation of the left ventricle. Both of these were corrected without an adverse effect on the patient.

We use several methods of reopening the chest, each depending on the individual situation. We have used the Stryker saw, sternal saw, and Luebsche knife, or a combination of the above. With our earlier reoperation cases we used normothermic perfusion and anoxic myocardial arrest. More recently we have changed to hypothermic potassium arrest at $5^{o}C$. We do not routinely close the pericardium at first surgery and have not encountered any difficulties at reoperation attributable to this.

Results

One patient died in the perioperative period at 4 weeks of congestive heart failure, for an operative mortality rate of 1.3%. One patient died at 9 months and the cause of death is unknown. The 77 patients included in this study received, at initial operation, an average of 2.4 grafts per patient and at second operation an average of 1.9 grafts per patient. There was no significant difference in the number of vessels grafted per patient in the symptomatically improved group as compared to those patients who remained in the same New York Heart Association Classification postoperatively (excluding the patients who were asymptomatic preoperatively).

Of the surviving patients 68 of 75 have been followed up at a mean of 22.5 months (6 weeks - 60 months). Using the NYHA classification system, 40 patients are asymptomatic, 19 are Class II, 8 are Class III and 1 is Class IV. Excluding those who were asymptomatic prior to the operation, 16 patients have improved by one class, 2 patients have improved by two classes and 10 patients have improved by three classes. Nine patients have remained in the same class.

The work status is known on 62 of the patients receiving follow-up. Forty-five patients are working fulltime and one is working part-time, this one is a housewife who requires assistance in heavier housekeeping duties. Of the remaining 16 patients, 9 are not working because of disabling angina, 1 Class IV and 8 Class III. One patient who is not employed due to no work being avialable is capable of working. Six patients are retired and their mean age is 61.5 years (range 51-66).

The incidence of perioperative infarction at first operation was four (5.2%) and at second operation was eight (10.4%). Seventeen patients (22%) had myocardial infarctions during the interval between the two surgical procedures.

Forty-one patients (53%) with 62 grafts received routine postoperative angiography. The patency rate was 76% (47/62). These grafts were widely patent with good distal runoff. The remaining 15 grafts were occluded. This figure of 76% is significantly lower than our total patency rate of 89% of 1,400 grafts studied postoperatively.

At first operation, the mean graft flow recorded intra-operatively was 74 ml/min for patent grafts and 71 ml/min for occluded grafts, resulting in an overall mean rate of 72.5 ml/min. The graft flow was highest (97 ml/min) in those with a technical error.

The mean flow in patients reoperated for graft occlusion was 70 ml/min and for patients who had progression of disease and graft occlusion, the mean flow was 69 ml/min.

At second operation, the mean flow recorded intra-operatively was 64.6 ml/min. Of the 62 grafts studied postoperatively, the mean flow in the 47 patent grafts was 72 ml/min as compared to a mean flow of 65 ml/min for the 15 occluded grafts. Although there are differences in the blood flows, they are not statistically significant. It is interesting to note that four of eight patients having perioperative infarcts at reoperation had one occluded graft at angiographic follow-up. One of these patients is in NYHA Class IV and is not working. The other three patients are all working, two are NYHA Class I and the third is NYHA Class II.

Discussion

The number of reoperations for myocardial revascularization performed at our unit has increased in recent years. It has progressed from 1.2% of the cases done in 1972 to 3.5% of the cases done in 1977. This is not unexpected since the total postoperative population from which the reoperation candidates are derived is cumulative. The rate is slightly higher than the 2%-3% reported by the Cleveland Clinic [4].

There is no denying that the hazards of performing repeat myocardial revascularization are very real [6,7,9,10]. They are normally attended by a higher surgical mortality although this is not the case with our own experience with an operative mortality of 1.3%. There is also a risk of damaging functioning grafts, the native coronary circulation, or the heart musculature itself. We had only one case of damaging the functioning graft and this was repaired without incident. On one occasion the left ventricle was perforated on opening the chest and this also was repaired without incident. It would appear that most complications arise on opening the sternum. Various precautions such as requesting the aneasthetist to deflate the lungs, dividing the sternum from the lower xyphisternal and upward, gentle dissection of the heart from the under surface of the sternum, and retrograde dissection of the functioning grafts to their origin at the aorta can assist in reducing technical problems. Certainly, the anticipation of technical problems at second operation is not sufficient reason to deny a patient second surgery particularly if that patient is incapacitated with angina.

It should be noted that at most institutions the primary indication for cardiac catheterization in reoperation was recurring disabling angina [4-7]. Approximately 30% of the surgical caseload in our Unit is referred by the National Defence Medical Centre where follow-up angiography is done on a routine basis at 3 weeks and 1 year postoperatively. Table 4 illustrates the advantages of routine angiography. Of the 607 patients referred to us from the National Defence Medical Centre, 37 (6%) have had reoperation. The late mortality for the 607 patients has been only 1.1%. The reoperation rate for the remaining patients is only 2.5% or 37 of 1,437 patients. The late mortality for this group of patients is 7.3%. Of the 77 patients presented in this series, 58 (75%) had angina of varying degrees. However, 19 (25%) patients had conditions which indicated the necessity for reoperation (Table 3) and these were discovered at routine follow-up angiography. The considerable increase in late mortality (6.2%) on those patients not having routine postoperative angiography

Table 4. Angiographic follow-up[a]

Referred from	# of patients	Reoperations #	Reoperations %	Late mortality #	Late mortality %
NDMC	607	37	6	7	1.1
OCH	1437	37	2.5	105	7.3

[a] Excludes 3 patients who had their first surgery at another center

and the fact that 25% of the patients requiring reoperation were asymptomatic underlines the importance of routine follow-up angiography. It is not only valuable in assessing the results of surgery but it leads to an early diagnosis of inadequacies resulting from the first operation. In this way, a second operation is not unduly delayed until symptoms are present and therefore, the late mortality decreases.

The major dilemma with routine follow-up angiography remains. That is, that some asymptomatic patients will have evidence of a defective operation (2 of 77). This leaves them at serious risk of infarction and/or death. We have reported on these two patients in an attempt to diminish these risks. We also believe that adequate assessment of the effect of initial revascularization on late mortality can not be made unless the operation is satisfactory from a technical point of view, and that the criteria defining "satisfactory technical operation" will require further study.

It has become well accepted that initial direct revascularization procedures result in complete relief or marked reduction of angina [1]. Our clinical results of reoperation suggest that it also is successful. Of 68 patients available for follow-up, 78% of those who were symptomatic prior to reoperation improved postoperatively. In addition, the rate of return to work is 74%.

It has been reported that most graft failures occur within the first few weeks postoperatively [11,12]. In our series of patients, it appears that when graft occlusion occurs, it is in the early stages postoperatively. The interval between operations for the patients with occluded grafts was 9.2 months as compared to 36.8 months and 55.2 months respectively for those patients with occlusion or stenosis of grafts in addition to progression of disease and those patients with progression of disease alone. There was no direct correlation between blood flow recorded intra-operatively at either first or second operation and subsequent occlusion of the graft. This gives support to our earlier theory [8] that low flows at operation are not necessarily indicative of future graft occlusion.

Conclusions

In summary, we conclude that an aggressive approach is necessary when patients whose follow-up angiography, whether routine or necessitated by recurrent symptoms, indicates a vascular deficit that is potentially correctable. Despite the fact that reoperation is technically challenging, repeat surgery for myocardial revascularization can be performed without undue morbidity or mortality and is justified by the improved clinical conditions observed in previously symptomatic patients. The results presented here also indicate that effective rehabilitation can be accomplished. In addition, we suggest that routine postoperative angiography should be considered. Even though it increases the rate of reoperation, it appears to reduce the late mortality following initial aortocoronary bypass grafting by revealing indications for reoperation in those patients who are asymptomatic and who may be at serious risk of sudden death.

References

1. Mundth, E.D., Austen, W.G.: Surgical measures for coronary heart disease. N. Engl. J. Med. *293*, 13, 75, 124 (1975)
2. Alderman, E.L., Matlof, H.J., Wexler, L. et al.: Surgery for the treatment of angina pectoris. N. Engl. J. Med. *288*, 535 (1973)
3. Cannon, D.S., Miller, D.C., Shumway, N.E. et al.: Long-term follow-up of patients undergoing saphenous vein bypass surgery. Circulation *49*, 77 (1977)
4. Irarrazaval, H.J., Cosgrove, D.M., Loop, F.D. et al.: Reoperations for myocardial revascularization. J. Thorac. Cardiovasc. Surg. *73*, 181 (1977)
5. Allen, R.H., Stinson, E.B., Dyer, P.E. et al.: Predictive variables in reoperations for coronary artery disease. J. Thorac. Cardiovasc. Surg. *75*, 186 (1978)
6. Stiles, Q.R., Lindesmith, G.G., Tucker, B.L. et al.: Experience with fifty repeat procedures for myocardial revascularization. J. Thorac. Cardiovasc. Surg. *72*, 849 (1976)
7. Norwood, W.I., Cohn, L.H., Collins, J.J.: Results of reoperation for recurrent angina pectoris. Ann. Thorac. Surg. *23*, 9 (1977)
8. Keon, W.J., Bedard, P., Akyurekli, Y. et al.: Experience with reoperation following coronary bypass grafting. Can. J. Surg. *28*, 142 (1977)
9. Skow, J.R., Carey, J.S., Plested, W.G. et al.: Saphenous vein bypass as a second cardiac procedure. Arch. Surg. *107*, 34 (1973)
10. Johnson, W.D., Hoffman, J.F. (Jr.), Flemma, R.J. et al.: Secondary surgical procedure for myocardial revascularization. J. Thorac. Cardiovasc. Surg. *64*, 523 (1972)
11. Alderman, E.L., Harrison, D.C., Shumway, N.E.: Longevity and symptom relief in four year follow-up of coronary surgical patients. Proceedings of the 2 Henry Ford International Symposium on Cardiac Surgery. Detroit, 1975. (in press) (1978)
12. Lesperance, J., Bourassa, M.G., Saltiel, J. et al.: Changes in aortocoronary vein grafts: Lack of progression of disease beyond the first year. Circulation *48*, 633 (1973)

6. What Can be Done to Improve Long-Term Results and Vocational Rehabilitation?

Recent Changes in Incidence and Course of Hepatitis After Heart Surgery

M. Kaltenbach, L. Krehan, K. Wolf, and P. Satter

In this report I would like to comment very briefly on a type of hepatitis about which still very little is known. The disease is often mild and remains sometimes even unrecognized. However, in a certain percentage a chronic form develops which impairs considerably the rehabilitation following heart surgery. Therefore, it seems justified to discuss the problem at this occasion.

In the past 8 years hepatitis B was observed in our institution with an incidence of about 5% (Fig. 1). In the 1 year period from spring 1976 to 1977 a different form of hepatitis was observed. This disease occurred with an incidence of about 30%, the clinical entity of the disease being consistently different from hepatitis B (Table 1).

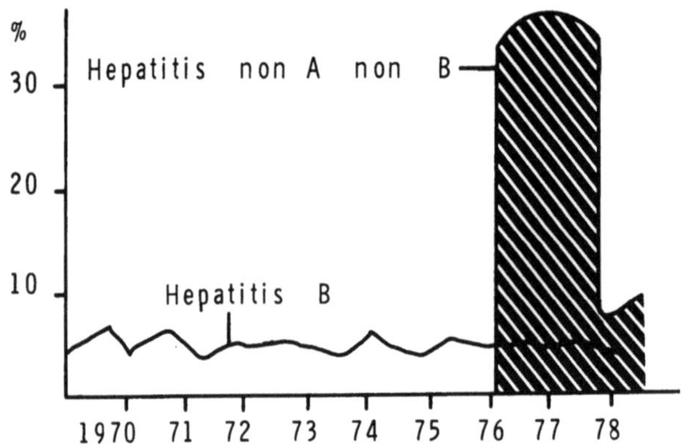

Fig. 1. Incidence of the two different forms of hepatitis between 1970 and 1978 in Frankfurt

Table 1. Incidence and main symptoms of hepatitis B and the new form of hepatitis

1970 - 1978	1976 - 1977
~5% Hepatitis B	~30% Hepatitis non A non B
Onset 4 weeks to 6 months after surgery	2-8 weeks after surgery
SGOT~400-1000 U/l SGPT~200- 500 U/l	SGOT~20-150 U/l SGPT~20-250 U/l
Bilirubin 10-30 mg%	Bilirubin~1-2 mg%
Australia antigen +	Australia antigen - Austrailia antibody ±

Table 2. Serum enzyme levels of 19 patients suffering from hepatitis non-A non-B

n = 19	$\bar{x}$	range	normal
GOT	51 mU/ml	8-168	4-19
GPT	77 mU/ml	10-297	6-19
AP	260 mU/ml	60-428	<190
γGT	103 mU/ml	14-267	<28

The patients had usually no clinical distress. The rise in enzyme levels started 2-8 wekks after surgery, the values returning to normal within 6-12 months (Table 2). In 10%-20% of patients a chronic form of hepatitis persisted over a period of more than 1.5 years. Among a total of about 150 affected patients, so far no deaths were reported.

In 1977 a questionnaire was sent to 12 other heart centers in Germany. Nine reported somewhat similar findings. Three rehabilitation centers observed the disease in one group of their patients, while the other group was free. The difference dependet on where the patients had been previously operated; thus, it is clearly established that the higher incidence is real, and not the consequence of a more careful observation in certain groups of patients.

In our own experience a clear change in epidemiology was found in so far as the disease started in early 1976 and finished more or less 1 year later. However, it still occurs in a smaller percentage. A similar observation with an outburst and a disappearance of the disease after several months was made in at least one other place in Germany. The appearance and disappearance of the disease was not related to any measure which we could define. The absolute number of operated patients in our hospital had steadily increased during the past 10 years.

No specific prophylaxis for this type of hepatitis was introduced, although the prophylaxis against hepatitis B consists in our institution of autolog retransfusion. Since 1970 most patients receive retransfusion of 0.4-1.2 liter blood which is taken from the patients in the preoperative period, i.e., within 30-10 days prior to surgery. This type of prophylaxis was found to be helpful in keeping the incidence of serum hepatitis low, but apparently had no influence on the new type of hepatitis.

In conclusion it seems that in many heart centers in Germany an undefined type of hepatitis is observed. The disease is usually anicteric and different from hepatitis A and hepatitis B and might therefore be called hepatitis non-A non-B. The clinical course is mostly mild, however, a chronic form can result, producing long morbidity. The pathogenesis of the disease is unclear. No findings were obtained pointing towards any known viral infection or any toxic or allergic mechanism. An infectious nature of the disease in relation to blood transfusion seems most likely.

Contributing Factors Preventing Return to Work of Cardiac Surgery Patients

P. David

This paper presents the preliminary results of a very recent study to determine the factors associated with the return to work of patients who have had successful coronary bypass operation.

From 31 January 1973 to 1977, a total of 1,534 patients have had such an operation at the Montréal Heart Institute. We eliminated 33 male patients who were 65 years or older, 79 known deaths, 235 female and 268 patients who had not returned their questionnaire by 15 January. The results of the remaining 919 male survivors were tabulated (Table 1).

The patients were divided into three groups (Table 2): those who were working at the time of the survey (W), those who had worked and stopped (WS), and those who had never returned to work (NW).

Of the working patients 98% stated that their health was good, as compared to 90% of those who had stopped, and 84% who had never worked. This last percentage is surprising and indicates that the subjective feeling of the patient is not a major factor.

In this series, 63% were working at the time of the survey, 13% had worked and stopped and 24% had never worked (Table 3).

Table 1. Coronary bypass surgery Jan. 1973 - Aug. 1977 (4.8 years)

No.	Patients	%
33	Male ≥65 y.	2
79	Known deaths	5
235	Female	15
268	Have not answered	18
919	Studied	60
1534	Total	100

Table 2. Subjective evaluation of health in 909 patients

	No.	Good	Poor
W	581	98%	2%
WS	112	90%	10%
NW	216	84%	16%

Table 3. Percentage of patients working or not working at time of inquiry and after surgery

At time of inquiry	919 Male survivors under 65 years at operation	After operation
63%	584 are working	76%
37%	113 have worked and stopped	
	222 have never worked	24%
53.4 years	50.7 years	Mean age

Table 4. Attitude of employer

	No.	Positive	Negative
W	472	96%	4%
WS	98	90%	10%
NW	142	75%	25%
Total	712	91%	9%

With a mean age of 53.4 years at the time of the follow-up, it was upsetting to find 37% of nonworking patients in whom more than 90% declared themselves in good health. In a previous study, we did an objective evaluation of the nonworking patients. There was a close correlation between the subjective and objective evaluation. Therefore, we must conclude that other factors than health play a major role in the return to work.

In the questionnaire, we tried to determine the attitude of the employer, and surprisingly, in 91% of the 712 patients who had an employer, it was described as positive (Table 4).

In 646 patients who felt that the employer had a positive attitude, 70% were working at the time of inquiry. When the attitude of the employer was felt as negative, the same percentage of patients were not working (Table 5).

In 869 patients, the description of the work done before operation was divided into two main categories: light and hard. The two groups were about equal. In the category of light work, 70% were working and 20% had not returned to work, as compared to 55% and 30%, in the group of hard work. The working prognosis was better for patients who had light work before operation (Table 6).

We divided our population into three groups: 362 patients who were less than 50 years old, 441 patients who were between 50 and 59 years of age, and 116 who were between 60 and 64 years of age (Table 7).

Table 5. Attitude of employer according to 712 patient replies

	No.	W	WS	NW
Positive	646	70%	14%	16%
Negative	66	30%	15%	55%

Table 6. Type of work before operation (869 patients)

	No.	W	WS	NW
Light	455	70%	10%	20%
Hard	414	55%	15%	30%

Table 7. Age at time of operation

	No.	W	WS	NW
20-49 yrs.	362	74%	11%	15%
50-59 yrs.	441	53%	12%	25%
60-64 yrs.	116	32%	18%	50%
All ages	919	64%	12%	24%

Table 8. Education (908 patients)

	No.	W	WS	NW
Lower	735	59%	14%	27%
Higher	173	83%	5%	12%

In the 20-49 years range of patients, 74% were working, as compared to 63% in the 50-59 years range and 32% in those who were 60-64. In this last group, 50% of the patients had never worked.

The importance of age in returning to work is not only logical, but also well documented: the younger, the better. It remains bothersome that 26% of the younger group and 37% in the middle age group were not working.

At the age of 60, there is only one chance out of two to bring a patient back to work.

Regarding education, 908 patients were divided into two categories. Lower education included patients who had anywhere from 0-10 years of education. Higher education included 11 years or more. With such a classification, 735 patients (81%) had lower education and 173 a higher education. With a higher education, 83% of the patients were working, as compared to 59% in the second group. Subgroups demonstrated a clear relation between the degree of education and the return to work (Table 8).

Table 9. Preoperative period of inactivity in 865 patients

	No.	0-3 mo	4-6 mo	7+ mo
W	546	66%	16%	18%
WS	108	58%	17%	25%
NW	211	21%	15%	64%

Table 10. Preoperative period of inactivity in 865 patients

	No.	W	WS	NW
0-3 mo	467	77%	13%	10%
4-6 mo	134	64%	13%	23%
7+ mo	264	39%	10%	51%

Table 9 illustrates a very important factor. In the 546 workers, 66% had a preoperative period of inactivity of 3 months or less, 16% a 4-6 months delay and 18% a 7 months or more period of inactivity. In the 211 patients who had never worked, these data were strictly reversed and 64% of the patients had a preoperative inactivity lasting 7 months or more.

In 467 patients (54%) who had a preoperative inactivity of 3 months or less, 77% are working as compared to only 39% in the 264 patients who had a preoperative inactivity of 7 months or more. From these data, we can assume that the prognosis of working for a patient who has stopped working for 7 months or more before the operation is very poor (Table 10).

In the 572 patients who were working, the postoperative convalescence was less than 6 months in 87%. In those who had worked and stopped, this percentage was 70%. In the patients who had a convalescence of 7 months or more, only 13% were still working and 30% had worked and stopped. The return to work must then be settled within a maximum of 6 months after operation (Table 11).

The overall results can be seen in Table 3. The few articles written on this subject have given a range of return to work which varies from 50%-80%. Our own data can fit in both directions.

A percentage of 76% is obtained if we limit our study to patients who have effectively returned to work after operation. It drops to 63% if we analyse the photographic situation at the time of the survey.

Table 11. Postoperative convalescence

	No.	0-3 mo	4-6 mo	7+ mo
W	572	44%	43%	13%
WS	108	26%	44%	30%
Both	680	41%	44%	15%

This preliminary report was prepared for this meeting as a task force effort with the help of our social workers and Dr. Daniel Fagret. Though 93% of the patients feel well, only 63% were working at the time of the survey. The reasons for such a discrepancy were shown. They were mostly psychological, social, and economical. By increasing order of importance, we classified them as follows: attitude of the employer, type of work, age, education, and duration of inactivity before and after operation.

If we consider the cost of these 919 coronary bypass patients, the social results are not satisfactory. With the fast growing number of coronary patients who are operated upon, we must find ways and means to enable our patients to remain working citizens. To avoid premature invalidism, we must promote new rehabilitation programs and convince health authorities, physicians, related professionals, and the patients themselves. Then, and only then, the beneficial effects of this surgical procedure will become rewarding for the individual and the society. Specialized and multidisciplinary programs of rehabilitation working closely with cardiac surgery departments seem a logical and practical approach.

Clinical Results and Social Implications in Patients After Coronary Bypass Surgery

G. Blümchen, E. Scharf-Bornhofen, D. Brandt, C. van den Bergh, and G. Bierck

The medical system in Germany differs from that of the United States. It is therefore difficult to compare the rates of patients returning to work after aortocoronary bypass surgery (ABC).

Approximately 90% of the German population is insured by goverment policy. The insurance is subdivided into "blue-collar" and "white-collar" workers. 10% of the population is insured independently, mainly professionals, e.g., lawyers, architects, doctors.

When severe disease prohibits working, blue- and white-collar workers are 18 months paid for 80% of their last income. Coronary artery disease and bypass surgery are considered by many patients and many doctors such a case. Most of these patients therefore wait for 18 months before returning to work or before applying for retirement.

In the German literature [1-4] about 50% of patients are found to return to work after aortocoronary bypass surgery, compared to about 80% in the United States [5]. This retrospective study was begun in order to find determinants for this discrepancy.

The following figures refer to the follow-up study of 314 patients: 207 blue-collar-, 97 white-collar workers, and 10 professionals.

We compared the results of the early postoperative period - up to 6 weeks after operation - with the social long-term outcome 18 months after operation (Fig. 1). On the left side of the figure, pre- and postoperative exercise tolerance and subjective data with respect to angina pectoris (AP) and dyspnea (D) are shown (better, same, worse after operation). The right side of the figure shows the long-term social outcome: pension, not working, working.

In all 314 patients before and shortly after surgery submaximal exercise-test, exercise tolerance was almost the same, although angina pectoris improved markedly. Symptoms of 13 patients did not change and 4 patients deteriorated postoperatively.

Eighteen months after surgery 20% received a pension, 25% returned to work, and the future of the remaining 55% remained undecided.

Postoperatively the "return-to-work" rate of aortocoronary bypass patients is disappointing. It is doubtful whether many of these patients will return to work, since they have become accustomed over a long period of time to the so-called benefits of a "tied social network."

We observed 207 blue-collar workers for 16 months after bypass operations. Pre- and postoperative (6 weeks after operation, submaximal test) exercise tolerance was almost the same. Subjective date improved (Fig. 2). Sixteen months after surgery 12% of the workers received a pension, 27% returned to work and the future of the remaining 61% remains undecided.

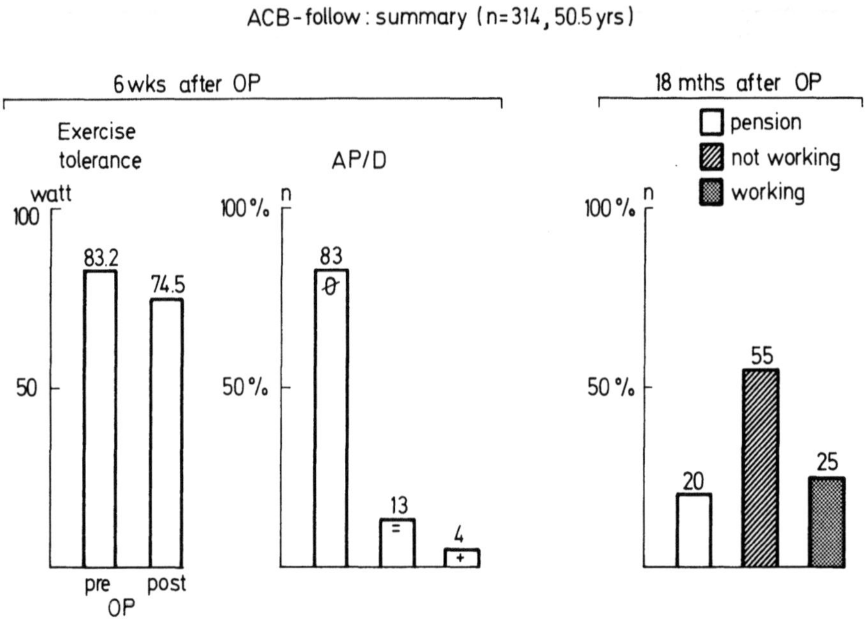

Fig. 1. Clinical results (6 weeks after surgery) after ABC in 314 patients (*left*) and the long-term outcome (18 months after surgery) with respect to "return to work" (*right*). Exercise tolerance: supine position; *AP* angina pectoris; *D* dyspnea; + better; = same; Ø worse

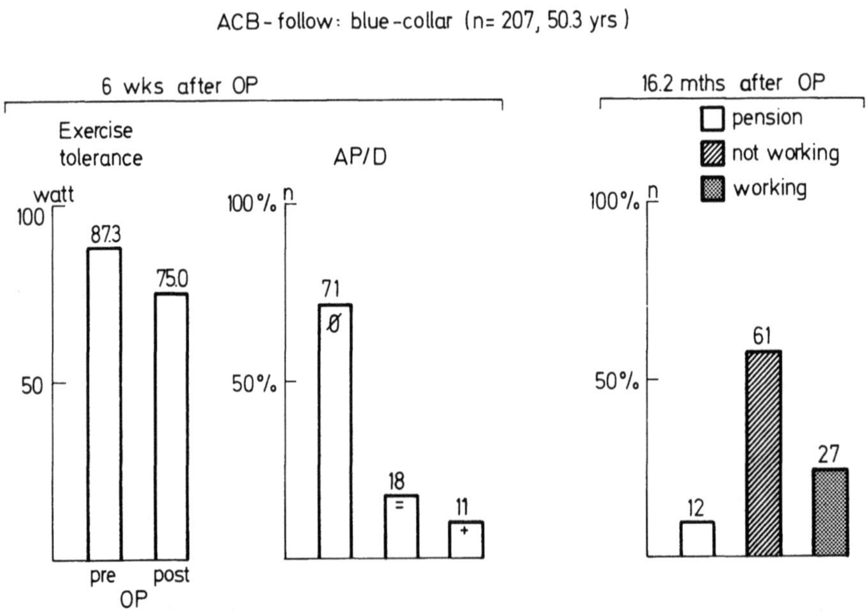

Fig. 2. Clinical results (6 weeks after surgery) after ABC in 207 blue-collar workers (heavy work) and the long-term outcome (16.2 months after surgery) in respect to "return to work." Exercise tolerance: supine position; *AP* angina pectoris; *D* dyspnea; + better; = same; Ø worse

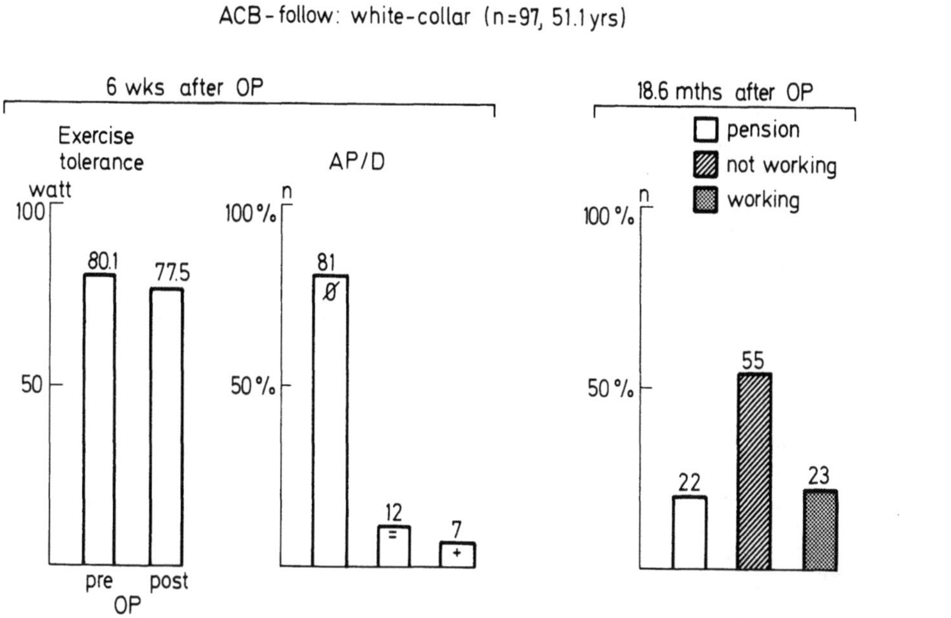

Fig. 3. Clinical results (6 weeks after surgery) after ACB in 97 white-collar workers (light work) and the long-term outcome (18.6 months after surgery) in respect to "return-to-work." Exercise tolerance: supine position; *AP* angina pectoris; *D* dyspnea; + better; = same; Ø worse

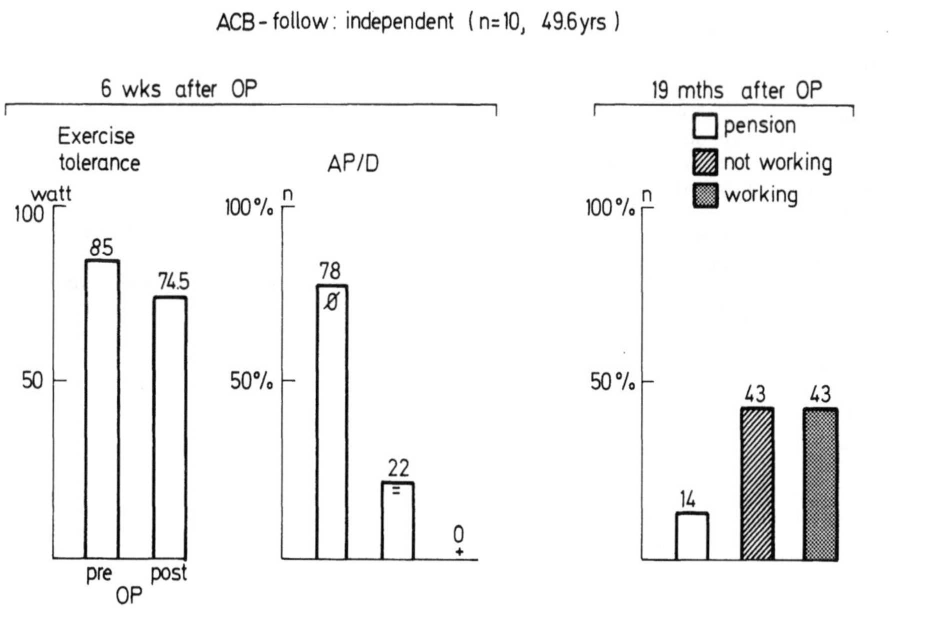

Fig. 4. Clinical results (6 weeks after surgery) after ACB in 10 professionals and the long-term outcome (19 months after surgery) in respect to "return-to-work". Exercise tolerance: supine position; *AP* angina pectoris; *D* dyspnea; + better; = same; Ø worse

Ninety-seven white collar workers were observed for 18.6 months after operation. Exercise tolerance before and 6 weeks after operation submaximal-test remained the same, although symptoms decreased markedly.

Of these workers 22% received a pension, 23% returned to work, and the future of the remaining 55% remains undecided. For a light-working population this is a disappointing longterm social result (Fig. 3).

Figure 4 shows the results of 10 professionals, who were privately insured. Exercise tolerance and symptoms 6 weeks after surgery did not differ from blue and white collar workers. Nineteen months after surgery 14% received a pension, 43% returned to work and the future of the remaining 43% remained undecided. The "return-to-work" rate of professionals was higher than that of blue- and white-collar workers, although the clinical findings shortly after operation (submaximal-test) do not differ in the three groups.

In summary, the long-term social outcome is not determined by the short-term medical results after aortocoronary bypass surgery. Good exercise tolerance and marked improvement of symptoms 6 weeks after aortocoronary bypass surgery do not guarantee a high "return to work" rate. The rate of patients returning to work is determined only to a small degree by medical results.

The main determinants for the long-term social outcome are the medical insurance system, the motivation of the patients, and - at least in Germany - the high rate of unemployment. Officials deciding about a pension or a "return to work" would rather give a 50-year-old man after aortocoronary bypass surgery a pension than send him back to work. This is especially true for patients performing heavy work. But this is also true for patients performing light work.

References

1. Gleichmann, U., Faßbender, D.: Probleme der Früh- und Spätrehabilitation nach Herzinfarkt. International Symposium: Der Herzinfarkt. Wien, 31.3.-2.4.1977
2. Lichtlen, P., Liese, W., Leit, K., Borst, H.G.: Postoperative Klinik nach aortokoronarem Venenbypass in Relation zum Ausmaß der Revaskularisation. Z. Kardiol. *67*, 83 (1978)
3. Neuhaus, L.: Probleme der Berufsaufnahme nach koronarchirurgischen Eingriffen. Med. Welt (in press) (1977)
4. Rothlin, M., Senning, A.: Indikationen, Risiko und Spätergebnisse der Koronarchirurgie. Internist *18*, 322 (1977)
5. Lawrie, G.M., Morris, G.C., Howelly, J.F., Spencer, W.H., Winters, W.L., Chapman, D.W., Ogura, J.W., Lie, J.T.: Clinical, angiographic and treadmill results of coronary bypass surgery, 5 to 7 years after operation. Am. J. Cardiol. *39*, 270 (1977)

Clinical Results and Return to Work After Coronary Heart Surgery

L. Benesch, K. L. Neuhaus, J. Rivas-Martin, and F. Loogen

Knowing that the return-to-work process after coronary heart surgery is influenced by many factors of medical, psychological and sociologic origin, we wanted to elucidate the influence of medical factors.

A questionnaire was sent to all patients who underwent coronary heart surgery in Düsseldorf, F.R.G. The replies and case histories were analyzed. The criteria for admission to this study were surgery between 1970 and September 1976, younger than 60 years of age, and no vascular heart disease or other disease limiting functional capacity. The shortest interval between surgery and this study was 9 months, the mean interval 22 months.

This study included 191 patients; 36 of these were self-employed, 102 office workers, and 53 laborers. The mean age of the entire group was 49 years of age. The self-employed patients and the laborers averaged 48, the office workers 50 years of age.

Only 20% of the patients worked up to 8 weeks or less before surgery and again postoperatively (Fig. 1). About one-third were preoperatively unable to work but resumed working postoperatively. The largest group, 44%, did not work pre- or postoperatively. Many of these patients were retired preoperatively because of coronary heart disease or for social reasons. Five percent of the patients were preoperatively employed but did not resume work postoperatively.

The average time of preoperative inability to work was 10 months, excluding the patients who were retired. The mean time for resumption of work postoperatively was 7 months; for the group of the selfemployed and the office workers 6; for the laborers 11 months.

Within the 3 vocational groups, the rate of those returning to work was the highest in the group of the self-employed patients (78%). The percentage for the office workers was 57, whereas only 21% of the laborers went back to work (Fig. 2). More than 50% of the laborers were retired preoperatively, excluding these, 44% of the laborers resumed working. With respect to their medical status, the retired workers followed the same pattern as all the patients taken together.

The criteria for the subjective postoperative result were the comparisons between the pre- and postoperative state concerning angina, functional capacity, and consumption of nigroglycerin. As objective criteria the number of diseased vessels, the number and function of aortocoronary bypass grafts, and the postoperative pulmonary artery pressure during exercise were examined in relation to the resumption of work.

Seventy-five percent of the patients stated that they were relived of angina (Fig. 3). This result is comparable to the observations of other groups. Of these patients 56% had resumed working. Within the

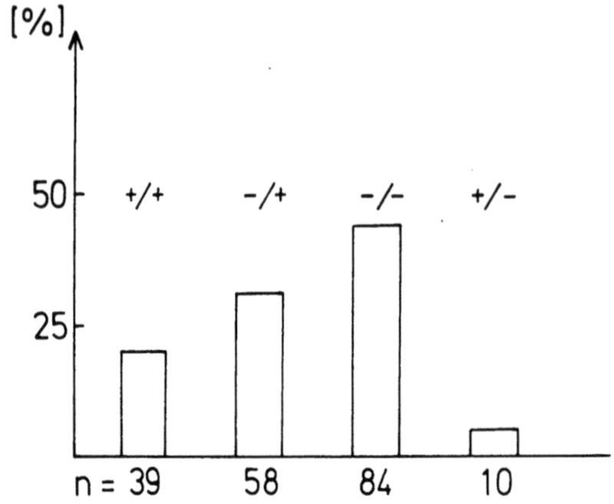

Fig. 1. Capability of work before and after surgery. +/+ working up to 8 wks. or less preop., regularly working postop.; -/- unemployed more than 8 wks. preop., unemployed postop.

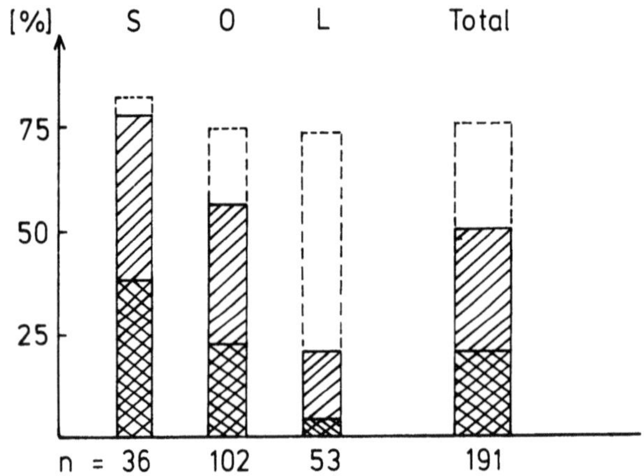

Fig. 2. Rate of return to work of the 3 vocational groups. *S* self-employed; *O* office worker, *L* laborer, preop. retired workers are indicated by broken lines. *Diagonally striped areas* pre- and postop. employed; *crisscrossed areas* preop. not working, postop. employed; *white area* postop. unemployed

subgroups, 78% of the self-employed, 64% of the office workers, and 24% of the laborers had returned to work.

Subjectively, the functional capacity of 68% of the patients had improved. Of these, 55% had resumed working; within the subgroups, 77% of the self-employed, 64% of the office workers and 16% of the laborers (Fig. 4).

To verify the symptomatic improvement, we inquired about nitro consumption. Eighty percent of the patients admitted to taking a small amount or none at all. Of these, 58% had returned to work; within the subgroups, 74% of the self-employed, 64% of the office workers and 26% of the laborers (Fig. 5). In summary, the symptomatically improved patients as a whole and as subdivided groups showed only a slightly higher rate of return to work than all the patients together.

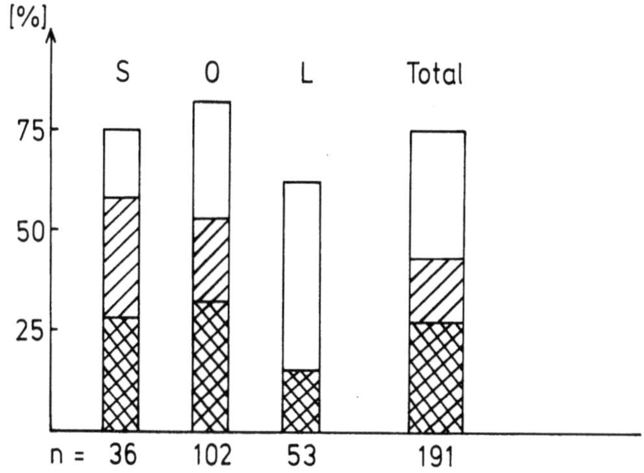

Fig. 3. Relief of angina and resumption of work. *Diagonally striped areas* pre- and postop. employed; *crisscrossed areas* preop. not working, postop. employed; *white area* postop. unemployed

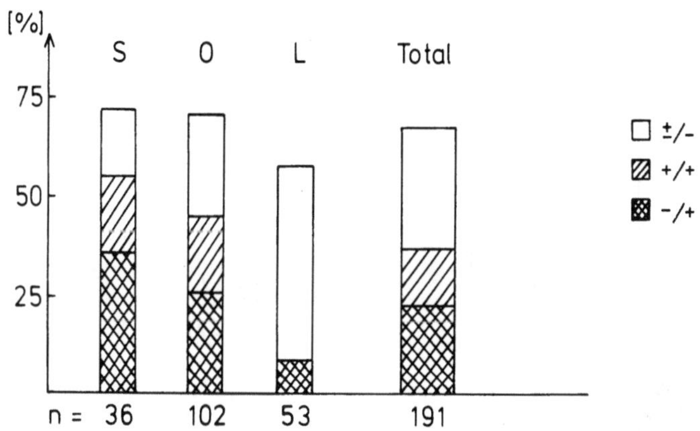

Fig. 4. Increase of functional capacity and resumption of work. *Diagonally striped areas* pre- and postop. employed; *crisscrossed areas* preop. not working, postop. employed; *white area* postop. unemployed

We studied the relation between the severity of coronary artery disease expressed as one-, two-, or three-vessel disease and the resumption of work. In all 3 subgroups, about 50% of the patients had returned to work (Fig. 6).

We found a similar situation in complete and incomplete revascularization (Fig. 7). Complete revascularization means the bypass grafting of all vessels with significant stenosis. The apparently high incidence of incomplete revascularization, about 47%, is due to the stenosed vessels not being bypassed because of technical or anatomic reasons and the rate of occluded grafts. In our group, the overall patency rate was 79%. Complete and incomplete revascularization appeared to have no influence on the resumption of work. In both groups, about 50% of the patients were postoperatively working.

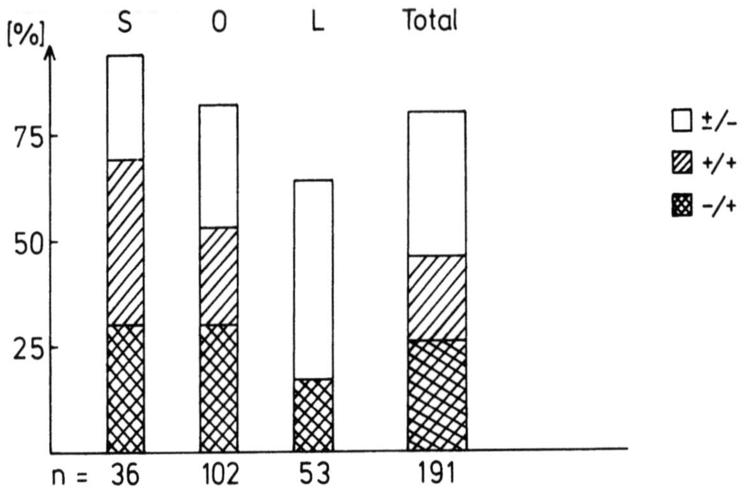

Fig. 5. Decrease of nitroglycerin consumption and resumption of work. *Diagonally striped areas* pre and postop. employed; *crisscrossed areas* preop. not working, postop. employed; *white area* postop. unemployed

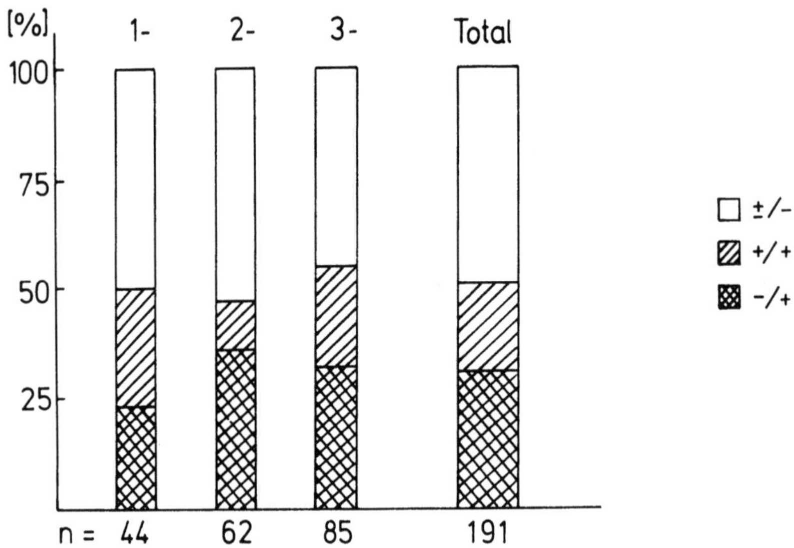

Fig. 6. One-, two-, or three-vessel disease and resumption of work. *Diagonally striped areas* pre- and postop. employed; *crisscrossed areas* preop. not working, postop. employed; *white area* postop. unemployed

In addition to the severity of coronary artery disease and the completeness of revascularization, we expected the level of the pulmonary artery pressure during exercise to have a significant influence on the resumption of work (Fig. 8). The mean pulmonary artery pressures during moderate exercise of 60 W were almost equal for the postoperatively employed and unemployed patients. The significance of this finding is limited because only one-third of the patients had

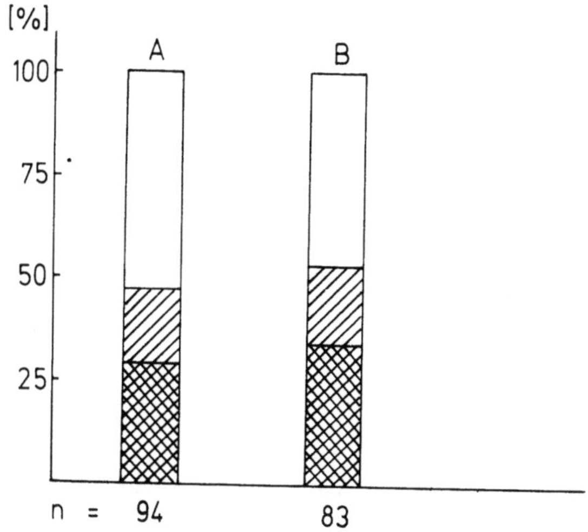

Fig. 7. Completeness of revascularization and resumption of work. *Diagonally striped areas* pre- and postop. employed; *crisscrossed areas* preop. not working, postop. employed

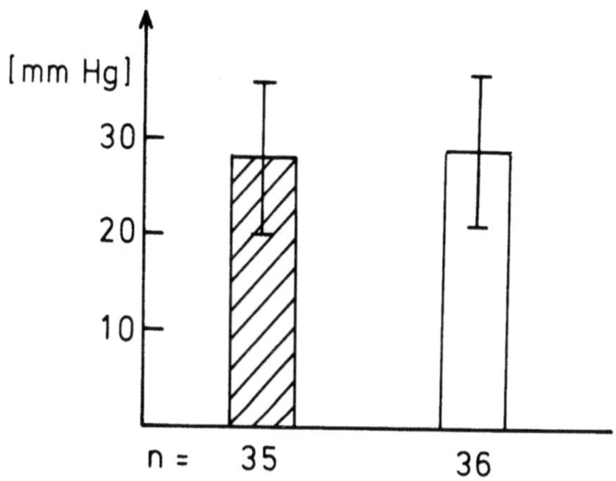

Fig. 8. Pulmonary artery pressure and resumption of work. *Striped area* postop. employed; *white area* postop. unemployed

an exercise test with measurement of the pulmonary artery pressure postoperatively.

In summary, we can say that the relation between the medical status and the postoperative resumption of work is surprisingly insignificant. The postoperative medical condition was not the determining factor in the return-to-work process in our group of patients.

In this context we tried to obtain information about the influence of rehabilitation programs (Fig. 9). As far as resumption of work is concerned, there was no recognizable advantage in having been in a rehabilitation center. The rate of those returning to work was higher in the patients who were not involved in a special rehabilitation program. The significance of this finding requires further investigation.

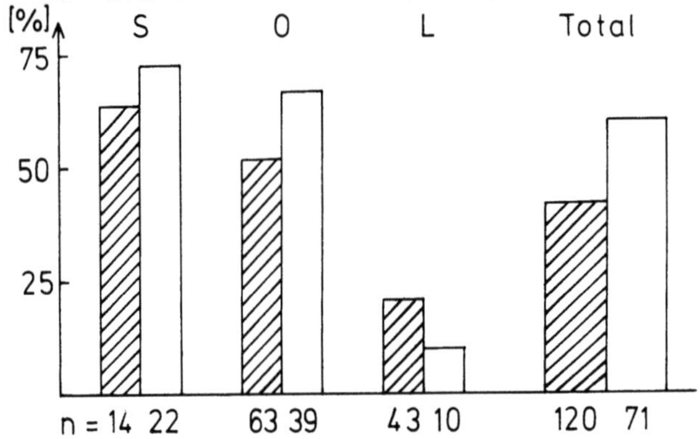

Fig. 9. Rehabilitation program and resumption of work. *Striped area* patients who spent some time in a rehabilitation center; *white area* patients who returned to work without having been in such a center

References

1. Tremblay, G., Biron, P., Pelletier, L.-C., Cossette, R., Dontigny, L., Proul, A.: Retour au travail après pontage aorto-coronarien. Union Méd. Can. *105*, 1206-1208 (1977)
2. Hollender, M.C., Abram, H.S.: Coronary artery bypass operation: psychological and medical problems. Int. J. Psychiatry Med. *5*, 67-80 (1974)

Need for Coronary Bypass Surgery in Europe

E. Varnauskas

There are several reasons for asking the question about the need for coronary bypass surgery (CABG). The medical rationale for the explosive spread of coronary bypass surgery in the United States is not entirely clear. It is questioned whether rapid and uncontrolled development has created demands which exceed the need.

The increasing proportion of the national budget spent for health care has, during recent years, reached in some countries a level which is causing considerable concern. Introduction of new methods of treatment requiring considerable expansion of budgets is met with demands for solid motivation. The available funds are more limited than before and the competition from many fields of medical care is hard.

The present situation of coronary bypass surgery in Europe is illustrated in Fig. 1. This graph includes approximate numbers of operations performed per year during the period 1976-1977 per million inhabitants in some selected European countries and in the United States. The numbers were provided by fellow cardiologists of renowned centers of the respective countries and do not represent official statistics. Although the absolute numbers are not necessarily correct they are acceptable for the purpose of comparison. The amount of coronary bypass surgery varies considerably from country to country. The United States represents the tallest column of the graph. The question arises which of the columns best represents the real need for bypass surgery or do they all represent a pattern of uncontrolled adaptation of a new surgical method?

There might be several approaches to evaluate the need for CABC in the community. A working group, convened by the World Health Organisation November 1977 in The Hague [1] adopted the approach based on the prevalence and incidence of angina pectoris meeting the criteria for surgery. I will give an account of this approach including the result of calculations.

It was considered that the indications for surgery are either definitely established or less well established. Only definitely established indications were considered to form the basis for assessment of the need. The less well established indications are under continuous investigation, which will hopefully provide the evidence for accepting these indications as definite or rejecting them completely.

Definitely established indications for CABG:
1) Severe stable angina not responding to optimal medical therapy
2) Unstable angina not responding to optimal medical therapy
3) Symptomatic left main coronary artery disease
4) Angina pectoris of any degree in patients with a cardiac lesion for which surgery is indicated.

Review of the epidemiologic evidence disclosed that adequate information is not available on the prevalence and incidence of angina pec-

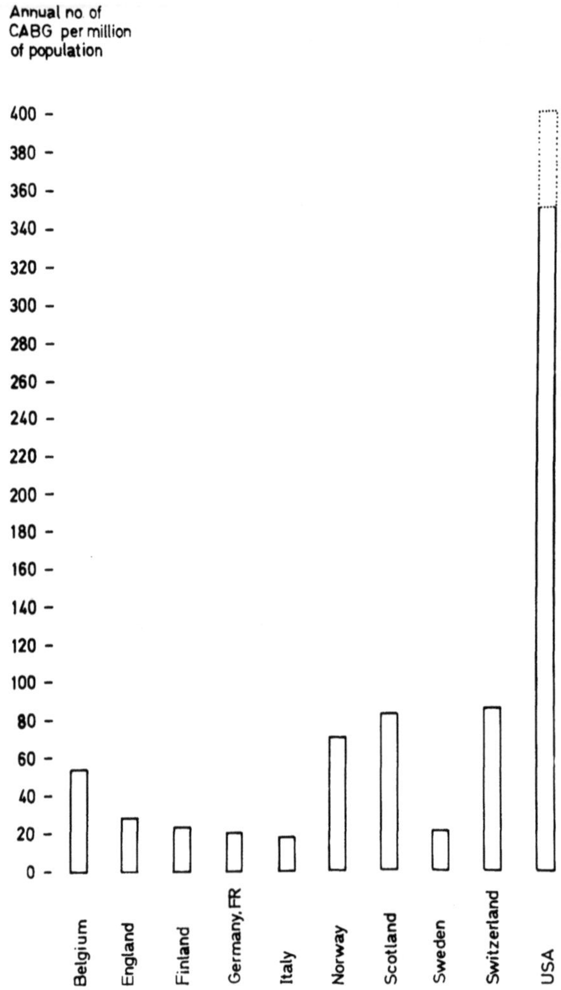

Fig. 1

toris in many communities. It appears that angina pectoris is not the most accessible symptom for epidemiologic studies, because of its highly variable intensity, duration, and course. The methods of diagnosis are burdened by false negatives and false postives. Consequently, the conclusions which can be considered today are necessarily tentative and limited to the available data. New developments, including more accurate and detailed epidemiologic information on patients, in whom CABG is indicated, may well require subsequent revision of the presently assessed needs.

For the purpose of the present demonstration I will limit myself to the prevalence and incidence data available form Great Britain.

The rate of incidence of angina pectoris is 0.2% in male subjects 30-64 years of age, according to a study by Fulton et al. [2]. Male subjects of this age represent 20% of the total population and thus a 0.2% incidence rate corresponds to 400 new cases of angina pectoris per year per million of the total population. There are no studies available on the incidence of severe angina pectoris not responding to optimal medical therapy. Clinical experience suggests that approximately 10% or 40 of 400 new annual cases may present themselves severe stable or unstable angina mereting coronary surgery. The validity of this assumption is supported by the data from a randomized coronary bypass surgery study [3]; approximately 10% of patients with moderate angina pectoris allotted medical treatment developed severe angina pectoris in spite of optimal therapy during an observation period of 1 year.

Another 10% (40 cases) requiring surgery should be added to the account of increment of severe angina cases from previous years.

The proportion of patients with left main disease among the 400 cases is assessed to be approximately 5% (20 cases).

Altogether there will be 100 patients requiring CABG of 400 new cases of angina pectoris (40 + 40 + 20).

It is assumed that approximately 100 patients will develop angina after myocardial infarction annually in the male population of 30-64 years of age per million of inhabitants. Approximately 25% or 25 patients may experience worsening of angina to a level which merits surgery.

Females requiring surgery are appreciably less, i.e., approximately 20% of male surgical cases (= 25 cases) which corresponds to the proportion of female patients operated at the present time.

Thus, the total annual need of CABG approximates 150 cases of both sexes (100 + 25 + 25).

There is a backlog of patients with angina requiring surgery. This backlog should be taken into consideration when defining the final annual number of operations during the first years of activity. An increased amount of surgery will be needed until backlog is eliminated or reduced to a reasonable stable level. The backlog is assessed on the basis of angina prevalence in the community. In England this prevalence is 3.6% of males 35-64 years of age [4] or 0.8% of total population according to the registry of a British general practice of 2500 subjects. Thus the 0.8% prevalence will result in 8000 cases of angina per million inhabitants. The fraction of the population below 65 years of age amounts to 50% giving 4000 cases of angina. The 10% proportion requiring surgery will correspond to 400 cases. Assuming that this backlog of 400 cases will be dealt with at the rate of 25-50 cases per year the total annual need of bypass surgery will then be 175-200.

It must be kept in mind that the above assessed need applies only to Great Britain and other countries exhibiting similar prevalence and incidence of angina. The need might be appreciably higher or lower in other countries; it is well documented that both prevalence and incidence of coronary heart disease varies considerably between some European countries suggesting similar variation regarding angina pectoris.

It might be appropriate to reemphasize the limitations of the above assessment. The calculations do not take into account patients older than 65 years of age. These patients may also develop severe angina requiring surgery. The need for CABG may increase if proven that it saves life in other circumstances than currently believed (main stem disease). Improved operative results and increased incidence of coronary heart disease will also tend to augment the need.

On the other hand, there are factors acting in the opposite direction, i.e., diminishing the need for CABG. These factors include spontaneous disappearance of angina at least for a period of time, inevitable mortality, improvement in nonsurgical management, decreased incidence of coronary heart disease, etc.

At times a marked increase of resources for CABG is demanded without elaborated analysis to enforce the demands. It should be recognized that several factors may markedly influence the demands.
These factors include attitude of the physician, attitude of the patient, and available resources.

The attitude of the physician as to the benefits and limitations of coronary bypass surgery is an important factor. Since all aspects of CABG are not sufficiently well substantitated by the objective evidence, principally two categories of physicians can be recognized: the conservative and the aggressive. There is good reason to believe that a conservative physician, who refers patients for surgery only for relief of angina that does not respond to medical treatment, will produce demand which is considerably less than the aggressive physician, referring patients for surgery on the basis of a significant obstructive coronary lesion. The ratio for demand caused by conservative versus aggressive physician is assessed to be 1:4.

The attitude of the patients towards bypass surgery is also extremely important. This is primarily affected by the opinion of the physician. Information obtained from friends, patients, and massmedia also has a great impact on the patients' attitude. The level of disability that is accepted as tolerable is also important and likely to vary from community to community.

The available resources for coronary bypass surgery may increase or decrease the demand. Limited resources generally have a restraining effect on the demand while the overprovison of facilities (both investigative and operative) may lead to exaggerated demands in order to justify the investment.

Considering all positive and negative aspects of the above assessment of the need for CABG it is reasonable to conclude that the American CABG production of approximately 350-400 operations per million inhabitants per year is most likely too high a standard for Europe. On the other hand, the number of CABG performed in the majority of the European countries are most likely too small in relation to actual needs. The truth lies most likely somewhere between the two continents. An appreciable increase is to be expected in most European regions in the near future.

References

1. Report on a working group "The long-term effects of coronary bypass surgery." The Hague, 1.-4. Nov. 1977. Who.
2. Fulton, M., Duncan, B., Lutz, W. et al.: Natural history of unstable angina. Lancet *1972/I*, 860
3. Varnauskas, E., Olsson, S.B.: The European Multicenter CABG Trial. Progr. Cardio. Cardiol. *6*, 83 (1977)
4. Rose, G.A.: Chest pain questionnaire. International Conference on Comparability in Epidemiological Studies. Millbank Memorial Fundation. Princeton (N.J.), 1964. p. 32

Subject Index

MIX
Papier aus verantwortungsvollen Quellen
Paper from responsible sources
FSC® C105338

If you have any concerns about our products,
you can contact us on
ProductSafety@springernature.com

In case Publisher is established outside the EU,
the EU authorized representative is:
Springer Nature Customer Service Center GmbH
Europaplatz 3, 69115 Heidelberg, Germany

Printed by Libri Plureos GmbH
in Hamburg, Germany